D1516331

DATE DUE

NOV 5 1997	
DEC 23 1997	
MAY 5 1998	
MAY 2 1998	
DEC 19 1998	
2271212	AUG 2 6 1999
8519304	MAY 1 2 2000
DEC 14 2000	
APR 2 8 2001	6779572
DEC 6 2001	
DEC 6 2001 AUG 2 0 2002	

GAYLORD   PRINTED IN U.S.A.

Bipolar Disorder

Medical Psychiatry

Series Editor

William A. Frosch, M.D.

Cornell University Medical College
New York, New York

1. *Handbook of Depression and Anxiety: A Biological Approach*, edited by Johan A. den Boer and J. M. Ad Sitsen
2. *Anticonvulsants in Mood Disorders*, edited by Russell T. Joffe and Joseph R. Calabrese
3. *Serotonin in Antipsychotic Treatment: Mechanisms and Clinical Practice,* edited by John M. Kane, H.-J. Möller, and Frans Awouters
4. Handbook of Functional Gastrointestinal Disorders, *edited by Kevin W. Olden*
5. Clinical Management of Anxiety, *edited by Johan A. den Boer*
6. Obsessive-Compulsive Disorders: Diagnosis • Etiology • Treatment, *edited by Eric Hollander and Dan J. Stein*
7. Bipolar Disorder: Biological Models and Their Clinical Application, *edited by L. Trevor Young and Russell T. Joffe*

ADDITIONAL VOLUMES IN PREPARATION

Dual Diagnosis and Treatment: Substance Abuse and Comorbid Medical and Psychiatric Disorders, *edited by Henry R. Kranzler and Bruce J. Rounsaville*

Geriatric Psychopharmacology, *edited by J. Craig Nelson*

Bipolar Disorder

Biological Models and Their Clinical Application

edited by

L. Trevor Young
Russell T. Joffe

McMaster University
Hamilton, Ontario, Canada

SETON HALL UNIVERSITY
WALSH LIBRARY
SO. ORANGE, N.J.

MARCEL DEKKER, INC.   NEW YORK · BASEL · HONG KONG

RC
516
.B526
1997

Library of Congress Cataloging-in-Publication Data

Bipolar disorder: biological models and their clinical application /
edited by L. Trevor Young, Russell T. Joffe.
    p. cm. -- (Medical psychiatry; 7)
    Includes bibliographical references and index.
    ISBN 0-8247-9872-4 (hardcover : alk. paper)
    1. Manic-depressive illness--Pathophysiology. 2. Biological
psychiatry. 3. Biological models. I. Young, L. Trevor.
II. Joffe, Russell T. III. Series.
    [DNLM: 1. Bipolar Disorder--physiopathology. 2. Models,
Biological. 3. Models, Psychological. W1 ME421SM v. 7 1997 / WM
207 b616 1997]
RC516.B526   1997
616.89'507--dc21
DNLM/DLC
for Library of Congress   97-22826
                                                               CIP

The publisher offers discounts on this book when ordered in bulk quantities. For more information, write to Special Sales/Professional Marketing at the address below.

This book is printed on acid-free paper.

Copyright © 1997 by MARCEL DEKKER, INC. All Rights Reserved.

Neither this book nor any part may be reproduced or transmitted in any form or by any means, electronic or mechanical, including photocopying, micro-filming, and recording, or by any information storage and retrieval system, without permission in writing from the publisher.

MARCEL DEKKER, INC.
270 Madison Avenue, New York, New York 10016
http://www.dekker.com

Current printing (last digit):
10 9 8 7 6 5 4 3 2 1

PRINTED IN THE UNITED STATES OF AMERICA

Series Introduction

Psychiatry has long prided itself on its attempts to understand the psycho-pathologies of individual patients. Bleuler, Freud, and others led the way to the recognition that there were idiosyncratically interpreted life experiences behind the "ravings" of the insane, that distortions and delusions were meaningful, and that these meanings were potentially discoverable. Three decades ago, however, interest turned from meanings to molecules. Madness was increasingly seen as the simple result of a shifted balance of neurotransmitter(s) or of a twisted molecule leading to a twisted brain and, in turn, to a twisted mind. The individuality of patients became an epiphenomenon of little interest.

Young and Joffe's book on the biological models of bipolar disorder is an appropriate welcome to the new millennium. It moves us from the simple and simplistic era of "too much of this" or "too little of that" toward the complex world of multiple transmitters, families of receptors, cascades of messenger systems, and interacting systems; it also moves us from *a biology* toward *the biologies* of a particular illness. While this complexity may, at first, bewilder the clinician, it also holds the promise of improved treatments tied to individuals' specific biologies; their unique hormonal statuses; or the nature of their circadian, circalunar, or circannual cycles, thereby leading us back to an appreciation of the importance of the differences as well as of the similarities between our patients.

William A. Frosch

iii

Preface

Bipolar affective disorder, or manic-depressive illness, is a common disorder that affects approximately 1.5% of the population. It frequently has an onset at an early age and a chronic and recurrent course resulting in considerable suffering and dysfunction. Despite advances in the diagnosis and treatment of this illness over the last 25 years, there are still substantial limitations to the various options for treatment; thus, many patients struggle with the illness and have a difficult course of life. There is little doubt that a greater understanding of the neurobiology of bipolar illness will lead to the development of more effective treatments and better patient management techniques that will greatly alleviate the suffering of patients with this chronic disorder.

There is an impressive body of literature, dating back more than 40 years, that examines the neurobiology of bipolar illness. In many respects, bipolar disorder is one of the psychiatric illnesses that best lend themselves to study. This common illness has discrete episodes with periods in between of general well-being and optimal function, and appears to have greater diagnostic homogeneity then many other psychiatric illnesses. It does, however, have many of the same difficulties that present in all biological studies of patients with psychiatric disorders. These include the absence of a "gold standard" to establish diagnosis and the relative inaccessibility of the brain to direct study—and consequently the need to use biological materials such as blood, urine, and even cerebrospinal fluid to serve as proxies for the direct study of the affected brain. Furthermore, as with many other psychiatric disorders, these illnesses are likely to have complex etiologies involving the confluence of biological, social, and psychological factors.

Approximately a quarter of a century ago, the introduction of lithium as a specific treatment for bipolar disorder revolutionized the treatment and prognosis of this illness. It also renewed hope that the study of the pharmacology and biological effects of lithium would give direct clues to and an understanding of the biological basis of manic-depressive illness. However, lithium is a small and relatively simple molecule that has ubiquitous effects on a wide range of chemical systems. Consequently, although clinically invaluable, lithium has not yet helped to clarify the specific biological factors involved in the pathogenesis of bipolar disorder that remain elusive. This is further complicated by the fact that, over the last 20–30 years, the concept of manic-depressive illness has been broadened with the recognition and identification of specific subtypes such as mixed manic states and rapid-cycling bipolar disorder. These subtypes may have a distinct pharmacological response profile and possibly unique biological features.

In this book, we have attempted to provide a comprehensive, critical, and clinically useful overview of the current knowledge about the biological basis of bipolar affective disorder. We have assembled a group of authors that includes many of the leading international authorities on the subject. All the authors responded admirably to our charge to provide a critical overview of their topic and to ensure that their discussion had clinical applicability and relevance. They offer insight with their descriptions of the importance of their findings for the pathophysiology, symptomatology, course of illness, and pharmacotherapy of the disorder when appropriate. Each chapter summarizes the current state of research as well as future directions for investigation.

Some chapters—such as that on monoaminergic mechanisms—are broad in historical scope, reflecting the concerted research effort to examine the role of classic neurotransmitter systems implicated in mood disorder. Others describe more recent research efforts, such as the chapter on postreceptor signal transduction mechanisms in the pathophysiology of bipolar disorders and their relevance to mood-stabilizing treatments. Some chapters also address advances in techniques for gaining more direct access to the diseased brain, such as the chapter on neuroanatomical models and brain imaging studies. Still other chapters provide a conceptual and theoretical framework for understanding how biological mechanisms may affect the clinical presentation, course of illness, and response to treatment of this complex disorder.

The later chapters attempt to synthesize the specific research findings in several ways. Results from various fields are collated to form the basis for specific hypotheses about the underlying biological disturbances in bipolar disorder. The authors then delineate the ways in which the biology of bipolar disorder differs from that of other psychiatric disorders, including mood and anxiety disorders and schizophrenia. In the final chapter, we place the specific findings into context with current pharmacotherapy (and other treatments) of bipolar disorder, and illustrate how these findings may direct the development of new treatment strategies.

The book is intended in part as a resource and a reference for those involved in the treatment of bipolar disorder. However, it is also intended to provide a readily accessible and useful guide to a richer understanding of the biological basis of this common illness that will facilitate readers' clinical management of their bipolar patients.

L. Trevor Young
Russell T. Joffe

Contents

Series Introduction   William A. Frosch   *iii*

Preface   *v*

Contributors   *xi*

1   Monoaminergic Systems   1
    Husseini K. Manji and William Z. Potter

2   Signal Transduction Abnormalities in Bipolar Disorder   41
    Jun-Feng Wang, Peter P. Li, Jerry J. Warsh,
    and L. Trevor Young

3   Hormones and Bipolar Affective Disorder   81
    Russell T. Joffe and Stephen T. H. Sokolov

4   Kindling and Stress Sensitization   93
    Robert M. Post and Susan R. B. Weiss

5   The Chronobiology of Mood-Related Disorders   127
    Meir Steiner and Diana Ingram

6 Neuropeptides in Bipolar Disorder 161
   Emile D. Risby, Kelly Hartline, Michael J. Owens,
   and Charles B. Nemeroff

7 Neuroanatomical Models and Brain-Imaging Studies 179
   Terence A. Ketter, Mark S. George, Tim A. Kimbrell,
   Mark W. Willis, Brenda E. Benson, and Robert M. Post

8 Linkage Studies of Bipolar Syndromes 219
   Wade H. Berrettini

9 Toward an Integrated Biological Model of Bipolar Disorder 235
   Charles L. Bowden

10 Is Bipolar Depression a Specific Biological Entity? 255
    Alan C. Swann

11 Biological Models and Pharmacotherapy of Bipolar Disorder: 287
    Summary
    L. Trevor Young and Russell T. Joffe

Index *297*

Contributors

Brenda E. Benson, B.S. Biological Psychiatry Branch, National Institute of Mental Health, National Institutes of Health, Bethesda, Maryland

Wade H. Berrettini, M.D. Department of Psychiatry, University of Pennsylvania, Philadelphia, Pennsylvania

Charles L. Bowden, M.D. Department of Psychiatry, The University of Texas Health Science Center at San Antonio, San Antonio, Texas

Mark S. George, M.D. Departments of Psychiatry, Radiology, and Neurology, Medical University of South Carolina, Charleston, South Carolina, and National Institute of Mental Health, National Institutes of Health, Bethesda, Maryland

Kelly Hartline, B.S. Department of Psychiatry and Behavioral Sciences, Emory University School of Medicine, Atlanta, Georgia

Diana Ingram, M.D. Department of Psychiatry, McMaster University, Hamilton, Ontario, Canada

Russell T. Joffe, M.D. Department of Psychiatry, McMaster University, Hamilton, Ontario, Canada

Terence A. Ketter, M.D. Department of Psychiatry and Behavioral Sciences, Stanford University School of Medicine, Stanford, California

Tim A. Kimbrell, M.D. Biological Psychiatry Branch, National Institute of Mental Health, National Institutes of Health, Bethesda, Maryland

Peter P. Li, Ph.D. Department of Psychiatry and Pharmacology, University of Toronto, Toronto, Ontario, Canada

Husseini K. Manji, M.D. Departments of Psychiatry and Behavioral Neurosciences and Pharmacology, Wayne State University School of Medicine, Detroit, Michigan

Charles B. Nemeroff, M.D., Ph.D. Department of Psychiatry and Behavioral Sciences, Emory University School of Medicine, Atlanta, Georgia

Michael J. Owens, Ph.D. Department of Psychiatry and Behavioral Sciences, Emory University School of Medicine, Atlanta, Georgia

Robert M. Post, M.D. Biological Psychiatry Branch, National Institute of Mental Health, National Institutes of Health, Bethesda, Maryland

William Z. Potter, M.D., Ph.D. Department of Nervous System Disorders, Lilly Research Laboratories, Indianapolis, Indiana

Emile D. Risby, M.D. Department of Psychiatry and Behavioral Sciences, Emory University School of Medicine, Atlanta, Georgia

Stephen T. H. Sokolov, M.D. Department of Psychiatry, McMaster University, Hamilton, Ontario, Canada

Meir Steiner, M.D., Ph.D. Department of Psychiatry and Biomedical Sciences, McMaster University, Hamilton, Ontario, Canada

Alan C. Swann, M.D. Department of Psychiatry, University of Texas Medical School at Houston, Houston, Texas

Jun-Feng Wang, Ph.D. Department of Psychiatry, McMaster University, Hamilton, Ontario, Canada

Jerry J. Warsh, M.D., Ph.D. Departments of Psychiatry and Pharmacology, University of Toronto, Toronto, Ontario, Canada

Susan R. B. Weiss, Ph.D. Unit of Behavioral Biology, Biological Psychiatry Branch, National Institute of Mental Health, National Institutes of Health, Bethesda, Maryland

Mark W. Willis, M.Engr. Biological Psychiatry Branch, National Institute of Mental Health, National Institutes of Health, Bethesda, Maryland

L. Trevor Young, M.D., Ph.D. Department of Psychiatry, McMaster University, Hamilton, Ontario, Canada

Bipolar Disorder

1

Monoaminergic Systems

Husseini K. Manji
Wayne State University School of Medicine, Detroit, Michigan,

William Z. Potter
Lilly Research Laboratories, Indianapolis, Indiana

I. INTRODUCTION

Bipolar affective disorder (manic-depressive illness) is a common, severe, chronic, and often life-threatening condition with a lifetime prevalence of 1.2% (Weissman et al., 1988). The cumulative effects of recurring bouts of mania and depression lead to an increased rate of marital and family breakdown, unemployment, impaired career progress, and consequent financial difficulties. The effect on the broader community is highlighted by one estimation that the use of lithium saved the United States $4 billion in the period 1969–1979, by reducing associated medical costs and restoring productivity (Reifman and Wyatt, 1980). Approximately 6% of bipolar patients commit suicide, and mortality rates due to physical disorders are also increased (Angst, 1986). Although there is undoubted evidence for significant genetic transmission of bipolar disorder (Gershon, 1990), segregation analyses have been unable to determine the particular mode of transmission of this condition (Cox et al., 1989). Additionally, despite extensive research, there is a dearth of knowledge concerning the etiology and/or pathophysiology of this disorder.

The stimulus for the study of the biogenic amines in patients with manic-depressive illness was provided by the discovery of effective pharmacological treatments for depression and mania. These treatments led to the formulation of the so-called pharmacological bridge between depressive illness and neurotransmitter systems in the brain. The foundation for the pharmacological bridge was the observation that reserpine use was associated with an unexpected high incidence of depression; this antihypertensive was later shown to deplete amine neurotransmitters in animals. Methyldopa, now believed to act via stimulation of presynaptic receptors that inhibit norepinephrine release, can also precipitate depression (Whitlock and Evans, 1978).

Table 1 summarizes the major known drug-amine-behavioral associations relevant to manic-depressive illness. We will only briefly discuss this extensive literature since it has been well reviewed and critiqued elsewhere (Goodwin and Jamison, 1990). The specific drug effects listed in Table 1 are those generally reported as the acute effects in most animal species. Amphetamine, a stimulant in normals, is generally not thought to be an effective antidepressant agent. Cocaine, also a powerful stimulant in normals, is a potent inhibitor of catecholamine reuptake at the synapse, an effect similar to that of the tricyclic antidepressants. L-dopa, primarily a precursor of dopamine (DA) and secondarily of norepinephrine—acutely, at least— increases the output of both. It is not an effective "broad-spectrum" antidepressant, however, although it may be of benefit to some patients (Goodwin et al., 1970). It has been reported to be activating, as evidenced by increased anger and psychosis ratings in some patients, and hypomanic episodes superimposed on depression in a high proportion of bipolar patients (Murphy et al., 1971).

An imbalance in the noradrenergic and cholinergic transmitter systems that regulate affect—a relative predominance of noradrenergic over cholinergic tone associated with mania and the reverse with depression—was a specific hypothesis that emerged in the 1970s from such pharmacological observations (Janowsky et al., 1972). Evidence for a pharmacological bridge to manic-depressive illness was provided by studies demonstrating the ability of intravenous physostigmine, a central cholinesterase inhibitor, to briefly but dramatically reduce symptoms in manic patients (Janowsky et al., 1973) and to precipitate depression in euthymic bipolar patients maintained on lithium (Oppenheim et al., 1979). However, the therapeutic activity of antidepressant and antimanic drugs does not consistently parallel effects on the cholinergic system, and a number of these agents, including monoamine oxidase inhibitors (MAOIs) and various "second-generation" antidepressants, lack any interaction with cholinergic receptors (Rudorfer et al., 1984). Together these results suggest that, although manipulation of the cholinergic system is *capable* of modulating affective state, it does not appear to represent a relevant therapeutic action of a currently available agent. Interestingly, one of the most consistent pharmacological findings in manic-

Table 1 The Pharmacological Bridge: Drug-Neurotransmitter Relations and Behavioral Effects in Humans

Drug	Acute effects on the functional output of neurotransmitters	Predisposed to affective illness	Depressed patients	Manic patients	Normals
MAOI	(NE, DA)	Can ppt mania	AD	Aggravates mania	?
Tricyclic antidepressants	(NE, 5HT)	Can ppt mania	AD	Aggravates mania	?
Amphetamine	(NE, DA)	Can ppt mania (?)	Poor AD	Stimulant	
Cocaine	(NE, DA)	Can ppt mania	Poor AD	Stimulant	
L-dopa	(DA, ?NE)	Can ppt hypomania	Activation—no AD effect		No effect
Reserpine	(NE, 5-HT, DA)	Can ppt depression	?	Partial antimanic	Can ppt depression
Lithium	?	Does not ppt depression	AD (some patients)	Antimanic	Mild sedation
Neuroleptics	(DA)	?	?	Partial antimanic	Sedation
AMPT	(DA, NE)	?	Does not reverse imipramine	Antimanic	Sedation (?)
Piribedil	(DA)	Can ppt mania	? Antidepressant	?	?
Bromocriptine	(DA)	Can ppt mania	?	Euphorogenic	
Physostigmine	(AcH)	Can ppt depression in euthymic bipolars	Worsens	Transiently antimanic	Transient depressive symptoms

ppt = precipitate; MAOI = monoamine oxidase inhibitors; NE = norepinephrine; DA = dopamine; 5-HT = serotonin; AMPT = α-methylparatyrosine; AcH = acetylcholine; ? = insufficient data available to make any judgment.
Source: Adapted from Goodwin and Sack, 1973.

depressive illness is that direct or indirect norepinephrine and dopamine agonists precipitate episodes of mania or hypomania in patients with underlying
manic-depressive illness. This effect is usually observed as a switch from
depression to mania or hypomania (since the compounds that produce it are
given as antidepressants), although it can also occur from the euthymic state.

Many of the "classic" biochemical effects outlined in Table 1 are based
on the ability of drugs to alter the so-called turnover of the neurotransmitter.
High turnover has traditionally been thought to represent a higher level of
functions—low turnover, the reverse—although we have learned that there
are many exceptions to this rule. Table 1 characterizes the net action of a
drug on an amine system, rather than dealing with the complexities of drug
effects on different measures of these systems.

Where relevant data in humans or primates exist, they are consistent
with the simple formulations outlined in Table 1, and thus there are now
drug-amine relationships established directly in patients. They lend support
to an association between a hyperadrenergic and/or hyperdopaminergic state
and the onset of hypomania or mania. This interpretation is also consistent
with longitudinal studies of norepinephrine and its metabolites in body fluids
(discussed later), which are generally low in bipolar depression and high in
mania.

II. THE EXTENDED BRIDGE

There remain, however, even more striking pharmacological findings going
beyond effects on a single episode of depression or mania, that is, the effects
of drugs on the long-term course of bipolar illness (Goodwin and Jamison,
1990). As discussed elsewhere, antidepressants in general, and tricyclic
antidepressants (TCAs) in particular, may increase the frequency of cycles
and worsen long-term outcome. MAOIs can precipitate mania, apparently
with about the same frequency as TCAs, and may be associated with an
increased frequency of cycles. The data on cycle induction after MAOIs, and
compared to TCAs, are relatively sparse, although it seems to occur. There is
presently some data to suggest that, unlike the other selective serotonin-
reuptake inhibitors (SSRIs), paroxetine may be less likely to induce switches
into mania; however, double-blind studies are needed to confirm this clinical
observation. Interestingly (and perhaps somewhat counterintuitively), the
most putatively "dopaminergic" of the antidepressants available in the
United States—bupropion—has also been reported to have marked efficacy
in bipolar depression, and a lower propensity to induce switches into mania
than the TCAs. Although speculative, it is quite plausible that a moderate,

Table 2 Drugs with Three Classes of Actions on Bipolar Illness

Classes of action	Drug types (relative potency)				
	TCA	MAOI	Lithium	VPA	CBZ
Single episode (weeks to months)					
Antidepressants	+++	+++	++	?+	?+
Precipitate depression	0	0	0	0	0
Precipitate mania	+++	+++	0	0	0
Antimanic	0	0	+++	+++	+++
Long-term (years)					
Increase cycle frequency	++	0/+[a]	0	?0	0
Reduce cycle frequency	0	0/+[a]	++	?+	?+

[a] Action may be related to balance MAO type A versus B inhibition.
0 = no effect; + = weak effect; ++ = moderate effect; +++ = strong effect.
Source: Adapted from Goodwin and Jamison, 1990.

sustained enhancement of dopaminergic drive by bupropion may, in fact, protect against more dramatic changes in dopaminergic "throughput" (e.g., by alteration of dopamine (DA) receptor sensitivity), and thereby be less likely to induce mania.

These various clinical actions in bipolar patients are summarized in Table 2, along with potencies of the three most common treatments with multiple effects. Six fundamental categories of actions on the illness can be identified: four relating to effects on a given episode (precipitate or reverse depression, precipitate or reverse mania) and two relating to the long-term course of the illness (increase or decrease cycle frequency). In Table 2, an attempt has been made to roughly quantify the overall relative potency and/or range of effectiveness among compounds for each class of action. Keep in mind that this is an attempt to examine the question of whether there is a general pattern, and we must necessarily ignore individual differences, gray areas, and clinically important distinctions. For example, we have listed MAOIs and TCAs as having approximately equal antidepressant activity in bipolars; this is, of course, a complex question, the answer to which may depend on such things as the severity of the depressive episode. Abundant data suggest that both TCAs and MAOIs are more potent than lithium for most depressive episodes, and lithium may be more potent than carbamazepine or valproate. Interestingly, another anticonvulsant, lamotrigine, appears to have potent antidepressant efficacy in preliminary open studies (Calabrese et al., 1996). Lithium is firmly established as reducing cycle frequency, and carbamazepine and valproate appear to be capable of this as well; whether these three "stabilizers" really have their effects on different ranges of cycle frequency remains to be seen. TCAs and MAOIs appear to be equipotent in their ability to precipitate a manic episode, and lithium and valproate may be equipotent in treating mania. Only TCAs are well established as increasing the frequency of cycles, although other agents, including nonspecific MAOIs (Kukopoulos et al., 1980), may have such effects as well.

Given these compelling pharmacological data, it is not surprising that investigators have postulated that dysregulation of the major monoaminergic systems may also play some primary role in the pathophysiology of manic-depressive illness. The multiple functions of central neurotransmitter systems, however, make it difficult to conceptualize, let alone demonstrate, true specificity of detected abnormalities. We now review the biological studies that can be directly or indirectly related to the hypotheses generated by various pharmacological bridges.

III. BIOLOGICAL STUDIES IN DETAIL

A. Caveats in the Interpretation of Biological Data

Two major problems in the interpretation of biological data are the diagnostic specificity of patient populations and the lack of comparability of state of patients across studies even in those who truly have the same diagnosis. Are they studied at the same point of their recurrent illness? Are the effects "primary" to the illness, or do they represent the individual's compensatory adaptations to the illness? How long have they been drug-free? It is now clear, for instance, that withdrawal from the high therapeutic doses of antidepressants currently employed produces biochemical changes that persist for at least 3 and up to 8 weeks following discontinuation. For more than a decade, the bulk of psychiatric patients available for biochemical studies have recently been or are on medication at the beginning of an investigation. None of the studies below specifies a minimum withdrawal over 3 weeks, and most involve only a 1- to 2-week drug-free period. There are, however, a few studies in which a parameter is followed longitudinally over different states in one or two untreated subjects. From a research point of view, such studies are particularly valuable—although they clearly must be generalized with caution, since investigated patients are those who are able and willing to tolerate prolonged periods without drugs and therefore may be atypical.

Many other factors, such as age, sex, and body size, as well as assay variability—too often taken for granted—can contribute to the lack of consensus across studies. In general, however, it is our contention that unrecognized differences in diagnosis, assessment of severity of illness, and failure to allow for an adequate period free of medications are the major sources of variance.

With these caveats in mind, we now move to a critical review of the research studies of biogenic amines in manic-depressive illness.

B. Norepinephrine

Originally proposed a quarter century ago, the catecholamine hypothesis of affective disorders posited a deficiency of norepinephrine (NE) at critical sites in the central nervous system (CNS) depression and an excess of functional NE in mania (Schildkraut, 1965; Bunney and Davis, 1965). This postulate has been extensively investigated but has proven difficult to study experimentally, at least in part because of the formidable methodological difficulties in assessing CNS noradrenergic function in humans.

Nevertheless, we attempt here to briefly review, critically appraise, and integrate the research findings in an attempt to present a coherent summary of the present status of findings on NE in affective illness.

1. Studies of Norepinephrine and MHPG in Plasma

During the 1980s there was a series of investigations of plasma norepinephrine (NE), with the majority revealing some degree of elevation interpreted as evidence of increased peripheral sympathetic nervous system activity in patients with major depression (Barnes, 1983; Maas et al., 1987; Roy et al., 1985, 1987, 1988; Rudorfer et al., 1985; Wyatt et al., 1971; de Villiers et al., 1987; Louis et al., 1975; Veith et al., 1988; Koslow et al., 1983). Several studies using radioenzymatic and radiotracer assay techniques have demonstrated elevated plasma NE concentrations at presumed rest in patients with major depression, although there is considerable overlap. These elevations appear to be largely attributable to unipolar depressives, in particular those who fulfill criteria for melancholia (Roy et al., 1985; Veith et al., 1985). Similarly, unipolar dexamethasone nonsuppressors have significantly higher lying plasma NE concentrations than dexamethasone suppressors (Roy et al., 1985; Barnes, 1983). The variance in plasma NE has also been reported to be greater in depressed patients than normal controls in the absence of differences between the means (Siever et al., 1986).

However, since plasma NE is determined by a variety of factors, including release, reuptake, and degradation (Kopin, 1985), NE "spillover rates" have been determined in an attempt to control for clearance. This involves repeated blood sampling following an infusion of tritiated NE to a plateau concentration. Esler et al. (1982) demonstrated that depressed patients had elevated spillover rates, theoretically representing the rate of entry of NE to plasma from peripheral sympathetic nerves. It is likely, however, that uptake-1 is much more important for the removal of endogenously released NE than for removal of circulating (and infused) NE, which may preclude definitive interpretation of the results.

This caveat notwithstanding, another study found that endogenously, but not nonendogenously, depressed patients show a selective increase in NE "spillover," with no intergroup differences in clearance rate when compared to controls (Veith et al., 1985). Rosenblatt et al. (1969) had earlier infused labeled NE and measured the ratio of amines to oxidized metabolites. Depressed patients excreted relatively more NE and less oxidized metabolites. Attempting to control for a number of confounding variables, including period off prior medications, baseline activity level, and assay methodology, it appears that plasma NE may be heterogeneously abnormal in depressed patients under conditions of limited rest (supine for 30–60 minutes prior to blood drawing), with a significant subgroup—particularly unipolar, anxious, melancholic patients with dexamethasone nonsuppression—showing elevated plasma NE. A subgroup of bipolar depressed patients may, however, actually show reduced supine NE (Rudorfer et al., 1985).

Going beyond the study of plasma NE levels under resting conditions, studies of the responsiveness of plasma NE to various provocative challenge tests provide evidence for dysregulation of the NE system in depression. Thus, using an orthostatic challenge paradigm, we have previously demonstrated that the increase in plasma NE produced by standing up is consistently greater in depressed unipolar or bipolar patients vs. age- and sex-matched controls (Rudorfer et al., 1985). This has also been demonstrated in several other studies (Roy et al., 1985; Rubin et al., 1985; Veith et al., 1988). Depressed patients also show significantly higher plasma NE levels following a cold pressor test than age- and sex-matched controls, with the unipolar melancholic DST nonsuppressors showing a trend toward higher plasma NE than suppressors (Roy et al., 1987). Taken together, the studies of plasma NE provide strong evidence for dysregulation of peripheral release of NE in affective illness, with a difference in the pattern of dysregulation between unipolar and bipolar patients. Stated another way, bipolar patients appear to have a reduced to average resting output of NE with a highly exaggerated NE response to standing, while unipolar patients have an average to elevated resting NE with a moderately exaggerated response to standing (and perhaps "stressors" in general).

Studies of plasma MHPG have yielded variable results and do not generally support the concept of a unipolar–bipolar distinction (discussed in Goodwin and Jamieson, 1990). Plasma MHPG in unipolar depressives tends to be similar to that of controls, albeit with greater variance (Siever et al., 1984a). Similar to the association with plasma NE, depressed DST nonsuppressors have higher levels of plasma MHPG (Jimerson et al. 1983; Roy et al., 1986). Plasma MHPG levels tend to be lower in bipolar than unipolar depressed patients (for review, see Goodwin and Jamieson 1990; Siever 1987) and, interestingly, are higher in bipolars when manic than when depressed (Halaris et al., 1978; Jimerson et al., 1981). In a recent study of 18 manic patients, plasma MHPG correlated with their manic symptoms (in particular, grandiosity and elation) but not with anxiety, depression, motor behavior, acute psychosis, or severity of illness. The mechanism(s) through which MHPG is elevated in mania remains to be determined.

2. Studies of Norepinephrine and MHPG in CSF

For some years, measures of NE and its metabolites in cerebrospinal fluid (CSF) were thought to directly reflect brain NE "activity." This assumption is problematic, however, since high correlations have been found between plasma and CSF NE and MHPG (Kopin, 1985; Goldstein et al., 1987). Pharmacological studies in dogs reveal parallel changes in plasma and CSF NE following ganglion blockade, suggesting that sympathetic outflow may determine (at least in part) NE concentrations in both compartments (Goldstein et al., 1987). Plasma MHPG is the major source of CSF MHPG, which readily crosses the blood–brain barrier (Kopin, 1985). Using the high correlation between plasma and CSF MHPG observed in comparisons of high and low catecholamine output states, an equation has been derived to "correct" for the contribution of plasma MHPG to that of CSF (Kopin, 1985; Goldstein et al., 1987). However, in the relatively narrow range of values observed in depressed patients and controls, the utility of such an equation to identify "brain MHPG" is questionable (Linnoila et al., 1986) and, to date, has not revealed new insights in studies of depression.

Certain other methodological problems are unique to CSF measures. Standards for obtaining spinal fluid, such as elapsed time between needle insertion and sample collection, have not been established. Therefore, subjects may not have the same degree of accommodation to the stress of the needle stick. Moreover, sampling at a single point in time may not reflect the biochemical process of depression or mania but rather a state-dependent fluctuation from a recent external or internal stress.

Four of the seven studies of CSF concentrations of NE that compare depressed patients and control subjects in the same study report elevations, one a decrease, and the other two no significant change. Since the 1980s, there has been an overall lowering of the absolute values reported for NE subsequent to quantification by HPLC with electrochemical detection. CSF concentrations of NE have been reported to be elevated in depressed patients with an atypical presentation, higher scores for nurse-rated anxiety, and a longer duration of hospitalization (Post et al., 1984). Earlier, investigations had shown that CSF NE was higher in mania than in depression (Post et al., 1978). Perhaps the most novel finding has been in dysphoric mania, defined by the coexistence of high depression ratings: NE in CSF correlates modestly but significantly ($r \approx 0.5$) with ratings of dysphoria and anxiety but not with ratings of mania (Post et al., 1989). These authors suggest that CSF NE may be positively correlated with the degree of anxiety across a variety of psychopathological syndromes, including depression, mania, and perhaps anxiety.

CSF MHPG in depressed patients is consistently reported as not different from that in controls, except for higher levels in postmenopausal women (Koslow et al., 1983). Within the depressed group, however, significant subgroup differences emerge in some reports, suggesting lower CSF MHPG in bipolar I than in unipolar patients (Potter et al., 1987). As was the case for CSF NE, variables other than overall diagnosis may influence values. For instance, within a group of depressed patients, those with increased anxiety, agitation, somatization, and sleep disturbance had significantly elevated levels of CSF MHPG (Redmond et al., 1986). CSF MHPG has also been reported to be elevated in manics compared to controls (Post et al., 1984; Swann et al., 1986; Redmond et al., 1986). Swann et al. (1987) also noted that in their population CSF MHPG concentration correlated with several dysphoric elements of the manic syndrome, namely, total manic severity and hostility. Moreover, this study found a significant reduction in CSF MHPG with lithium treatment, even when treatment was unsuccessful.

Taken together, the CSF studies of NE and its metabolite MHPG suggest that NE output is higher in mania than in depression and that there may be relatively higher values in unipolar versus bipolar depression. Relative elevation within patient groups may, in turn, be related to anxiety or the overall severity of the condition. As noted previously, it is possible that the CSF findings reflect events occurring in the sympathetic nervous system as much as events occurring in the brain, and it is therefore not surprising that the pattern of findings is similar in CSF and plasma. Nevertheless, in recent studies CSF NE or MHPG was correlated with dysphoric elements of the manic syndrome, while urinary measures tended to be associated with euphoric components (Post et al., 1989; Swann et al., 1986), suggesting that studies examining multiple measure/components of the norepinephrine system(s) allow for the most meaningful interpretations.

3. Studies of Norepinephrine and Its Metabolites in Urine

Since the catecholamine hypothesis of affective disorders was proposed, attempts to characterize output of the norepinephrine system in depressed patients have focused on measurements of MHPG in urine more than any other single parameter (see Potter et al., 1987; Filser et al., 1988). These studies were fueled (at least to some extent) by the early interpretations of data suggesting that about 50% of MHPG in the urine was derived from the CNS. However, subsequent work indicated that MHPG readily crosses the blood–brain barrier to the CSF; earlier estimates of CNS contribution to urinary MHPG have thus been revised to approximately one-third (reviewed in Kopin, 1985). Nevertheless, as discussed already, peripheral and central NE systems interact, and thus even a "primarily peripheral" measure such as urinary MHPG can theoretically provide useful information.

Detailed reviews of the literature differ in their conclusions, but some emphasize that there is decreased (albeit modestly) 24-hour urinary excretion of MHPG in depressed patients compared to controls. When one examines the studies in more detail, it appears that the MHPG reduction is accounted for exclusively by bipolars, although a recent study of ours, in which subsequent patients in the same center were examined, does not replicate this finding, perhaps suggesting a change in the patient population (unpublished observations). Reduced urinary MHPG may be present only in bipolar I and not in bipolar II patients (Muscettola et al., 1984). Average urinary MHPG is not reduced in unipolar populations taken as a whole; rather, there may be a subgroup of unipolar patients who have elevated MHPG compared to controls and bipolar subjects (Schatzberg et al., 1982). Investigators have also attempted to use this variance to subtype patients within the unipolar group and to try to predict treatment response based on pretreatment urinary MHPG values (Schildkraut et al., 1978; Goodwin et al., 1978). Indeed, several reports supported the notion that in unipolar depression, lower urinary MHPG predicts favorable responses to antidepressants that primarily block NE reuptake (imipramine, desipramine, nortriptyline, maprotiline) (Maas et al., 1972, 1982); others, however, could find no evidence for such a prediction (Muscettola et al., 1984; Janicak et al., 1986). Again, these different findings may represent the shifting patient profile studied at tertiary referral centers.

Low levels of urinary MHPG in depressed patients have been reported to approach normal values with clinical improvement, suggesting that this measure may be state-dependent (Pickar et al., 1978). Similarly, longitudinal studies of bipolar patients suggest increased MHPG excretion in the manic compared to depressed state (Post et al., 1984; Potter et al., 1987). A more recent study (Swann et al., 1987) noted that manic patients responding to lithium had decreased MHPG and increased NE excretion relative to the total excretion of NE and its metabolites, suggesting that lithium response was associated with an alteration of catecholamine metabolism pathways. Overall, urinary MHPG by itself has not proven to be a sufficiently robust and consistent measure to be generally accepted as a useful tool in diagnosis or prediction of treatment response (Davis and Bresnahan, 1987).

In recent years, investigators have attempted to go beyond the "too little or too much" hypotheses of affective disorders; one approach has been to measure the 24-hour concentrations of urinary catecholamines and their metabolites in order to identify possible abnormalities in the relative activity of NE metabolic pathways in depression and mania. As discussed elsewhere (Manji et al., 1994), one can obtain reliable information about the average output of NE and its metabolites within an individual in a stable mood state from only two consecutive 24-hour urine collections. Furthermore, since all major metabolites are measured, 24-hour urinary measures of NE and of its metabolites can account for interindividual differences in the relative metabolism of NE as well as its turnover (amount formed and excreted per 24 hours at steady state).

Consistent with the findings of elevated basal and/or stress-induced plasma NE, several investigators have observed elevated urinary excretion of NE and of its major extraneuronal metabolite normetanephrine (NMN) in depressed patients (Roy et al., 1985, 1986; Maas et al., 1987; Davis et al., 1988; Roy et al., 1988). Moreover, the finding appears more impressive when the excretion of NE and NMN in depression is examined *relative* to total NE excretion—in the study by Maas and associates (1987), a modest increase in total urinary catecholamine excretion (16%) was accompanied by marked increases in urinary NE (57%) and NMN (42%) in depressed patients. These results suggest a shift toward extraneuronal metabolic pathways and are consistent with the suggestions of increased NE release and "spillover" in depression. Indeed, experimental data in humans indicate that a greater pulsatile release of NE is associated with a relative increase in NE excretion and a relative decrease in MHPG excretion (Maas et al., 1970, 1971).

We have recently analyzed data collected from over a decade of studies on an inpatient unit at the National Institute of Mental Health. We compared baseline excretion of urinary NE and its metabolites and the fractional extraneuronal concentration of NE (NE+NMN/ΣNE) in unmedicated unipolar and bipolar depressed patients and healthy volunteers. Consistent with previously reported results, urinary NE, as well as the urinary NE and NMN relative to total turnover, were elevated in the depressed patients as a whole compared to healthy volunteers. In contrast to previous studies, we found significantly elevated concentrations of urinary NE in bipolar but not unipolar depressed patients compared to healthy volunteers, and a trend toward decreased MHPG in both patient groups (unpublished observations). Several possible methodological factors may account for these differences, including differences in assay and length of inpatient drug-free duration (a minimum of 4–8 weeks). Interestingly, total turnover of NE (NE+NMN+MHPG+VMA) was significantly lower in unipolar and bipolar patients compared to healthy volunteers, suggesting a reduction of tyrosine hydroxylase activity in sympathetic neurons.

C. Clinical Studies of Adrenergic Receptors

The future development of selective receptor ligands for positron emission tomography (PET) studies may soon permit the direct assessment of CNS adrenergic receptors in humans. To date, studies of NE receptors in affective disorders have been limited to indirect research strategies. The most commonly utilized strategies include:

1. Characterization of receptor number and function in readily accessible blood elements
2. Pharmacological "challenge" strategies whereby alterations in biochemical neuroendocrine, cardiovascular, or behavioral parameters in response to various receptor agonists and/or antagonists are measured

D. Receptor Studies on Blood Cells

Due to the accessibility of platelets and lymphocytes, both α_2- and β_2-adrenergic receptors have been extensively studied in affective disorders, frequently generating elaborate hypotheses about CNS adrenergic receptor dysfunction based solely on studies of these tissues. There are several problems with the assumption that changes in adrenergic receptors on peripheral cells reflect similar alterations in the CNS. First, receptors on blood cells, by definition, are noninnervated, exist in a markedly different environment, and may therefore poorly reflect central, innervated adrenergic receptors.

Another major (often overlooked) consideration when interpreting studies of dynamic receptor regulation in blood cells is the fact that white blood cell counts and the relative proportions of subsets of lymphocytes may vary. Recruitment into the circulation of cells with different characteristics may frequently explain altered receptor function. Precisely such a mechanism appears to be operative in the studies demonstrating the seemingly paradoxical *increase* in lymphocyte β-adrenergic receptor (βAR) density and responsiveness during short-term isoproterenol infusion, mental arithmetic, and dynamic exercise (procedure that stimulate the sympathetic nervous system) (Van Tits et al., 1990; Maisel et al., 1990a,b). The mechanism appears to be a release of subsets of "fresh" lymphocytes from the spleen into the circulation (see Van Tits et al., 1990; Werstuik et al., 1990). These fresh, activated lymphocytes express enhanced βAR responsiveness, and this probably accounts for the exercise- and catecholamine-induced increases in βAR responsiveness. Indeed, a recent study reported a "normalization" of previously blunted lymphocyte βAR responsiveness in depressed patients following electroconvulsive therapy (ECT) (Mann et al., 1990a). Given the increase in plasma catecholamine produced acutely by ECT (Mann et al., 1990b) and the intermittent "phasic" nature in which ECT is administered (i.e., three times per week), the exchange of lymphocyte subsets from the spleen to the circulation may explain the apparent "resensitization" of circulating β-receptors.

1. Platelet α_2-Adrenergic Receptors

Based on the assumption that postulated alterations in CNS α_2-adrenergic receptors may also be reflected in peripheral tissues, numerous studies have measured the binding of α_2-agonist or -antagonist ligands to platelets obtained from patients with affective illness and normal individuals. However, although human platelets and cerebral cortex contain homogeneous populations of the same α_2A-receptors (Bylund et al., 1988), radioligand studies across groups are confounded by numerous methodological problems, such as varying patient populations, sex, age, clinical state, drug-washout period, and assay technique (see review by Piletz et al., 1986). A review of 13 studies using yohimbine-alkaloid radioligands reveals no significant differences in the B_{max} of platelet α_2-receptors between depressed patients and controls (see Piletz et al., 1986; Kafka and Paul 1986; Katona et al. 1987). Most of the studies using partial or full agonists, however, have observed increased B_{max} in the platelets of depressed patients as compared to controls (Garcia Sevilla 1986, 1990; Pandey et al., 1989; Piletz et al., 1990). These results have frequently been interpreted as evidence for the α_2-hypersensitivity theory of depression (Garcia-Sevilla et al., 1986, 1990; Piletz et al., 1990).

These studies, however, have utilized the imidazoline compounds, clonidine, para-aminoclonidine (PAC), and UK-14,304 as radioligands, and there are problems with the use of these radioligands that go beyond reproducibility of measures across groups. Thus, it is now clear that a variety of compounds (e.g., clonidine, PAC, idazoxan, and UK-14,304) previously considered to be selective α_2-ligands, also bind with high affinity to nonadrenergic catecholamine-insensitive sites (Meeley et al., 1986; Bricca et al., 1988a,b; Boyajian and Leslie, 1987). These sites, termed imidazoline sites, appear to mediate the hypotensive effects of clonidine (Bousquet and Feldman, 1987) and are also present on human platelets (Michel et al., 1990). Furthermore, the ratio of imidazoline sites to α_2-receptors in human platelets varies widely among healthy volunteers (Michel et al., 1990), making it difficult to arrive at any meaningful inferences about α_2-adrenergic receptors on the basis of these agonist-binding studies. Indeed, a recent report even suggests that the elevated platelet para aminoclonidine binding in depressed subjects is due solely to increases in the catecholamine-insensitive (imidazoline) sites (Piletz et al., 1990, 1991, 1995). If anything, the results of some (but not all) studies examining α_2 inhibition of platelet adenylyl cyclase (AC) activity are more supportive of subsensitive α_2-receptors in depression (reviewed in Pandey et al., 1990; Kafka and Paul, 1986; Garcia-Sevilla et al., 1996). As discussed already, however, receptor number and sensitivity on circulating blood cells may be significantly regulated by plasma catecholamines. In support of this, Freedman et al. (1990) have demonstrated stress-induced desensitization of α_2-adrenergic receptors in human platelets, accompanied by significant increases in plasma catecholamines and subjective anxiety.

E. Mononuclear Cell βARs

The well-documented decrease in the number of cortical βARs and reduced sensitivity of βAR-stimulated adenylyl cyclase found in rodent brain following chronic administration of all classes of antidepressant drugs and repeated electroconvulsive shocks (Sulser, 1978; Banerjee et al., 1977; Bergstrom and Kellar, 1979) suggest that such changes may be related to the therapeutic action of antidepressant treatments. Peripheral β-receptors, which mirror changes in central βARs would clearly represent useful tools for defining the role of βARs in depressive illness and in the effects of treatment. However, alterations in βAR density in the rat brain induced by antidepressants appears to be restricted to the β_1 subtype (Minneman et al., 1979), while human mononuclear cells (MNLs) contain only the β_2 subtypes (Meurs et al., 1982).

Despite these caveats, several groups have investigated the density of βARs in untransformed lymphocytes or leukocytes of untreated depressed patients. The studies have yielded fairly inconsistent results. Many groups report a decrease in βAR number (Extein et al., 1979; Pandey et al., 1986, 1990; Carstens et al., 1988; Magliozzi et al., 1989), while others describe an increase or no change when compared to healthy volunteers (Pandey et al., 1985; Sarai et al., 1982; Healy et al., 1985; Mann et al., 1985; Zohar et al., 1983; Cooper et al., 1985). These studies and possible methodological sources of the differences in results (e.g., methods of tissue preparation, type of ligand used, subtypes of patient populations, length of drug-free interval) have been discussed in a very thorough critical appraisal (Werstuik et al., 1990).

In contrast to the inconsistent results from binding studies described above, most studies measuring MNL βAR-stimulated AC activity report decreased responsiveness in depressed patients compared to healthy volunteers (Pandey et al., 1979; Extein et al., 1979; Mann et al., 1985; Healy et al., 1983; Ebstein et al., 1988; Halper et al., 1988; Klysner et al., 1987). The consistently observed decrease in leukocyte βAR function in depression could reflect an inherited abnormality of the βAR/Gs/AC complex, as suggested by the findings of Wright et al. (1984), utilizing Epstein-Barr virus (EBV)-transformed lymphocytes from manic-depressives and controls. However, these findings need to be replicated, and a number of additional confounding factors need to be considered. In this context, twin studies do not show a significant variability of isoproterenol (ISO)-stimulated cAMP production, suggesting that variations in ISO-stimulated cAMP production are most likely due to "environmental" effects on the number or sensitivity of βARs (Ebstein et al., 1986). As discussed already, elevated catecholamine-induced changes in MNL βAR sensitivity may be due to alterations in the subsets of lymphocytes. Additionally, elevated circulating catecholamines and glucocorticoids may exert significant effects on βAR sensitivity (Westeruik et al., 1990), perhaps via their effects at the level of the stimulatory G-protein, Gs (Malbon et al., 1990; Manji, 1992). Thus, additional studies are clearly needed to ascertain if the consistent differences in MNL βAR sensitivity in depression truly reflect comparable differences in the brain.

F. Pharmacological Challenge Strategies

Pharmacological challenge paradigms, which utilize agents known to directly or indirectly stimulate receptor sites, have been extensively utilized for testing pathophysiological hypotheses about noradrenergic dysfunction in affective illness (Siever, 1987). The α_2-adrenergic agonist clonidine (which may also exert effects at imidazoline sites; see above) has been administered to depressed patients, and the response of plasma MHPG, blood pressure, heart rate, sedation, growth hormone (GH), and cortisol has been measured. Clonidine-induced decreases of plasma MHPG have been found to be somewhat more marked (Siever et al., 1984a,b,c) or unchanged (Charney et al., 1983), when using either oral or i.v. clonidine, respectively. Similarly, the plasma MHPG response to yohimbine is unchanged in depressed patients (Heninger et al., 1988). Clonidine-induced decreases in blood pressure and increases in sedation have been found to be not significantly different in depressives compared to normals (Charney et al., 1982; Checkley et al., 1981). Similarly, responses of cortisol and ACTH to acute clonidine administration in depressed patients vary, with levels increased, decreased, or unchanged (Siever, 1987).

In contrast, a series of studies have consistently shown a significantly reduced GH response to clonidine (presumably mediated by postsynaptic hypothalamic α_2-receptors) in depressed patients (Matussek et al., 1980; Checkley et al., 1981, 1984, 1985; Charney et al., 1982; Siever et al., 1982; Lechin et al., 1985; Boyet et al., 1986; Hoehe et al., 1986; Uhde et al., 1986; Ansseau et al., 1988). These findings have generally been interpreted as evidence for subsensitive central postsynaptic α_2-receptors in depression, perhaps secondary to elevations in norepinephrine. However, it is clear that this response is not specific for depression, since a blunted GH response to clonidine has been reported in patients with panic disorder (Uhde et al., 1986; Charney and Heninger, 1986; Nutt, 1989), generalized anxiety symptoms, obsessive-compulsive disorder (Siever et al., 1983), and even in mania (Dinan et al., 1991). Thus, a blunted α_2 response may be observed in any condition characterized by tonic or episodic abnormally elevated central NE.

It is also possible that factors distal to the α_2-receptors in the hypothalamus, such as growth hormone–releasing hormone (GHRH) or somatostatin may underlie the blunted GH response to clonidine. Attempts to address this by the use of GHRH challenge tests have thus far proved unsuccessful, with conflicting results reported (Laakman et at., 1990). Adding to the difficulty in interpreting the blunted GH responses to clonidine are findings suggesting that the major GH-releasing effects of clonidine are exerted via inhibition of hypothalamic release of somatostatin rather than by stimulating GHRH secretion (Devesa, 1990). To date, the direct study of CNS adenergic receptors has been limited to the comparison of receptor density and affinity in suicide victims (generally unipolar depressives) to "appropriate controls."

The numerous methodological pitfalls associated with the study of post-mortem tissues (including postmortem delay, cause of death, morbid and premorbid drug history, etc.) notwithstanding, preliminary data suggest alterations in the density and/or affinity of β- and possibly α_2-adrenergic receptors in depressed suicide victims. Similar to the findings observed in platelets, there are elevations in the binding of the imidazolinic "α_2-ligands" such as clonidine and UK 14,304 (Meana and Garcia-Sevilla, 1987). However, whether these sites represent α_2-receptors or imidazoline sites remains to be established, although very recent data indicate that both classes of receptors/sites are elevated (Garcia-Sevilla et al., 1996). By contrast to the findings with lymphocytes, postmortem analysis of frontal contex from depressed suicide victims show an *elevation* in the density of β-receptors (Arango et al., 1990).

G. Summary of Findings of the Noradrenergic System in Mood Disorders

Considerable evidence suggests that depressed patients excrete disproportionately greater amounts of NE and its major extraneuronal metabolite, normetanephrine (NMN), relative to total catecholamine synthesis compared to controls. This is particularly true of melancholic, unipolar depressed subjects, but our recent data suggest that under adequately controlled, drug-free (>4 weeks) study, bipolar depressed subjects may exhibit a similar dysregulation of the noradrenergic system. At least with regard to mania, the original catecholamine hypothesis has withstood the test of time, with increased noradrenergic function consistently observed in mania—although this finding may ultimately reflect a secondary effect. The intriguing recent findings that CSF and urinary NE measures may be associated with the dysphoric and euphoric components of the manic syndrome, respectively, deserve further investigation and suggest that something other than mania *per se* may be producing the changes.

Findings of increased fractional urinary output of urinary NE and NMN and of an exaggerated raise in plasma NE upon orthostatic challenge in depressed patients are compatible with those of Esler et al. (1982) and Veith et al. (1985) of increased "leakiness" of presynaptic NE terminals. One possible mechanism for this is a subsensitivity of nerve-terminal α_2-autoreceptors. These receptors operate as "thermostats" and depress NE release upon activation (Starke et al., 1989). They do not directly influence the firing rate of the neuron but attenuate the release of neurotransmitters when an action potential depolarizes the varicosity or terminal or may even prevent the action potential from "invading" the nerve terminal (Starke et al., 1989).

Indeed, preclinical studies have demonstrated that blockade of presynaptic α_2-receptors on sympathetic neurons markedly increases the amount of neurotransmitters released per impulse (Starke et al., 1989). Subsensitive peripheral α_2-autoreceptors would be expected to result in a greater fractional excretion of NE and an exaggerated NE release upon any activation of the sympathetic nervous system (e.g., orthostatic stress, cold stress, "early hospitalization stress," etc). The suggestion of a subsensitivity of α_2-receptors receives additional support from the blunted GH responses to clonidine and attenuated platelet α_2 function (as assessed by inhibition of AC activity). One might justifiably argue that the subsensitive α_2-receptors may be the sequelae, not the cause, of increased NE release in depression. While this is probably true of the platelet (circulating) α_2-receptors, such a mechanism is difficult to reconcile teleologically for the nerve-terminal α_2-receptors. If these autoreceptors do down-regulate in the presence of increased NE, it would suggest the potential for an escalating feed-forward cycle, generally not seen in biological systems.

Another putative peripheral mechanism to explain the findings seen in depressed patients is that of an attenuation of the reuptake mechanism. The pattern of the relative excretion of NE and its metabolites in urine from depressed patients as compared to that from controls is strikingly similar to the further shift in the pattern observed during treatment with NE-reuptake blockers. Although considerable evidence suggests that depression is associated with reduced platelet *serotonin*-reuptake sites, this has not been adequately investigated for NE because of the absence of suitable peripheral tissues. Nevertheless, there is some evidence that there may be physiological regulation of the reuptake process (Lee et al., 1983), a possibility that requires further study in animal models or appropriate cultured cells.

H. The Serotonergic System

As with the noradrenergic system, interest in the role of the serotonergic system in mood disorders derived from a long-standing tradition of research into the role of this indoleamine in the therapeutic mechanisms of action of antidepressants and lithium.

It should be noted that of the three monoamine neurotransmitters most extensively evaluated in preclinical studies, two—serotonin and dopamine—have been studied in depressed patients almost exclusively in terms of concentrations of their respective *metabolites*, 5-hydroxy-indoleacetic acid (5-HIAA) and hormovanillic acid (HVA) in CSF. Under carefully controlled conditions, the neurotransmitter metabolites will, in part, reflect relative differences in the output and metabolism of dopamine and serotonin in the brain regions that contribute most to CSF concentrations. However, in humans, the relative contribution of different brain areas is not well understood. Moreover, it is not really possible to study the responsiveness of 5-HT and dopamine neuronal systems using a single-point measure of transmitter metabolite in CSF; at most, longer-term changes can be reflected in CSF studies. Thus, CSF studies of HVA and 5-HIAA in untreated depressed patients can identify some relative differences but cannot directly address the source of any alteration, even to the extent of distinguishing changes of output from those of metabolism and/or elimination. When considering actual studies, it is also important to recognize that limitations of assay methodology make it difficult to feel confident about many earlier studies. The technique of performing two lumbar punctures within a few days of each other—before and after the administration of probenecid to block the active acid transport of 5-HIAA and HVA out of the CSF—was an ingenious approach to obtaining an estimate of 5-HT and DA function and release (that is, the amount of accumulation of 5-HIAA and HVA between the period of probenecid administration and the lumbar tap). Such probenecid-induced accumulations sometimes revealed group differences not observed in using so-called baseline measures (Goodwin et al., 1973).

Earlier findings on 5-HIAA in CSF are also in the direction of reductions in depressed patients, but with much less consistency, perhaps because of reliance on a fluorometric assay. There is also a trend in this data for bipolar patients to have lower 5-HIAA than unipolars (reviewed in Goodwin and Jamison, 1990). Investigators have been unable to demonstrate convincing evidence for group differences in the CSF levels of 5-HIAA (with or without probenecid) of either unipolar or bipolar patients; there appears, however, to be a subgroup of patients with low levels of 5-HIAA, which may be associated with certain illness characteristics (impulsivity, aggression, and suicide attempts [reviewed in Meltzer and Lowy, 1987]). Interestingly, unlike the HVA pattern observed in comparison of mania with depression, 5-HIAA concentrations are not different in the two states. In fact, 5-HIAA may be reduced in mania as compared to controls to the same extent as observed in depression. More recent studies of baseline 5-HIAA in CSF of unmedicated depressed patients are inconsistent: the NIMH Collaborative Study reports *increased* 5-HIAA in depressed women (Koslow et al., 1983). In 83 patients with melancholia diagnosed and treated at the Karolinska Institute in Sweden, 5-HIAA was modestly, but significantly, reduced (Asberg et al, 1984). In the former study there was a trend for female bipolar patients to have lower 5-HIAA than unipolars; in the latter study, there were no differences between unipolars and bipolars in this measure.

Table 3 Evidence Implicating Dopamine in Depression

Depression in parkinsonism (up to 40% of cases)
Requirement for intact relationships of dopamine, serotonin, and norepinephrine for
   AD response
Reduced HVA, the major DA metabolite, in CSF from depressed patients
Action of many AD drugs on DA function

I. Dopamine

A relevant preclinical model derives from the crucial role of mesoaccumbens DA in the neural circuitry of reward and/or incentive motivational behavior (Wise, 1989). Loss of motivation is one of the central features of depression; indeed, anhedonia is one of the defining characteristics of melancholia. A deficiency of DA systems thus stands out as a prime candidate for involvement in the pathophysiology of depression (Willner et al., 1990) (see Tables 3 and 4).

The strongest finding from clinical studies implicating DA in depression is reduced homovanillic acid (HVA, the major DA metabolite) in the CSF; this is one of the most consistent biochemical findings in depression (Asberg et al., 1984; Potter et al., 1987). There is also evidence for a decreased rate of CSF HVA accumulation in subgroups of depressed patients, including those with marked psychomotor retardation versus agitation (Willner, 1983).

1. Antidepressants and Dopamine Function

Increasingly, preclinical studies show that chronic administration of antidepressants and electroconvulsive shock (ECS) enhances mesolimbic DA functioning (Willner et al., 1990). Thus, in some animal models of depression the efficacy of antidepressants involves increased transmission through DA synapses, particularly in the mesolimbic system (Willner et al., 1990; Koob, 1989). Similarly, d-amphetamine-induced locomotor activity, a behavior dependent on the integrity of the mesoaccumbens DA neurons, is enhanced

Table 4 Antidepressant Treatments and Dopamine Function

Enhanced mesolimbic function in preclinical studies of responses to DA agonists
Efficacy of ECT in parkinsonism
Enhanced postsynaptic DA receptor sensitivity following ECS in animals
Increased HVA in CSF of patients treated with ECT

following chronic antidepressants. Since the responses to either DA or apomorphine (direct-acting agonists) are also enhanced following chronic antidepressants, they appear to be due at least in part to increased postsynaptic DA-receptor sensitivity (Maj, 1990; Maj and Wedzony, 1985). In humans, ECT appears to increase DA-receptor responsiveness, as indexed by apomorphine's effect on plasma prolactin (Balldin et al, 1982; Modigh et al., 1984). Moreover, chronic ECT increases both CSF HVA and 5-HIAA, suggesting increased DA and 5-HT turnover. These findings are particularly striking, since a significant *reduction* in 5-HT turnover is observed after TCAs and MAOIs (Rudorfer et al., 1989).

The mechanism(s) by which antidepressants enhance postsynaptic DA function in the accumbens remain unknown, and binding studies have failed to reveal consistent alterations in the density of either D_1- or D_2-receptors. However, elegant studies on chronically stressed animals suggest that the effect may involve both D_1- and D_2-receptors or an interaction between them (Willner et al., 1990) Despite the opposite effects of D_1- and D_2-receptors on adenylyl cyclase (AC) activity, these receptors can also couple to multiple G-proteins and effectors such that D_1- and D_2-receptor stimulation may be required for maximal production of vigilance, alertness, and more sensitive control of reactivity (Ongini and Longo, 1989).

It appears that direct or indirect facilitation of dopamine function is necessary in at least some depressed patients to achieve therapeutic response. As articulated already, there is also considerable evidence that the administration of directly and indirectly acting DA agonists is capable of inducing hypomania or mania in susceptible individuals.

Interestingly, MAOIs constitute the only pharmacological monotherapy reported to be effective in 50% or more of patients who fail to respond to the full range of tricyclic antidepressants. Nolen et al. (1988) reported a controlled trial pointing to the superior efficacy of tranylcypromine (average dose of approximately 80 mg/day) in such patients. Tranylcypromine is superior to imipramine in chronic, mild unipolar patients (McGrath et al., 1987) in "anergic" bipolar depression (Himmelhoch et al., 1991; Thase et al., 1992), and phenelzine is superior in unipolar patients refractory to imipramine (McGrath et al., 1993). An open-label study of high-dose tranylcypromine (average 120 mg/day) in 14 unipolar patients who had "a clear history of non-response to at least two prior medication treatments" yielded an impressive 50% "complete" (21-item HDRS <10) response rate (Amsterdam, 1991). It was speculated that at higher plasma concentrations of tranylcypromine, the inherent "sympathomimetic (amphetamine-like) activity of the drug emerges." In other words, at higher doses one may actually recruit a pharma

Table 5 Cerebrospinal Fluid Studies of Neurotransmitters and/or Their Metabolites in Depression and Mania

	HVA, 5-HIAA, and MHPG		
Substance and comparison[a]	Review of world literature (Post et al., 1980) 1969–1979 $n = 352\ (120)^b$	Karolinska series (Asberg et al., 1984) 1970–1980 $n = 83\ (0)^b$	NIMH Collaborative Study (Koslow et al., 1983) 1975–1980 $n = 92\ (14)^b$
HVA			
D vs. C	↓	↓	↓
BP vs. UP	=	=	=
M vs. BP	?↑	N/A	↑
5-HIAA			
D vs. C	?↓	↓	=
BP vs. UP	=	=	=
M vs. BP	=	N/A	=
MHPG			
D vs. C	=	=	=
BP vs. UP	?	?c	=
M vs. BP	?↑	N/A	↑

	Norepinephrine	
	Radioenzymatic method (Post et al., 1978) $n = 20\ (8)^b$	HPLC-EC method (Rudorfer et al., 1983) $n = 21\ (0)^b$
NE		
D vs. C	=	N/A
BP vs. UP	***	↓
M vs. D	↑	N/A

[a] D = depressed (unipolars+bipolars); C = control; BP = bipolar depressed (includes types I and II); UP = unipolar depressed; M = mania (includes hypomania).

[b] n = total population of depressed patients in whom HVA or 5-HIAA was available; number in parentheses indicates size of manic sample.

[c] Insufficient depressed and BPs studied or specified; two BPI patients in Karolinska series.

↑ = increased; ↓ = decreased; + = data supporting both increased and decreased; — = no differences; ? = insufficient data available to make any judgment; ?↑ or ?↓ trend toward increase or decrease, but data preliminary or questionable; N/A = not applicable.

codynamic effect of the drug beyond MAO inhibition. Identifying multiple specific effects in humans, however, is not simple.

As should be clear from the discussion in the preceding sections, despite extensive research, the roles of the biogenic amines in the pathophysiology and treatment of manic-depressive illness remain to be clearly established; this is perhaps not surprising since clinical studies have generally dealt with individual monoaminergic measures as if they existed in isolation. However, there is considerable preclinical evidence that monoamine systems interact with one another (Bourne and Nicoll, 1993; Nicoll et al., 1989; Goldman-Rakic et al., 1990; McCormick and Williamson, 1989), and it has become increasingly more apparent in recent years that most effective drugs do not work on any given system in isolation, but rather affect the functional *balance* between interacting systems. It might be speculated that drugs designed to affect the functional balance between systems (e.g., those acting at intracellular sites) may be more effective than those exerting their effects only indirectly (e.g., those via specific neurotransmitter projections). However, this may result in a loss of the anatomical specificity necessary. With these caveats in mind, we review the data on the known interactions between the major monoaminergic systems (Table 5).

IV. NEUROTRANSMITTER INTERACTIONS IN THE CNS

A. Interactions Between Norepinephrine and Serotonin

Noradrenergic and serotonergic systems appear to interact at several different levels in the central nervous system (CNS). Early studies showed that serotonin-mediated behaviors were enhanced by β-adrenergic agonists (Cowen et al., 1982; Ortmann et al., 1981), as was the density of 5-HT2-binding sites in cortex (Scott and Crews, 1985), while β-antagonists reduced 5-HT activity (Hallberg et al., 1982). Interpretation of these studies must be tempered, however, as we have come to realize that a wider range of receptors are affected by what were previously identified as "selective" β-agonists and antagonists; other lines of evidence also demonstrate that noradrenergic and serotonergic systems interact with one another. There are data to show that α_2-adrenoreceptors modulate 5-HT release in the hippocampus (Benkirane et al., 1985), and that firing of cell bodies in the dorsal raphe is modulated by a central noradrenergic system (Gallager and Aghajanian, 1976). Finally, NE and 5-HT in dorsal raphe and locus ceruleus covary in a circadian fashion (Agren et al., 1986b), and there is direct histological evidence for noradrenergic terminals in the dorsal raphe (Baraban and Aghajanian, 1981).

B. Serotonin-Dopamine Interactions

Biochemical, electrophysiological, and behavioral data demonstrate important functional interactions between brain serotonergic and dopaminergic systems. Moreover, a strong correlation between CSF homovanillic acid (HVA) and 5-hydroxyindole acetic acid (5-HIAA) is one of the most consistent findings in biological psychiatry (Agren et al., 1986), supporting the abundant preclinical literature on functional interactions between 5-HT and DA in the midbrain. Although the subject has been widely investigated, data do not allow for simple unequivocal interpretations of either exact mechanism(s) or direction of 5-HT–DA interactions. At least some of the confusion arises from 1) regarding midbrain serotonergic and dopaminergic systems as homogeneous and unitary, 2) the failure to account for receptor subtypes' often mediating opposite biochemical electrophysiological and behavioral effects, 3) the failure to recognize that some of the effects of the 5-HT–DA interaction may be phasic rather than tonic and therefore require appropriate experimental manipulations to be manifest, 4) the overinterpretation of monoamine metabolites (e.g., 5-HIAA) to reflect function, and 5) the failure to recognize that pharmacological specificity for agonists and antagonists used is only *relative*; indeed, there is considerable overlap of drugs binding affinities both within a system (e.g., 5-HT2 and 5-HT 1C) and between neurotransmitter systems (e.g., D_2 and 5-HT2).

With these caveats, we briefly review the strongest evidence for 5-HT–DA interactions.

In general, serotonin appears to *inhibit* mesolimbic DA activity while *facilitating* that in the nigrostriatal system. Thus, amphetamine- or DA-induced hyperactivity in animals is suppressed by administration of 5-HT to the nucleus accumbens, while depletion of 5-HT within the nucleus accumbens potentiates amphetamine hyperactivity (Lyness et al., 1979). Electrophysiological studies have demonstrated that stimulation of 5-HT neurons produces changes in DA neuronal activity (Dray et al., 1976; Park et al., 1982), and numerous behavioral studies (Green and Graham-Smith, 1974; Srebro and Lorens, 1975; Costall and Maylor, 1978; Carter and Pycock, 1979) also suggest an interaction of 5-HT and DA in the mesolimbic system at the level of both DA terminals and cell bodies.

In contrast to the inhibitory effects observed in the limbic system, both biochemical and behavioral evidence suggest a facilitory role of serotonin on striatal DA function. Thus, lesions of the dorsal or median raphe nuclei cause an elevation of nigral HVA, associated with increased DA concentration in the striatum, which would result from decreased release. Similarly, stereotyped behaviors induced by peripheral administration of DA agonists such as apomorphine are reduced by lesions of the raphe nuclei, suggesting a facilitory role of 5-HT on behaviors mediated by striatal DA. There is also evidence that the effects of 5-HT on DA function may be *modulatory* rather than simply excitatory or inhibitory.

If we turn to relevant clinical research, we are limited to neuroendocrine response data and measures of the dopamine (HVA) and serotonin (5-HIAA) metabolites in CSF. Whether such neuroendocrine probes really test selective amine function has been questioned. For example, the well-documented blunted prolactin response to 5-HT agonists in depression may reflect abnormalities at the level of the DA neuron rather than at serotonergic receptors or terminals (Meltzer and Lowy, 1987). Furthermore, the biochemical changes produced by chronic administration of 5-HT-uptake inhibitors suggest that they affect DA turnover in the human CNS. Thus, it is clearly an oversimplification to attribute therapeutic efficacy to a single neurotransmitter system.

As already noted, in human CSF the most replicated biochemical finding is a high correlation between the concentrations of HVA and 5-HIAA, a finding that cannot be explained simply by a common transport mechanism. When values from the literature are plotted as a frequency distribution of the regression of HVA on 5-HIAA, a single peak emerges in healthy volunteers and an extra peak is found in depressed populations (Gibbons and Davis, 1986). Another way of expressing the relationship in an individual is through the ratio of CSF HVA to 5-HIAA, which is found to be low in depression. Studies on how drugs affect this CSF ratio show that 5-HT-reuptake inhibitors markedly increase it (beyond what can be explained by any decrease in 5-HIAA), while NE-reuptake inhibitors, which significantly reduce 5-HIAA in CSF, do not alter the HVA/5-HIAA ratio (Risby et al., 1987). A tentative interpretation is that the effects of 5-HT-reuptake inhibitors in humans may be, at least in part, through dopamine, although the clinical consequences of any 5-HT–DA interaction therefore need to be more fully elucidated.

C. Functional and Biochemical Evidence for Norepinephrine–Dopamine Interactions

Antelman and Chiodo (1981) hypothesized that functional facilitation in the DA system occurs as a result of stressful stimuli to compensate for diminished intensity of noradrenergic activity and to maintain normal functioning. Evidence for interactions between NE and DA emerged from studying maintenance of behavior reward, a parameter in animals that may model a response that is significantly impaired in depression. Unilateral NE ventral bundle transection increased DA in the A10 region (mesolimbic dopamine cell bodies) and decreased DA in the nucleus accumbens, olfactory tubercle, and interstitial nucleus of the striae terminalis (mesolimbic terminal areas) (O'Donohue et al., 1979). Other studies demonstrated that the mesolimbic DA cell bodies and their projections are necessary for the production of the behavioral effects produced by i.v. self-administration of amphetamines (O'Donohue et al., 1979; Lyness et al., 1979).

A model has been formulated in which NE is a modulator that enhances signal/noise ratios in targeted brain areas, while DA is involved in the switching between channels of activity to different brain regions (Oades, 1985). In this model, smoothly working brain function would depend on both systems' being intact. Support for NE modulation of DA function is based on new studies that α_2-antagonists potentiate the locomotor effects of the D_2-agonist quinpirole. More importantly, we have recently demonstrated significant efficacy of the α_2-adrenergic antagonist idazoxan in schizophrenic patients stabilized with D_2-blockers. This finding is consistent with a modulation of DA-receptor function that might result from sustained alteration of the firing pattern of DA neurons or from α_2–D_2 interactions via common G-proteins/second messengers (Manji, 1992).

We have previously demonstrated that, in contrast to their absolute concentrations, it is the correlations between the monoamine metabolites in the CSF that differ considerably between antidepressant responders and nonresponders (Hsiao et al., 1987). In responders, the changes in metabolite concentration with antidepressant treatment moved together and were linked statistically. In contrast, in nonresponders, these changes occurred independent of one another. Similar findings have recently been reported by another laboratory, suggesting that in antidepressant nonresponders, normal adaptive synaptic changes induced by antidepressants are prevented by an "uncoupling" of monoamine systems. In this context, novel therapeutic agents working beyond the receptor may be ideally suited to affect the functional balance between neurotransmitter systems by their actions on second-messenger systems. Thus, the drugs can be therapeutic not because they are "noradrenergic" or "serotonergic" agents per se, but because they alter the postsynaptic signal generated in response to such endogenous neurotransmitters as NE, 5-HT, and DA. In this regard, the well-established use of lithium to augment partial or absent response to uptake inhibitors is particularly relevant. It is now well established that approximately 50% of nonresponding patients can be converted to responders within 2 weeks of addition of lithium (Price, 1989). Lithium is perhaps *the* drug used in psychiatry that clearly exerts significant effects on signal transduction pathways, and it is probably the effects on G-proteins and PKC isozymes (Manji et al., 1995), which alter the "throughput" of multiple neurotransmitter systems (and thereby the functional balance between them), that underlie its remarkable efficacy.

Given the preceding discussion, it is logical to question whether depressions involve various degrees of imbalance among multiple neurotransmitter systems. As a corollary, antidepressant effects might be achieved through initial effects on one or more neurotransmitters, setting off a cascade of biochemical events that after a couple of weeks establish a new balance or setpoint of and between the systems. This would suggest that, even if some modulation of DA function is involved in antidepressant efficacy, it might be achieved by drugs acting initially on NE or 5-HT. For instance, in patients refractory to standard TCAs, it may be necessary to alter DA function more directly and perhaps at multiple levels through addition of amphetamine or methylphenidate with MAOIs, lithium (to act at postreceptor sites), or DA-reuptake inhibitors.

In sum, several lines of evidence suggest a role for dopamine in affective states at the clinical level or reward-seeking and "motivational" behavior at the preclinical one. Most convincing are empirical clinical studies of antidepressant treatment in patients not responding to monoamine-uptake inhibitors, which utilize drugs or ECT that share the property of producing transient or sustained effects on dopamine function. There also appears to be a subgroup of depressed patients who have altered dopamine (and perhaps serotonin) function as evidenced by a low level of HVA (and 5-HIAA) in the CSF. Furthermore, interactions between all three monoamine systems implicated in antidepressant action—dopamine, norepinephrine, and serotonin—may be relevant to antidepressant action and/or response. Taken together, these considerations provide a rationale implicating dopamine in the pathophysiology of manic-depressive illness, and for the use of dopaminergic agents in bipolar depression.

V. SUMMARY

Biological findings in bipolar disorders have been reviewed in the context of findings in endogenous unipolar depression, as well as of the major biochemical effects of drugs used in the treatment of manic-depressive illness. A great number of studies implicating other substances, especially cholinergic ones, have not been included. Connections between the cholinergic and noradrenergic systems, particularly with regard to stress responses, are clearly widespread and likely to be involved in aspects of bipolar illness.

To even begin to do justice to the range of studies of the cholinergic and other systems is beyond the scope of this chapter. Thus, we have opted to avoid lists of all known findings accompanied by passing reference to each relevant series of hypotheses. Rather, the concentration has been on those classes of findings that have most often been claimed to distinguish bipolar from unipolar depression. One major integrative approach has then been selected: to understand the extent to which norepinephrine function is altered in bipolar versus unipolar depression, and the extent to which effects on the norepinephrine system explain the action of drugs used in the treatment of these conditions.

We conclude by emphasizing the importance of continuing to pursue the interface between biological findings and treatment. In general, looking for predictors of response has been frustrating and somewhat academic, since clinical criteria provide the "gold standard." Without a history of (hypo)mania, however, it is not possible to assess whether a depression is bipolar or unipolar. Thus, possible long-term adverse consequences of treating bipolar or "pseudo-unipolar" depression with mania- (or cycle-) inducing drugs gives a sense of urgency to the search for a biological test. In the foreseeable future, some combination of norepinephrine-related measures appears most likely to be able to identify the bipolar population most at risk. It is hoped that simpler and more robust measures will emerge, but we should try to find a means of better utilizing the knowledge that we already have.

ACKNOWLEDGMENT

The authors would like to thank Ms. Celia Knobelsdorf for her outstanding editorial assistance.

REFERENCES

Agren H, Mefford IN, Rudorfer MV, Linnoila M, Potter WZ. Interacting neurotransmitter systems: a non-experimental approach to the 5HIAA-HVA correlation in human CSF. J Psychiatr Res 1986; 20(3):175–193.

Amsterdam JD. Use of high dose tranylcypromine in resistant depression. In: Amsterdam JD, ed. Advances in Neuropsychiatry and Psychopharmacology. Vol 2. Refractory Depression. New York: Raven Press, 1991:123–130.

Angst J. The course of major depression, atypical bipolar disorder, and bipolar disorder. In: Hippius H, Klerman GL, Matussek N, eds. New Results in Depression Research. Berlin: Springer-Verlag, 1986:26–35.

Ansseau M, Von Frenckell R, Cerfontaine JL, Papart P, Franck G, Timsit-Berthier M, et al. Blunted response of growth hormone to clonidine and apomorphine in endogenous depression. Br J Psychiatry 1988; 153:65–71.

Antelman SM, Chiodo LA. Dopamine autoreceptor subsensitivity: a mechanism common to the treatment of depression and the induction of amphetamine psychosis? Biol Psychiatry 1981; 16:717–727.

Arango V, Ernsberger P, Marzuk PM, Chen JS, Tierney H, Stanley M, et al. Autoradiographic demonstration of increased 5HT-2 and β-adrenergic receptor binding sites in the brain of suicide victims. Arch Gen Psychiatry 1990; 47:1038–1047.

Asberg M, Bertilsson L, Martensson B, et al. CSF: monoamine metabolites in melancholia. Acta Psychiatr Scand 1984; 69:201–219.

Balldin J, Granerus AK, Lindstedt G, Modigh K, Walinder J. Neuroendocrine evidence for increased responsiveness of dopamine receptors in humans following electroconvulsive therapy. Psychopharmacology 1982; 76:371–376.

Banerjee SD, Kung LS, Riggi SJ, Chanda SK. Development of β-adrenergic receptor subsensitivity by antidepressants. Nature 1977; 268:455–456.

Baraban JM, Aghajanian GK. Noradrenergic innervation of serotonergic neurons in the dorsal raphe: demonstration by electron microscopic autoradiography. Brain Res 1981; 204:1–11.

Barnes RF, Veith RC, Borson S, et al. High levels of plasma catecholamines in dexamethasone-resistant depressed patients. Am J Psychiatry 1983; 140:1623–1625.

Benkirane S, Arbilla S, Langer SZ. A functional response to D-1 dopamine receptor stimulation in the central nervous system: inhibition of the release of (3H)-serotonin from the rat substantia nigra. Naunyn Schmeidebergs Arch Pharmacol 1987; 335:502–507.

Bergstrom DA, Kellar KJ. Effect of electroconvulsive shock on monoaminergic receptor binding sites in rat brain. Nature 1979; 278:464–466.

Bourne HR, Nicoll R. Molecular machines integrate coincident synaptic signals. Cell 1993; suppl 72:65–75.

Bousquet P, Feldman J. The blood pressure effects of alpha-adrenoceptor antagonists injected in the medullary site of action of clonidine: the nucleus reticularis lateralis. Life Sci 1987; 40:1045–1052.

Boyajian CL, Leslie FM: Pharmaoclogical evidence for α_2 adrenoceptor heterogeneity: Differential binding properties of [3H]rauwolscine and [3H]idazoxan in rat brain. J Pharmacol Exp Ther 241:1092–1098, 1987

Boyer P, Davila M, Schaub C, Kanowski S, et al: Growth hormone response to clonidine stimulation in depressive states. Part I. Psychiatr Psychobiol 1:189–195, 1986

Bricca G, Dontenwill M, Molines A, et al: Evidence for the existence of a homogenous population of imidazoline receptors in the human brainstem. Eur J Pharmacol 150:401–402, 1988a

Bricca G, Dontenwill M, Molines A, et al: The imidazoline preferring receptor: binding studies in bovine, rat, and human brainstem. Eur J Pharmacol 162:1–9, 1988b

Bunney WE, Davis JM: Norphinephrine in depressive reactions: a review. Arch Gen Psychiatry 13:483–494, 1965

Bylund DB, Ray-Prenger C, Murphy TJ. α_{2A} and α_{2B} adrenergic receptor subtypes: antagonist binding in tissues and cell lines containing only one subtype. J Pharmacol Exp Ther 1988; 245:600.

Calabrese JR, Fatemi SH, Woyshville MJ. Antidepressant effects of lamotrigine in bipolar rapid cycling. Am J Psychiatry. In press.

Carstens ME, Engelbrecht AH, Russell VA, et al. Biological markers in juvenile depression. Psychiatry Res 1988; 23:77–88.

Carter CJ, Pycock CJ. The effects of 4,7-dihydroxytryptamine lesions of extrapyramidal and mesolimbic sites on spontaneous motor behavior and amphetamine-induced stereotype. Naunyn-Schmiedebergs Arch Pharmacol 1979; 208:51–54.

Charney DS, Heninger GR. Abnormal regulation of noradrenergic function in panic disorders. Arch Gen Psychiatry 1986; 43:1041–1054.

Charney DS, Heninger GR, Sternberg DE, Hafstad KM, Giddings S, Landis DH. Adrenergic receptor sensitivity in depression. Arch Gen Psychiatry 1982; 39:290–294.

Charney DS, Heninger GR, Sternberg DE. Alpha$_2$ adrenergic receptor sensitivity and mechanism of action of antidepressant therapy. Br J Psychiatry 1983; 142:265–275.

Checkley SA, Glass TB, Thompson C, et al. The growth hormone response to clonidine in endogenous as compared to reactive depression. Psychol Med 1984; 14:773–777.

Checkley SA, Corn TH, Glass TB, et al. The responsiveness of central alpha adrenoceptors in depression. In: Deakin JFW, ed. The Biology of Depression. London: Gakell, 1985:110–119.

Checkley SA, Slade AP, Shur E. Growth hormone and other responses to clonidine inpatients with endogenous depression. Br J Psychiatry 1988; 138:51–55.

Cooper SL, Kelly JG, King DJ. Adrenergic receptors in depression effects of electroconvulsive therapy. Br J Psychiatry 1985; 147:23–29.

Costall B, Naylor RJ. Neuroleptic interactions with the serotonergic-dopaminergic mechanisms in the nucleus accumbens. J Pharm Pharmacol 1978; 30:257–259.

Cowen PJ, Grahame-Smith DG, Green AR, Heal DJ. β-adrenoreceptor agonists enhance 5-hydroxytryptamine-mediated behavioral responses. Br J Pharmacol 1982; 76:265–270.

Davis JM, Bresnahan DB. Psychopharmacology in clinical psychiatry. In: Hales RE, Frances AJ, eds. APA Annual Review. Vol 6. Washington, DC: American Psychiatric Press, 1987:159–187.

Davis JM, Koslow SH, Gibbons RD, Maas JW, Bowden CL, Casper R, et al. Cerebrospinal fluid and urinary biogenic amines in depressed patients and healthy controls. Arch Gen Psychiatry 1988; 45:705–717.

Devesa J, Arce V, Lois N, et al. α_2-adrenergic agonism enhances the growth hormone (GH) response to GH-releasing hormone through an inhibition of hypothalamic somatostatin release in normal men. J Clin Endocrinol Metab 1990; 71:1581–1588.

de Villiers AS, Russell VA, Carstens ME, Aalbers C, Gagiano CA, Chalton DO, et al. Noradrenergic function and hypothalamic-pituitary-adrenal axis activity in primary unipolar major depressive disorder. Psychiatry Res 1987; 22:127–140.

Dinan TH, Yatham LN, O'Keane V, Barry S. Blunting of noradrenergic-stimulated growth hormone release in mania. Am J Psychiatry 1991; 148:936–938.

Dray A, Gonye TJ, Oakley NR, et al. Evidence for the existence for raphe projections to substantia nigra in rat. Brain Res 1976; 113:45–57.

Ebstein RP, Lerer B, Bennett ER, Dayek DB, Newman Me, Shapira B, Kindler S. Second messenger function in lymphocytes and platelets: a comparison of peripheral and central mechanisms. Clin Neuropharmacol 1986; 9(suppl 4):350–352.

Ebstein RP, Moscovich D, Zeevi S, Amiri Z, Lerer B. Effect of lithium in vitro and after chronic treatment on human platelet adenylate cyclase activity: postreceptor modification of second-messenger signal amplification. Psychiatry Res 1987; 21:221–228.

Ebstein RP, Lerer B, Shapria B, Shemesh Z, Moscovich DG, Kindler S. Cyclic AMP second-messenger signal amplification in depression. Br J Psychiatry 1988; 152:665–669.

Esler M, Turbott J. Schwarz R, et al. The peripheral kinetics of norepinephrine in depressive illness. Arch Gen Psychiatry 1982; 39:295–300.

Extein I, Tallman J, Smith CC, Goodwin FK. Changes in lymphocyte β-adrenergic receptors in depression and mania. Psychiatry Res 1979; 1:191–197.

Filser JG, Spira J, Fischer M, et al. The evolution of 4-hydroxy-3-methoxy-phenyl-gylol sulfate as a possible marker of control norepinephrine turnover studies in healthy volunteers and depressed patients. J Psychiatr Res 1988; 22:171–181.

Freedman RR, Embury J, Migaly P, et al. Stress-induced desensitization of alpha$_2$-adrenergic receptors in human platelets. Psychosom Med 1990; 52:624–630.

Gallagher DW, Aghajanian GK. Effect of antipsychotic drugs on the firing of dorsal raphe cells. I. Role of adrenergic system Eur J Pharmacol 1976; 39:341–355.

Garcia-Sevilla JA, Padro D, Giralt MT, Guimon J, Areso P, Fuster MJ. Biochemical and functional evidence of supersensitive platelet α_2-adrenoreceptors in major affective disorder: effect of long-term lithium carbonate treatment. Arch Gen Psychiatry 1986; 43:51–57.

Garcia-Sevilla JA, Guimon J, Garcia-Vallejo P. α_2-adrenoceptor-mediated inhibition of platelet adenylate cyclase and induction of aggregation in major depression: effect of long-term antidepressant drug treatment. Arch Gen Psychiatry 1990; 47:125–132.

Gibbons JL, Davis JM. Consistent evidence for a biological subtype of depression characterized by low CSF monamine levels. Acta Psychiatr Scand 1986; 74:8–12.

Goldman-Rakic PS, Lidow MS, Gallager DW. Overlap of dopaminergic, adrenergic, and serotoninergic receptors and complementarity of their subtypes in primate prefrontal cortex. J Neurosci 1990; 10(7):2125–2138.

Goldstein DS, Zimlichman R, Kelly GD, Stull R, Bacher JD, Keiser HR. Effect of ganglion blockade on cerebrospinal fluid norepinephrine. J Neurochem 1987; 49:1484–1490.

Goodwin FK, Jamison KR. Biochemical and pharmacologic studies. In: Goodwin FK, Jamison KR, ed. Manic-Depressive Illness. New York: Oxford University Press, 1990:416–502.

Goodwin FK, Sack RL. Affective disorders: the catecholamine hypothesis revisited. In: Usdin E, Snyder S, eds. Frontiers in Catecholamine Research. New York: Pergamon Press, 1973.

Goodwin FK, Brodie HKH, Murphy DL, et al. L-dopa, catecholamines and behavior: a clinical and biochemical study in depressed patients. Biol Psychiatry 1970; 2:341–366.

Goodwin FK, Cowdry RW, Webster MH. Predictors of drug response in the affective disorders: toward an integrated approach. In: Lipton MA, Maschio AD, Killman KF, eds. Psychopharmacology: A Generation of Progress. New York: Raven Press, 1978:1277–1288.

Green AR, Grahame-Smith DG. The role of brain dopamine in the hyperactivity syndrome produced by increased 5-hydroxytryptamine synthesis in rats. Neuropharmacology 1974; 13:949–959.

Halaris AE. Plasma 3-methoxy-4-hyrdoxyphenylglycol in manic psychosis. Am J Psychiatry 1978; 135:493–494.

Hallberg H, Almgren O, Svensson TH. Reduced brain serotonergic activity after repeated treatment with β-adrenoceptor antagonists. Psychopharmacology 1982; 76:114–117.

Halper JP, Brown RP, Sweeney JA, Kocsis JH, Peters A, Mann JJ. Blunted β-adrenergic responsivity of peripheral blood mononuclear cells in endogenous depression. Arch Gen Psychiatry 1988; 45:241–244.

Healy D, Carney PA, Leonard BE. Monamine-related markers of depression: changes following treatment. J Psychiatr Res 1983; 17:251–260.

Healy D, Carney PA, O'Halloran A, Leonard BE. Peripheral adrenoceptors and serotonin receptors in depression: changes associated with response to treatment with trazodone or amitriptyline. J Affect Disord 1985; 9:285–296.

Heninger GR, Charney DS, Price LH. α_2-adrenergic receptor sensitivity in depression: the plasma MHPG, behavioral, and cardiovascular responses to yohimbine. Arch Gen Psychiatry 1988; 45:718–726.

Himmelhock JM, Thase ME, Mallinger AG, et al. Tranylcypromine versus imipramine in anergic bipolar depression. Am J Psychiatry 1991; 148:910–916.

Hoehe M, Valido G, Matussek N. Growth hormone response to clonidine in endogenous depressive patients: evidence for a trait marker in depression. In: Shagass C, Josiassen EC, Bridger WH, et al., eds. Biological Psychiatry Developments in Psychiatry. Amsterdam: Elsevier, 1986:862–864.

Hsiao JK, Agren H, Bartko JJ, Rudorfer MV, Linnoila M, Potter WZ. Monoamine neurotransmitter interactions and the prediction of antidepressant response. Arch Gen Psychiatry 1987; 44(12):1078–1083.

Janicak PG, Davis JM, Chan C, Altman E, Hedeker D. Failure of urinary MHPG levels to predict treatment response in patients with unipolar depression. Am J Psychiatry 1986; 143:1398–1402.

Janowsky DS, El-Yousef MK, Davis JM, et al. A cholinergic-adrenergic hypothesis of mania and depression. Lancet 1972; ii:632–635.

Janowsky DS, El-Yousef MK, Davis JM, et al. Parasympathetic suppression of manic symptoms of physostigmine. Arch Gen Psychiatry 1973; 28:542–547.

Jimerson DC, Nurnberger JI Jr, Post RM, Gershon ES, Kopin IJ. Plasma MHPG in rapid cyclers and healthy twins. Arch Gen Psychiatry 1981; 38:1287–1290.

Jimerson DC, Insel TR, Reus VI et al. Increased plasma MHPG in dexamethasone-resistant depressed patients. Arch Gen Psychiatry 1983; 40:173–176.

Kafka MS, Paul SM. Platelet α2-adrenergic receptors in depression. Arch Gen Psychiatry 1986; 43:91–95.

Katona CLE, Theodorou AE, Davies SL, et. al. [^{3}H]Yohimbine binding to platelet α_2-adrenoreceptors in depression. J Affect Disord 1987; 17:219–228.

Klysner R, Geisler A, Rosenberg R. Enhanced histamine and β-adrenoreceptor mediated cyclic AMP formation in leukocytes from patients with endogenous depression. J Affect Disord 1987; 13:227–232.

Koob GF. Anhedonia as an animal model of depression. In: Koob GF, Ehlers C, Kupfer DJ, eds. Animal Models of Depression. Boston: Birkhauser, 1989:162–183.

Kopin IJ. Catecholamine metabolism: Basic aspects and clinical significance. Pharmacol Rev 1985; 37:333–364.

Koslow SH, Maas JW, Bowden CL, et al. Cerebrospinal fluid and urinary biogenic amines and metabolites in depression and mania: a controlled, uivariate analysis. Arch Gen Psychiatry 1983; 40:999–1010.

Kukopoulos A, Reginalde D, Laddomada P, et al. Course of the manic depressive cycle and changes caused by treatments. Pharmkopsychiatry Neuropsychopharmakology 1980; 13:156–167.

Laakmann G, Hinz A, Voderholzer U, Daffner C, Muller OA, Neuhayser H. The influence of psychotropic drugs and releasing hormones on anterior pituitary hormone secretion in healthy subjects and depressed patients. Pharmacopsychiatry 1990; 23:18–26.

Lechin F, van der Dijs B, Jakubowicz D, Camero RE, Villa S, Arocha L, et al. Effects of clonidine on blood pressure, noradrenaline, cortisol, growth hormone, and prolactin plasma levels in high and low intestinal tone depressed patients. Neuroendocrinology 1985; 41:156–162.

Lee CM, Javitch JA, Snyder A. Recognition sites for norepinephrine uptake: regulation by neurotransmitter. Science 1983; 220:626–629.

Linnoila M, Guthrie S, Lane EA, et al. Clinical studies on norepinephrine metabolism: how to interpret the number. Psychiatry Res 1986; 17:229–239.

Louis WJ, Doyle AE, Anavekar SN. Plasma noradrenaline concentration and blood pressure in essential hypertension, phaeochromocytoma and depression. Clin Sci Mol Med 1975; 48:239S–242S.

Lyness WH, Friedele NM, Moore KE. Destruction of dopaminergic nerve terminals in nucleus accumbens: effect on D-amphetamine self-administration. Pharmacol Biochem Behav 1979; 11:553–556.

Maas JW, Benensohn H, Landis DH. A kinetic study of the disposition of circulating norepinephrine in normal male subjects. J Pharmacol Exp Ther 1970; 174:381–387.

Maas JW, Fawcett JA, Pekirmenjian H. Catecholamine metabolism, depressive illness, and drug response. Arch Gen Psychiatry 1972; 26:252–262.

Maas JW, Kocis JH, Bowden CL, Davis JM, Redmond DE, Hanin I, et al. Pretreatment on neurotransmitter metabolites and response to imipramine or amitriptyline treatment. Psychol Med 1982; 12:37–43.

Maas JW, Koslow SH, Davis J, Katz M, Frazer A, Bowden CL, et al. Catecholamine metabolism and disposition in healthy and depressed subjects. Arch Gen Psychiatry 1987; 44:337–344.

Magliozzi JR, Gietzen D, Maddock RJ, Haack D, Doran AR, Goodman T, et al. Lymphocyte β-adrenoreceptor density in patients with unipolar depression and normal controls. Bio Psychiatry 1989; 26:15–25.

Maisel AS, Knowlton KU, Fowler P, Rearden A, Ziegler MG, Motulsky HJ, Insel PA, Michel MC. Adrenergic control of circulating lympocyte subpopulations: effects of congestive heart failure, dynamic exercise, and tebutaline treatment. J Clin Invest 1990a; 85:462–467.

Maisel AS, Harris T, Rearden CA, et al. Adrenergic receptors in lymphocyte subsets after exercise: alterations in normal individuals and patients with congestive heart failure. Circulation 1990b; 82:2003–2010.

Maj J. Behavioral effects of antidepressant drugs given repeatedly on the dopaminergic systems. In: Gessa GL, Serra G, eds. Dopamine and Mental Depression (Advances in the Biosciences). Oxford: Pergamon Press, 1990:139–146.

Maj J, Wedzony K. Repeated treatment with imipramine or amitriptyline increases the locomotor response to rats to (+)-amphetamine given into the nucleus accumbens. J Pharm Pharmacol 1985; 37:362–364.

Malbon CC, Hadcock JR, Rapiejko PJ, et al. Regulation of transmembrane signaling elements: transcriptional, post-transcriptional and post-translational controls. Biochem Soc Symp 1990; 56:155–164.

Manji HK. G proteins: implications for psychiatry. Am J Psychiatry 1992; 149:746–760.

Manji HK, Lenox RH. Long-term action of lithium: a role for transcriptional and posttranscriptional factors regulated by protein kinase C. Synapse 1994; 16:11–28.

Manji HK, Rudorfer MV, Potter WZ. Affective disorders and adrenergic function. In: Cameron OG, ed. Adrenergic Dysfunction and Psychobiology. Washington, DC: American Psychiatric Press, 1994.

Manji HK, Potter WZ, Lenox RH. Signal transduction pathways: molecular targets for lithium's actions. Arch Gen Psychiatry 1995; 52:531–543.

Mann C. Meta-analysis in the breech. Science 1990; 249:476–480.

Mann JJ, Brown RP, Halper JP, Sweeney JA, Kocsis JH, Stokes PE, et al. Reduced sensitivity of lymphocyte β-adrenergic receptors in patients with endogenous depression and psychomotor agitation. N Engl J Med 1985; 313:715–720.

Mann JJ, Maevitz AZ, Chen JS, et al. Acute effects of single and repeated electroconvulsive therapy on plasma catecholamines and blood pressure in major depressive disorder. Psychiatry Res 1990; 34:127–137.

Matussek N, Ackenheil M, Hippius H, et al. Effect of clonidine on growth hormone release in psychiatric patients and controls. Psychiatry Res 1980; 2:25–36.

McCormick DA, Williamson A. Convergence and divergence of neurotransmitter action in human cerebral cortex. Proc Natl Acad Sci USA 1989; 86:8098–8102.

Meana JJ, Garcia-Sevilla JA. Increased α_2-adrenoceptor density in the frontal cortex of depressed suicide victims. J Neural Transm 1987; 70:377–381.

Meeley MP, Ernsberger PR, Granata AR, et al. An endogenous clonidine-displacing substance from bovine brain: receptor binding and hypotensive actions in the ventrolateral medulla. Life Sci 1986; 38:1119–1126.

Meltzer HY, Lowy MT. The serotonin hypothesis of depression. In: Meltzer HY, ed. Psychopharmacology: The Third Generation of Progress. New York: Raven Press, 1989:513–526.

Meurs H, van den Bogaard W, Kauffman HF, Bruynzeel PL. Characterization of (−) [3H] dihydroalprenolol binding to intact and broken cell preparations of human peripheral blood lymphocytes. Eur J Pharmacol 1982; 85:185–194.

Michel MC, Regan JW, Gerhardt MA, et al. Noradrenergic [3H]idazoxan binding sites are physically distinct from alpha$_2$-adrenergic receptors. Mol Pharmacol 1990; 37:65–68.

Minneman KP, Hegstrand LR, Molinoff PB. Simultaneous determination of beta-1 and beta-2 adrenergic receptors in tissues containing both receptor subtypes. Mol Pharmacol 1979; 16:34–46.

Modigh K, Balldin J, Eriksson E, Granerus AK, Walinder J. Increased responsiveness of dopamine receptors after ECT—a review of experimental and clinical evidence. In: Lerer B, Weiner RD, Belmaker H, eds. ECT: Basic Mechanisms. 1984:18–27.

Murphy DL, Brodie HKH, Goodwin FK, et al. Regular induction of hypomania by L-dopa in "bipolar" manic-depressive patients. Nature 1971; 229:135–136.

Muscettola G, Potter WZ, Pickar D, et al. Urinary MHPG and major affective disorders: a replication and new findings. Arch Gen Psychiatry 1984; 41:337–342.

Nicoll RA, Malenka RC, Kauer JA. Functional comparison of neurotransmitter receptor subtypes in mammalian central nervous system. Nature 1989; 87:741–746.

Nolen WA, Jansen GS, Broekman M. Measuring plasma levels of carbamazepine: a pharmacokinetic study in patients with affective disorders. Pharmacopsychiatry 1988; 21:252–254.

Nutt DJ. Altered central α_2-adrenoreceptor sensitivity in panic disorder. Arch Gen Psychiatry 1989; 46:165–169.

Oades RD. The role of noradrenaline in tuning and dopamine in switching between signals in the CNS. Neurosci Biobehav Rev 1985; 9(2):261–282.

O'Donohue TL, Crowley WR, Jacobwitz DM. Biochemical mapping of the noradrenergic ventral bundle projects sites: evidence for a noradrenergic-dopaminergic interaction. Brain Res 1979; 172:87–100.

Onginin E, Longo VG. Dopamine receptors subtypes and arousal. Int Rev Neurobiol 1989; 31:239–255.

Oppenheim G, Ebstein RP, Belmaker RH. The effect of lithium on the physostigmine-induced behavioral syndrome and plasma GMP. J Psychiatr Res 1979; 15:133–138.

Ortmann R, Martin S, Radeke E, Delini-Stula A. Interaction of β-adrenoceptor agonists with the serotonergic system in rat brain. Naunyn Schmied Arch Pharmacol 1981; 216:225–230.

Pandey GN, Dysken MW, Garver PL, et al. Beta-adrenergic receptor function in affective illness. Am J Psychiatry 1979; 136:675–678.

Pandey GN, Janicak PG, Javaid JI, Davis JM. Studies of beta-adrenergic receptors in leukocytes of patients with affective illness and effects of antidepressant drugs. Psychopharmacol Bull 1985; 21:603.

Pandey GN, Davis JM. Leukocyte β-adrenergic receptors: a marker for central β-adrenergic receptor function in depression. Clin Neuropharmacol 1986; 14(9 suppl):353–355.

Pandey GN, Janicak PG, Javaid JI, Davis JM. Increased ^{3}H-clonidine binding in the platelets of patients with depressive and schizophrenic disorders. Psychiatry Res 1989; 28:73–88.

Pandey GN, Pandey SC, Davis JM. Peripheral adrenergic receptors in affective illness and schizophrenia. Pharmacol Toxicol 1990; 3:13–36.

Park, MR, Gonzales-Vegas, JA, Kitai, JT. Serotonergic excitation from dorsal raphe stimulation recorded intracellularly from rat caudate-putamen. Brain Res 1982; 243:49–58.

Pickar D, Sweeney DR, Maas JW, Heninger GR. Primary affective disorder, clinical state change and MHPG excretion: a longitudinal study. Arch Gen Psychiatry 1978; 35:1378–1383.

Piletz JE, Halaris A. Noradrenergic imidazoline binding sites in platelets of depressed patients. Biol Psychiatry 1991; 29:167A.

Piletz JE, Schubert DSP, Halaris A. Evaluation of studies on platelet α_2 adrenoreceptors in depressive illness. Life Sci 1986; 39:1589–1616.

Piletz JE, Halaris A, Saran A, et al. Elevated ^{3}H-para-aminoclonidine binding to platelet purified plasma membranes from depressed patients. Neuropsychopharmacology 1990; 3:201–210.

Post RM, Lake CR, Jimerson DC, et al. Cerebrospinal fluid norepinephrine in affective illness. Am J Psychiatry 1978; 135:907–912.

Post RM, Jimerson DC, Ballenger JC, Lake CR, Uhde TW, Goodwin FK. Cerebrospinal fluid norepinephrine and its metabolites in manic-depressive illness. In: Post RM, Ballenger JC, eds. Neurology of Mood Disorders. Baltimore: Williams & Wilkins, 1984:539–553.

Post RM, Rubinow DR, Uhde TW, Roy-Byrne PP, Linnoila M, Rosoff A, et al. Dysphoric mania: clinical and biological correlates. Arch Gen Psychiatry 1989; 46:353–358.

Potter WZ, Rudorfer MV, Goodwin FK. In: Hales RE, Frances AJ, eds. APA Annual Review. Vol 6. Washington, DC: American Psychiatric Press, 1987:32–60.

Price LH. Lithium augmentation in tricyclic-resistant depression. In: Extein IL, ed. Treatment of Tricyclic-Resistant Depression. Washington, DC: American Psychiatric Press, 1989:49–80.

Redmond DE, Katz MM, Maas JW, Swann A, Casper R, Davis JM. Cerebrospinal fluid amine metabolites: relationships with behavioral measurements in depressed, manic, and healthy control subjects. Arch Gen Psychiatry 1986; 43:938–947.

Reifman A, Wyatt RJ. Lithium: a brake in the rising cost of mental illness. Arch Gen Psychiatry 1980; 37:385–388.

Risby ED, Hsiao JK, Sunderland T, Agren H, Rudorfer MV, Potter WZ. The effects of antidepressants on the cerebrospinal fluid homovanillic acid/5-hydroxyindoleacetic acid ratio. Clin Pharmacol Ther 1987; 42:547–554.

Rosenblatt S, Chanley JD, Leighton WP. The investigation of adrenergic metabolism with ^{3}H-norepinephrine in psychiatric disorders. II. Temporal changes in the distribution of urinary tritiated metabolites in affective disorders. J Psychiatr Res 1969; 6:321–333.

Roy A, Pickar D, Linnoila M, Potter WZ. Plasma norepinephrine level in affective disorders: relationship to melancholia. Arch Gen Psychiatry 1985; 42(12): 1181–1185.

Roy A, Jimerson DC, Pickar D. Plasma MHPG in depressive disorders and relationship to the dexamethasone suppression test. Am J Psychiatry 1986; 143:846–851.

Roy A, Guthrie S, Pickar D, Linnoila M. Plasma norepinephrine responses to cold challenge in depressed patients and normal controls. Psychiatry Res 1987; 21:161–167.

Roy A, Pickar D, DeJong J, Karoum F, Linnoila M. Norepinephrine and its metabolites in cerebrospinal fluid, plasma and urine: relationship to hypothalamic-pituitary-adrenal axis function in depression. Arch Gen Psychiatry 1988; 45:849–857.

Rubin AL, Price LH, Charney DS, Heninger G. Noradrenergic function and the cortisol response to dexamethasone in depression. Psychiatry Res 1985; 15:5–15.

Rubinow DR, Gold PW, Post RM, et al. CSF somatostatin in affective illness. Arch Gen Psychiatry 1983; 40:409–412.

Rudorfer MV, Potter WZ. Combined fluoxetine and tricyclic antidepressants. Am J Psychiatry 1989; 146:562–564.

Rudorfer MV, Ross RJ, Linnoila M, Sherer MA, Potter WZ. Exaggerated orthostatic responsivity of plasma norepinephrine in depression. Arch Gen Psychiatry 1985; 42(12):1186–1192.

Sarai K, Nakahara T, Kanagana K. Lymphocyte β-adrenergic receptor function in affective disorders. Adv Biosci 1982; 40:161–165.

Schatzberg AF, Orsulak PJ, Rosenbaum AH, et al. Toward a biochemical classification of depressive disorders. V. Heterogeneity of unipolar depressions. Am J Psychiatry 1982; 139:471–474.

Schildkraut JJ. The catecholamine hypothesis of affective disorders: a review of the supporting evidence. Am J Psychiatry 1965; 122.

Schildkraut JJ, Orsulak PJ, Schatzberg AF, Gudeman JE, Cole JO, Rohde WA, et al. Toward a biochemical classification of depressive disorders. I. Differences in urinary excretion of MHPG and other catecholamine metabolites in clinically defined subtypes of depression. Arch Gen Psychiatry 1978; 35:1427–1433.

Scott JA, Crews FT. Increase in serotonin$_2$ receptor density in rat cerebral cortex slices by stimulation of beta-adrenergic receptors. Biochem Pharmacol 1985; 34:1585–1588.

Siever LJ. Role of noradrenergic mechanisms in the etiology of the Affective Disorders. In: Meltzer HY, ed. Psychopharmacology: The Third Generation of Progress. New York: Raven, 1987:493–504.

Siever LJ, Uhde TW, Silberman EK, Jimerson DC, Aloi JA, Post RM, et al. Growth hormone response to clonidine as a probe of noradrenergic receptor responsiveness in affective disorder patients and controls. Psychiatry Res 1982; 6:171–183.

Siever LJ, Insel TR, Jimerson DC, Lake CR, Uhde TW, Aloi J, et al. Growth hormone response to clonidine in obsessive-compulsive patients. Br J Psychiatry 1983; 142:184–187.

Siever LJ, Uhde TW, Jimerson DC, Lake CR, Silberman ER, Post RM, et al. Differential inhibitory noradrenergic responses to clonidine in 25 depressed patients and 25 normal control subjects. Am J Psychiatry 1984a; 141:733–741.

Siever LJ, Uhde TW, Jimerson DC, et al. Plasma cortisol responses to clonidine in depressed patients and controls: evidence for possible alteration in noreadrenergic-neuroendocrine relationships. Arch Gen Psychiatry 1984b; 41:63–68.

Siever LJ, Kafka MS, Targum S, et al. Platelet alpha-adrenergic binding and biochemical responsiveness in depressed patients and controls. Psychiatry Res 1984c; 11:287–302.

Siever LJ, Uhde TW, Jimerson DC, Lake CR, Kopin IJ, Murphy DL: Indices of noradrenergic output in depression. Psychiatry Res 1986; 19:59–73.

Srebro B, Lorens SA. Behavioral effects of selective midbrain raphe lesion in the rat. Brain Res 1975; 89:303–325.

Starke CK, Gothert M, Kilbinger H. Modulation of neurotransmitter release by presynaptic autoreceptors. Physiol Rev 1989; 69:864–989.

Sulser F, Vetulani J, Mobley PL. Mode of action of antidepressant drugs. Biochem Pharmacol 1978; 27:257–271.

Swann AC, Secunda SK, Katz MM, Koslow SH, Maas JW, Chang S, Robins E. Lithium treatment of mania: clincal characteristics, specificity of symptom change, and outcome. Psychiatry Res 1986; 18:127–141.

Swann AC, Koslow SH, Katz MM, Maas JW, Javaid J, Secunda SK, et al. Lithium treatment of mania: cerebrospinal fluid and urinary monamine metabolites and treatment outcome. Arch Gen Psychiatry 1987; 44:345–354.

Thase ME, Mallinger AG, McKnight D, et al. Treatment of imipramine-resistant recurrent depression. IV. A double-blind crossover study of tranylcypromine for anergic bipolar depression. Am J Psychiatry 1992; 149:195–198.

Uhde TW, Vittone BJ, Siever LJ, Kaye WH, Post RM. Blunted growth hormone response to clonidine in panic disorder patients. Biol Psychiatry 1986; 21:1081–1085.

Van Tits LJ, Michel MC, Grosse-Wilde H, Happel M, Eigler FW. Catecholamines increase lymphocyte beta $_2$-adrenergic receptors via a beta $_2$-adrenergic, spleen-dependent process. Am J Physiol 1990; 258:E191–202.

Veith RC, Halter JB, Murburg MM, et al. Increased plasma NE appearance rate in dexamethasone resistant depression. Fourth World Congress of Biological Psychiatry, Athens, Greece, Oct 13–17, 1985.

Veith RC, Barnes RF, Villacres E, Murburg MM, Raskind MA, Borson S, et al. Plasma catecholamines and norepinephrine kinetics in depression and panic disorder. In: Belmaker R, ed. Catecholamines: Clinical Aspects. New York: Alan R Liss, 1988:197–202.

Weissman MM, Leaf PJ, Tischler GL, Karno M, Bruce ML, Florio LP. Affective disorders in five United States communities. Psychol Med 1988; 18:141–153.

Werstiuk ES, Steiner M, Burns T. Studies on leukocyte beta-adrenergic receptors in depression: a critical appraisal. Life Sci 1990; 47:85–105.

Willner P. Dopamine and depression: a review of recent evidence. I. Empirical studies. Brain Res Rev 1983; 6:211–224.

Willner P, Muscat R, Papp M, Sampson D. Dopamine, depression and antidepressant drugs. In: Willner, Scheel-Kruger, eds. The Mesolimbic Dopamine System: From Motivation to Action. Chichester, England: Wiley, 1990.

Wise RA, Rompre PP. Brain dopamine and reward. Annu Rev Psychol 1989; 40:191–225.

Wright AF, Crichton DN, Loudon JB, Morten JE, Steel CM. Beta-adrenoceptor binding defects in cell lines from families with manic-depressive disorder. Ann Hum Genet 1984; 48(pt 3):201–214.

Wyatt RJ, Portnoy B, Kupfer DJ, Synder F, Engelman K. Resting plasma catecholamine concentrations in patients with depression and anxiety. Arch Gen Psychiatry 1971; 24:65–70.

Zohar J, Bannet J, Drummer D, Fisck R, Epstein RP, Belmaker RH. The responses of lymphocyte β-adrenergic receptors to chronic propranolol treatment in depressed patients, schizophrenic patients, and normal controls. Biol Psychiatry 1983; 18:553–560.

2

Signal Transduction Abnormalities in Bipolar Disorder

Jun-Feng Wang and L. Trevor Young
McMaster University, Hamilton, Ontario, Canada

Peter P. Li and Jerry J. Warsh
University of Toronto, Toronto, Ontario, Canada

A neurobiological basis for bipolar disorder (BD) has long been postulated but has not yet been conclusively established. As reviewed in the Introduction and by other contributors to this volume, there are clear reasons to support this notion, including the heritability of the disorder, response to mood-stabilizing medications, and a recurrent clinical course with prominent neurovegetative features. Results of earlier studies on monoaminergic neurotransmitters (i.e., noradrenergic, dopaminergic, and serotonergic) have suggested that alterations may occur in these systems in BD, possibly due to changes in receptor sensitivity. These data have resulted in a recently burgeoning field of research investigating mechanisms regulating receptor responsivity and membrane receptor signal transduction.

In the following section, we highlight the major signal transduction pathways that have been studied in BD and review molecular pharmacological evidence implicating signal transduction processes as targets of mood-stabilizing agents, particularly lithium. A discussion of direct clinical findings on these mechanisms obtained in subjects with BD follows. As will be demonstrated, in BD there is evidence of dysfunction in several of the known signal transduction pathways, which may, at least in part, be compensated for by treatment with a mood stabilizer.

I. SIGNAL TRANSDUCTION PATHWAYS

Neurotransmitters, modulators, hormones, and other extracellular messengers bind to a family of membrane receptors that couple to intracellular events through guanine nucleotide-binding proteins (G-proteins). Neuroreceptor activation modulates ion flux through membrane channels in addition to the activity of a variety of cell membrane "effector" enzymes such as adenylyl cyclase (AC) and phospholipase C (PLC) that catalyze production of intracellular second messengers, in turn regulating cell function. Second messengers, including cyclic AMP, calcium, diacylglycerol, and the inositol polyphosphates, are part of an extensive array of cascading transduction processes that act on yet another level of signaling targets comprising a number of protein kinases. These play a role in regulating a number of physiological responses. Equally important, protein kinases also regulate gene expression by activating a variety of transcription factors. The latter are DNA-binding proteins found in nuclei of cells that bind to specific "consensus" sequences in the 5' noncoding but regulatory regions of target genes. For example, the immediate early genes, c-fos and c-jun, are two well-characterized transcription factors coupled to second messengers. These intricate signal transduction systems result in transduction and amplification of the original extracellular signal to a vast network of intracellular mechanisms and pathways.

A. Guanine Nucleotide-Binding Proteins

G-proteins are a family of signal transduction proteins that play a critical role in the transduction of information across the plasma membrane by coupling receptors to effectors (Gilman, 1987; Birnbaumer et al., 1990). G-proteins are heterotrimers consisting of two functional entities that are tightly associated in plasma membranes: an α subunit, which binds and hydrolyzes guanosine triphosphate (GTP), and a dimer composed of regulatory β and γ subunits (Backlund et al., 1991; Federman et al., 1992; Spiegel et al., 1992; Birnbaumer, 1993). Recent cloning and sequencing studies have demonstrated an extensive family of G-proteins based on α subunit diversity. These have been classified into four main categories: $G_s\alpha$, $G_i\alpha$ $G_q\alpha$, and $G_{12}\alpha$ subfamily (Hepler et al., 1992; Raymond, 1995). The multiplicity of α subunits provides for the coupling of a wide variety of neuromodulatory receptors to the same or different intracellular second-messenger systems and ion channels. It is generally assumed that the α subunits selectively regulate different effector proteins. For example, G_s stimulates AC and G_i inhibits AC. Some G-protein α subunits are substrates of bacterial toxin–catalyzed

ADP-ribosylation (Moss and Vaughan, 1988). Cholera and pertussis toxins can catalyze the transfer of the ADP-ribose moiety of nicotinamide adenine dinucleotide (NAD) to specific residues within the α subunits by ADP-ribo-syltransferase (Tamir and Gill, 1988). The major substrate for cholera toxin is α_s, and cholera toxin catalyzes ADP-ribosylation of Arg[187], inhibits GTPase activity, and leads to constitutive activation of α_s (Freissmuth and Gilman, 1989). Pertussis toxin catalyzes ADP-ribosylation at a cysteine residue fourth from the C-terminus of selected α subunits (e.g., α_i, α_o and α_t) (Moss and Vaughan, 1988; Ramdas et al., 1991).

The G-proteins have two conformations: an active GTP-bound form and an inactive form in which guanosine diphosphate (GDP) is bound. Receptor activation induces a conformational change in receptor-associated G-protein, resulting in dissociation of GDP on the α subunit, and GTP is bound. The GTP-bound α subunit activates intracellular effector enzymes. The intrinsic GTPase activity of the α subunit quickly hydrolyses GTP to GDP, which results in reassociation of G-protein subunits and termination of the interaction with the effector. The interconversion of GDP/GTP-bound state is a key step in regulating G-protein function (Neer, 1995; Raymond, 1995; Rens-Domiano and Hamm, 1995).

β and γ subunits act as a dimer. In most cases, agonist-occupied receptors cannot stimulate GTP/GDP exchange on an α subunit without the presence of the $\beta\gamma$ dimer. The $\beta\gamma$ subunit modulates GTP/GDP exchange directly, and also anchors α subunits to the plasma membrane (Birnbaumer et al., 1990). Recent evidence has also indicated important roles of β and γ subunits in signal transduction pathways. For example, $\beta\gamma$ subunit activates muscarinic K^+ channels and may also activate mitogen-activated protein kinase pathways through Ras (Logothetis et al., 1987; Clapham and Neer, 1993; Reuveny et al., 1994; Wickman et al., 1994; Crespo et al., 1994; Faure et al., 1994). It has also been shown that one AC subtype is activated synergistically by α and $\beta\gamma$ subunit, and another one is activated by α but inhibited by $\beta\gamma$ subunit (Iyengar, 1993). $\beta\gamma$ subunits can also activate PLCβ directly (Clapham and Neer, 1993; Smrcka and Sternweis, 1993).

B. Signaling Through Cyclic AMP (Figure 1)

Cyclic AMP is a ubiquitous second messenger that occurs in all cells and plays a critical role in intracellular signaling, regulating many cellular functions. The cytosolic concentration of cyclic AMP is determined by a balance between its rate of production by the action of AC on ATP and degradation by cyclic nucleotide phosphodiesterase. Cyclic AMP, in turn, activates several targets, primarily cyclic AMP–dependent protein kinase,

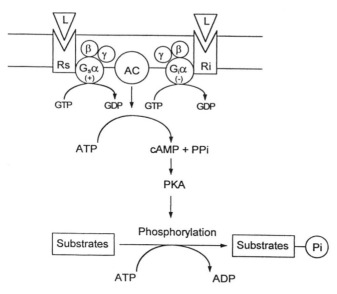

Figure 1 G-protein-coupled cyclic AMP system. Ligands (L) bind to receptors (Rs and Ri) that interact with G-proteins composed of α, β and γ subunits. Then G-protein stimulates (G$_s$) or inhibits (G$_i$) adenylyl cyclase (AC). Activation of AC converts ATP to cyclic AMP (cAMP). cAMP, as a second messenger, activates cAMP-dependent protein kinase (PKA), which in turn phosphorylates different substrates.

which in turn regulates cellular processes such as metabolism and gene transcription. Because cyclic AMP is rapidly hydrolyzed to 5'-AMP, the increase of cyclic AMP concentration is usually brief (seconds to minutes) when AC is activated (Strulovici et al., 1984; Bray, 1990).

A variety of neurohormones and neurotransmitters are coupled to AC through G-proteins (Gilman, 1987). At least nine isozymes of AC have been identified and characterized. Type I is stimulated by Ca^{2+}/calmodulin and inhibited by G-protein βγ subunits. Types III and VIII are also stimulated by Ca^{2+}/calmodulin. Types II and IV are Ca^{2+}-insensitive and highly activated by G-protein βγ subunits, but only in the presence of simultaneous Gα$_s$ activation. Types V and VI are Ca^{2+}-inhibited, but are not affected by G-protein βγ subunits. Type IX is not affected by Ca^{2+}/calmodulin and G-protein βγ subunits. Regulation of type VII is not clear yet (Tang and Gilman, 1991; Cooper and Brooker, 1992; Iyengar, 1993; Cali et al., 1994; Defer et al., 1994; Taussig and Gilman, 1995; Premont et al., 1996). The phosphodiesterases are also found in multiple forms, each with distinct kinetic characteristics and affinities for cyclic AMP and cyclic GMP. For example, a cyclic GMP–dependent form (types I and II) is sensitive to calmodulin and possesses high affinity for cyclic GMP and a lower affinity for cyclic AMP. An independent form (type IV) is insensitive to activation of calmodulin or cyclic GMP, but has high affinity and specificity for cyclic AMP. The cyclic GMP–inhibited form (type III) has little or low activity in the brain (Thompson and Appleman, 1971; Beavo and Reifsnyder, 1990).

Cyclic AMP–dependent protein kinase is the principal target enzyme regulated by cyclic AMP in eukaryotes (Beavo et al., 1974; Krebs and Beavo, 1980). Activation of this kinase phosphorylates proteins by transferring the γ phosphate from ATP to specific serine and threonine residues of substrate protein, thereby regulating protein functions. In the unstimulated state, cyclic AMP–dependent protein kinase is an inactive holoenzyme consisting of a dimeric regulatory subunit and two catalytic subunits, each of which is expressed in multiple isoforms in a tissue- and species-specific fashion (Beebe, 1994). Binding of cyclic AMP to the regulatory subunits causes the holoenzyme to dissociate, release, and active the catalytic subunits. The latter then phosphorylate cytoplasmic and nuclear substrates. One particularly important nuclear substrate is the transcription factor cyclic AMP–responsive element-binding protein (CREB), which regulates gene transcription by binding to the cyclic AMP–responsive element (CRE) of target gene promoter after CREB is phosphorylated by cyclic AMP–dependent protein kinase (Gonzalez and Montminy, 1989; Lee et al., 1990).

C. Polyphosphoinositide (PI)-Generated Second Messengers (Figure 2)

Many neurotransmitter receptors are coupled to phosphatidylinositol-specific phospholipase C (PLC) through G-protein (G_q)-dependent mechanisms. Activation of PLC catalyzes hydrolysis of phosphatidylinositol 4,5-biphosphate (PIP_2) to two second messengers, diacylglycerol (DAG) and inositol 1,4,5-trisphosphate [$Ins(1,4,5)P_3$] (Berridge et al., 1982; Strathman and Simon, 1990). $Ins(1,4,5)P_3$ binds to a specific receptor, which opens a calcium channel in the endoplasmic reticulum (ER) membrane, releasing Ca^{2+} into free cystolic pools (Berridge and Irvine, 1989). $Ins(1,4,5)P_3$ can undergo either phosphorylation to 1,3,4,5-inositol tetrakisphosphate [$Ins(1,3,4,5)P_4$] by 3-kinase or dephosphorylation to $Ins(1,4)P_2$ by 5-phosphatase. $Ins(1,3,4,5)P_4$ may mediate slower and more prolonged responses by enhancing external Ca^{2+} entry in the cell (Irvine, 1992). DAG and Ca^{2+} synergistically activate protein kinase C (PKC), another family of kinases

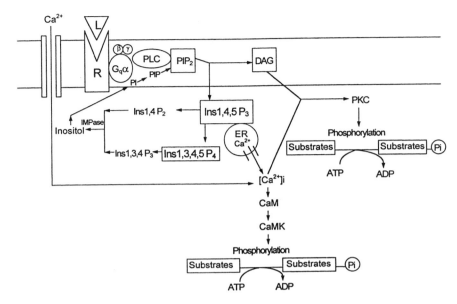

Figure 2 Phosphoinositide-generated second-messenger system. Other ligands bind to their receptors, which are coupled to a G-protein (G_q) composed of α, β, and γ subunits. Activation of PLC by $G_q\alpha$ catalyzes hydrolysis of phosphatidylinositol 4,5-biphosphate (PIP_2) to two second messengers, diacylglycerol (DAG) and 1,4,5-inositol trisphosphate ($Ins(1,4,5)P_3$). $Ins(1,4,5)P_3$ releases Ca2+ from endoplasmic reticulum (ER). Release of Ca2+ induces increment of intracellular free calcium concentration ([Ca2+]i). $Ins(1,4,5)P_3$ can undergo either phosphorylation to $Ins(1,3,4,5)P_4$ or dephosphorylation to $Ins(1,4)P_2$. $Ins(1,3,4,5)P_4$ can be dephosphorylated to $Ins(1,3,4,)P_3$. Inositol is produced by dephosphorylation of $Ins(1,4)P_2$ and $Ins(1,3,4,)P_3$ with inositol monophosphatase (IMPase). DAG and Ca2+ synergistically activate protein kinase C, which phosphorylates different substrates. Increased [Ca2+]i also binds to specific proteins, one of these proteins is calmodulin (CaM). Ca2+/CaM stimulate Ca2+/calmodulin-dependent protein kinase (CaMK), which in turn phosphorylates different substrates.

that play a major role in receptor-mediated signal transduction and are involved in a diverse range of cellular responses in the central nervous system (CNS) (Nishizuka, 1984). The maintainance and efficiency of the phosphoinositol signal system are dependent in part on its capacity to regenerate PIP_2 from myo-inositol. Because inositol crosses the blood–brain barrier poorly, in brain, in contrast to peripheral tissues, the action of the enzyme inositol monophosphate (IMPase) is crucial. In the CNS, the pool of free inositol depends strongly on recycling via dephosphorylation of inositol phosphates, IMPase being the rate-limiting step in inositol synthesis (Nahorski et al., 1992; Atack et al., 1995a,b).

Calcium-activated, phospholipid-dependent PKC participates in the regulation of a wide variety of physiological functions in the CNS. These are monomeric kinases consisting of an N-terminal regulatory region and a C-terminal catalytic region. Certain hydrophobic esters of the tumor promoter phorbol can diffuse through the membrane from the extracellular fluid and activate PKC by mimicking DAG. This property has led to their use as pharmacological agents to characterize the function of PKC in physiological events (Newton, 1995a,b). Molecular cloning has recently revealed the expression of multiple, closely related PKC isoforms. These have been categorized into three groups based on domain homology and biochemical properties: 1) conventional PKCs (α, β_I, β_{II}, γ), which are Ca^{2+}-dependent and phorbol ester–sensitive, 2) novel PKCs (δ, ϵ, η, θ), which are Ca^{2+}-independent and phorbol ester–sensitive; and 3) the atypical PKCs (ζ and λ), which are neither Ca^{2+}-dependent nor phorbol ester–sensitive (Nishizuka, 1988; Stabel and Parker, 1991; Hug and Sarre, 1993; Buchner, 1995).

PKC regulates cell function by phosphorylating a number of proteins. One of these proteins is myristolated alanine-rich C kinase substrate (MARCKS), which has been well studied. MARCKS is a widely distributed PKC substrate that is abundant in brain among other tissues. Recent evidence indicates that MARCKS may play an important role in transducing extracellular signals into changes in actin–membrane interactions that regulate processes such as neurotransmitter release (Hyatt et al., 1994). Differential tissue distribution of PKC isoforms and their coexistence in a single cell suggest that individual isoenzymes participate in distinct cellular responses, which may be important for fine-tuning the signaling properties of different neurons (Dekker and Parker, 1994; Newton, 1995a).

D. Intracellular Calcium

In addition to release by $Ins(1, 4, 5)P_3/Ins(1,3,4,5)Pa_4$, intracellular free Ca^{2+} levels are critically dependent on regulation by ion channels. As in other cells in the body, the concentration of intracellular free Ca^{2+} in the CNS is maintained at ~50 to 200 nM, approximately 10,000-fold lower than in the extracellular space (Resnik et al., 1986; Dubovsky et al., 1992). With cellular stimulation, cytosolic Ca^{2+} concentration increases rapidly to the μM range and shows oscillatory patterns. It is thought that the amplitude and frequency of the oscillations in intracellular Ca^{2+} entrain regulatory signals. Hormones, neurotransmitters, and electrical activity all regulate cytosolic Ca^{2+} concentration by influx of Ca^{2+} through Ca^{2+} channels into the cytosol and by release of Ca^{2+} from internal storage pools. Ca^{2+} influx across the plasma membrane is initiated by the opening of Ca^{2+} channels, which in neurons include voltage-dependent and ligand-gated subtypes (Palotta, 1987; Rink, 1988; Tsien et al., 1988; Sachs and Muallem, 1989). Release of Ca^{2+} from intracellular storage sites is regulated by second-messenger $Ins(1,4,5)P_3$, which is triggered by binding of various ligands to G-protein-coupled receptors on the cell surface that generate intracellular $Ins(1,4,5)P_3$, as described above (Reuter, 1983; Berridge, 1989; Snyder and Supattapone, 1989). Increased intracellular Ca^{2+} influences many cellular processes, including synthesis and release of neurotransmitters and receptor signaling.

To a large extent, intracellular Ca^{2+} binds to specific proteins, including calmodulin as well as other high-affinity Ca^{2+}-binding proteins (Burgoyne and Geisow, 1987; Kennedy et al., 1987). The Ca^{2+}/calmodulin complex regulates a wide variety of other proteins. Calmodulin participates in stimulation of many intracellular kinases, relaying the calcium-entrained signal to other target proteins. A number of other Ca^{2+}-binding proteins function as Ca^{2+} buffers, limiting the range of fluctuations in cytosolic free Ca^{2+} concentration.

Return of intracellular free Ca^{2+} to resting levels terminates many of its cellular effects. To reestablish the several-thousand-fold gradient of Ca^{2+} concentration across the plasma membrane, neurons, and other cells, calcium-dependent ATPase drives Ca^{2+} against its concentration gradient out of the cell as well as into intracellular calcium stores. Calcium may also be removed by Na^+/Ca^{2+} exchange, which pumps Ca^{2+} out and Na^+ into the cell through a Na^+-K^+-ATPase energy-dependent process (Carafoli, 1987; Blaustein, 1988).

E. Interactions Between Signal Transduction Systems

Although receptors can directly activate or inhibit specific second-messenger systems via coupling to primary effector enzymes, considerable evidence indicates that substantial *crosstalk* occurs between second-messenger systems. In this respect, second-messenger responses linked to one receptor may modulate effector responses linked to a different type of receptor, potentiating or attenuating response into the other system. For example, α_s-stimulated cyclic AMP formation by AC could be enhanced (or decreased) by $\beta\gamma$ subunits released from dissociation of α_i or by PKC in response to another inhibitory agonist binding to its receptor (Jacobowitz et al., 1993;

Lustig et al., 1993). Cyclic AMP–dependent protein kinase can inhibit the agonist-stimulated PPI hydrolysis, hence reducing production of the second messengers, $Ins(1,4,5)P_3$ and DAG (Jakobs et al., 1986). Cyclic AMP and calcium interact at multiple target sites. It has been reported that cyclic AMP can inhibit Ca^{2+} influx, desensitize $Ins(1,4,5)P_3$ receptor, or increase Ca^{2+} influx from cytosol by Ca^{2+}-ATPase (Burgess et al., 1991; Kennedy, 1993). Cyclic AMP can also regulate Ca^{2+} levels by phosphorylation of voltage-dependent Ca^{2+} channel. On the other hand, Ca^{2+} can also regulate cyclic AMP levels by activating Ca^{2+}/calmodulin-dependent phosphodiesterase (Sharma, 1995). Crosstalk between receptor-activated second-messenger systems may therefore be critical to processes such as signal integration and modulation and, accordingly, coordination of cell functions.

F. Regulation of Gene Expression (Figure 3)

Gene expression can be regulated by altering the rate of mRNA transcription initiated by RNA polymerase. The rate of transcription is regulated by *trans*-acting proteins (transcription factors) that bind to *cis*-acting DNA elements of target genes. Intracellular second messengers and related protein kinases can change transcription factor activity by altering the levels of these factors or through phosphorylation, which modifies their activity (Mitchell and Tjian, 1989; Berk and Schmidt, 1990). Two transcription factors, CREB and activating protein 1 (AP-1), and their regulation by intracellular signal pathways, have been intensively studied.

CRE is a binding site for the CREB transcription factor family, which includes CREB, CRE modulator (CREM), and activating transcription factors (ATF). The consensus CRE sequence is GTGACGc/aA. CREB contains a leucine zipper motif region that is responsible for dimerization and DNA binding. CREB can activate target gene transcription when it is phosphorylated at Ser-133 by cyclic AMP–dependent protein kinase or Ca^{2+}/calmodulin-dependent protein kinase, which are major signaling pathways (Sheng et al., 1991; Meyer and Habener, 1993; Lee and Masson, 1993).

Fos and Jun are transcription factors that can heterodimerize to form an AP-1 complex. There are several known Fos-related proteins called Fos-related antigens (FRAs), including FRA-1, FRA-2, and FosB, all of which form AP-1 complexes with Jun family protein. The AP-1 complex binds to the DNA regulatory element known as the AP-1 site, which shows the consensus sequence GTGAGTc/aA. The AP-1 site is also called phorbol or the 12-myristate 13-acetate (TPA) response element (TRE) because TPA, a potent tumor promoter, strongly activates PKC and induces expression of

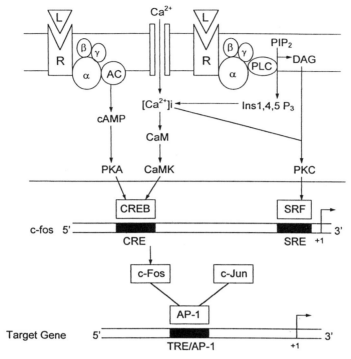

Figure 3 Regulation of gene expression by second-messenger systems. Second messengers, including cyclic AMP (cAMP), 1,4,5-inositol trisphosphate (Ins(1,4,5) P_3), diacylglycerol (DAG), and Ca^{2+}, lead to change in the activity of cAMP-dependent protein kinase (PKA), protein kinase (PKC), and Ca^{2+}/calmodulin-dependent protein kinase (CaMK), respectively, which phosphorylate the specific transcription factors. For example, the cAMP-responsive element-binding protein (CREB) binds to cAMP-responsive element (CRE), and serum-responsive factor (SRF) binds to serum-responsive element (SRE). This in turn regulates gene expression of c-fos and many others. Fos and Jun proteins can heterodimerize to form an AP-1 complex. The AP-1 complex binds to the DNA regulatory element known as the AP-1 site, also called the TPA response element (TRE), which regulates target gene expression.

genes that contain the TRE via the PKC pathway. The TRE/AP-1 site is found in the promoters of a large number of important genes such as preproenkephalin and tyrosine hydroxylase, and can negatively or positively regulate transcription (Angel et al., 1987; Curran and Vogt, 1992; Curran and Morgan, 1995).

Fos and Jun are induced in the CNS by a wide variety of extracellular stimuli and are thought to regulate gene expression by acting as third messengers in signal transduction cascades. In most cells, basal levels of Fos and Jun gene expression are very low, but are induced rapidly and transiently by a variety of extracellular stimuli. Extracellular signals activate intracellular second-messenger systems that induce the transcription of c-fos and c-jun mRNAs. Fos and Jun proteins are synthesized and translocated to the nucleus, where they form a heterodimeric protein complex that binds to the nuleotide sequence motif TRE/AP-1 site regulating gene transcription (Curran and Vogt, 1992; Curran and Morgan, 1995). The serum response element (SRE) and CRE have been identified within the c-fos promoter. The serum-responsive factor (SRF), platelet-derived growth factor (PDGF), epidermal growth factor (EGF), and interleukin-2 can induce c-fos gene expression by targeting SRE (Siegfried and Ziff, 1989; Fisch et al., 1987; Fisch et al., 1989; Janknecht et al., 1995).

Recently it has been reported that the 35 kDa Fos-related antigen protein can be expressed for an extended period, suggesting that some Fos-related antigen–Jun heterodimer combinations may activate long-term gene expression that is different from that of genes modulated by the acute factors (Sonnenberrg et al., 1989; Hope et al., 1994; Nye et al., 1995; Pennypacker, 1995).

II. MECHANISM OF ACTION OF MOOD-STABILIZER TREATMENT OF BIPOLAR DISORDER

Lithium and the anticonvulsants carbamazepine or sodium valproate are the primary treatments for BD, but the exact mechanisms that account for their mood-stabilizing effects remain unknown. Since lithium was established as a mood stabilizer long before these anticonvulsants, there is much more research on the molecular pharmacology of this agent than for carbamazepine or sodium valproate. Lithium has been shown to exert many effects on the CNS (Price et al., 1990; Odagaki et al., 1992). In animals, lithium increases the synthesis and turnover of 5-HT in presynaptic neurons, at least partly by increasing uptake of the 5-HT precursor tryptophan. The release of 5-HT into the synapse is also increased, particularly in hippocampus. Lithium diminishes the binding and function of postsynaptic 5-HT2 receptors, particularly in hippocampus, possibly reflecting compensation for primary presynaptic effects, and enhances electrophysiological and behavioral responses mediated by postsynaptic 5-HT1A receptors. This compound has no consistent effect on βAR binding, but it may alter βAR function as evidenced by decreased βAR-mediated stimulation of AC after lithium administration (Price et al., 1990). Many of these effects of lithium on brain serotonergic and noradrenergic systems occur at lithium concentrations higher than those that occur therapeutically (Bunney et al., 1987; Wood and Goodwin, 1987; Risby et al., 1991). The lack of a clear elucidation of the effect of lithium on neurotransmitter systems and receptors, together with the emerging understanding of the mechanisms involved in the coupling of receptors to cellular signal transduction systems, resulted in a shift of focus toward postreceptor events and mechanisms. In this regard, an increasing body of evidence has accumulated demonstrating effects of lithium (and possibly the mood-stabilizing anticonvulsants) on G-proteins and effectors, including AC^- and PI^- generated second messengers. These are reviewed in detail in the following section (Table 1).

A. The G-Protein-Coupled Cyclic AMP Signal System

Among the earliest evidence of lithium's action on signal transduction pathways were findings that it could blunt receptor-activated AC activity. Forn and Valdecasas (1971) reported that lithium in vitro attenuated norepinephrine-stimulated cyclic AMP acumulation. Following this study, much research demonstrated that in vivo treatment with lithium at therapeutic concentrations could blunt cyclic AMP signaling following stimulation with various neurotransmitters and hormones. For example, chronic lithium administration increased basal cyclic AMP and decreased noradrenaline- and isoprenaline-stimulated cyclic AMP production in rat brain, cultured renal epithelial cells, and human brain tissue (Forn and Valedcases, 1971; Goldberg et al, 1988; Mork and Geisler, 1989a,b; Masana et al., 1991, 1992). This effect is not limited to the noradenergic system, but has been shown for other neurotransmitter systems such as dopamine and 5-HT, which signal through cyclic AMP modulation (Mork and Geisler, 1989a,b; Newman et al., 1989, 1991; Carli et al., 1994). It has been hypothesized that lithium increases basal AC activity by stabilizing the inactive heterotrimeric form of G_i, thus reducing the inhibitory control of basal AC activity (Masana et al., 1992). Lithium may also act on AC by regulating the expression of specific AC isoforms (Colin et al., 1991) in rat brain. In vitro studies have also demonstrated an inhibitory effect of lithium on the accumulation of another cyclic nucleotide (cyclic GMP), while chronic in vivo treatment with lithium has been found to enhance cyclic GMP accumulation in rat cortex (Harvey et al., 1993). This latter effect was accompanied by an increase in total PDE activity and decrease in cyclic AMP. It was proposed that lithium may activate a cyclic GMP–stimulated PDE by increasing cyclic GMP levels, which in turn reduces cellular levels of cyclic AMP (Harvey et al., 1993).

A number of recent studies have implicated G-proteins as a possible target of lithium. In an early study employing transformed rat pheochromocytoma (PC-12) cells, Volonte (1988) found that lithium in vitro increased the density of [³H]GTP binding. Chronic lithium treatment of rats was also shown to reduce GTP-dependent isoprenaline activation as well as 5-HT inhibition of cyclic AMP production, which further implicated an effect of lithium at the G-protein level (Mork and Geisler, 1989a,b). In a much-cited work, Avissar and colleagues (1988) demonstrated that lithium blunted agonist-mediated increases in GTP binding in rat brain membrane. They concluded that this reflected lithium's effect to decrease G-protein functionality. This same group (Schreiber et al., 1991) found complementary evidence of such an effect in BD patients, demonstrating that βAR and muscarinic agonist-induced increases in [³H]guanosine imidodiphosphate (Gpp[NH]p) (a nonhydrolyzable GTP analog) binding to lymphocyte membranes obtained from manic BD subjects were greater than in control subjects and euthymic lithium-treated BD patients. They interpreted these data to be consistent with the notion that G-protein hyperfunctionality occurs in BD that is reduced by lithium treatment. This in turn is consistent with the findings of Risby et al. (1991), who found that lithium increased basal–, guanine nucleotide–, and cesium fluoride–stimulated AC activity (the latter two agents act directly on G-proteins) in platelets from healthy subjects. As discussed later, these observations of effects of lithium on G-protein were important in leading investigators to study G-proteins directly in patients with BD.

Several studies (Table 1) have attempted to clarify the exact mechanism(s) by which lithium modifies G-protein function (Lesch et al., 1991; Colin et al., 1991; Li et al., 1991, 1993a). Both Li et al. (1991) and Colin et al. (1991) found that chronic lithium treatment reduces rat cortical α_s and α_i mRNA levels, suggesting that lithium may also modify G-protein functionality through the regulation of the genes expressing these G-protein subtypes. This effect on G-protein expression, however, may be quite complex and accompanied by compensatory posttranslational biochemical changes, since some studies have found no changes in α_s, α_o, or β subunit levels in rat brain after chronic lithium treatment (Colin et al., 1991; Lesch et al., 1991; Li et al., 1993a). Li and Jope (1995), however, found that chronic lithium treatment reduced the ability of NGF to increase G-protein subunits (α_s, α_{o1}, α_{i1}, and β) in PC12 cells. In one study, carbamazapine had no effect on G-protein

Table 1 Effect of Mood Stabilizers on Intracellular Transduction Systems

Intracellular messengers	Tissue	Treatment	Effect	Ref.
G-protein-coupled cyclic AMP system	Rat cerebral cortex	In vitro incubation with LiCl 2–100 mM	↓NaF-induced AC activity; ↓NE-induced cAMP formation	Forn and Valdecases, 1971
	PC12 cells	Incubation with LiCl 1.1 mM for 3 min	↑[³H]GTP to PC12 binding to membrane	Volonte, 1988
	LLC-PK₁ cells	Incubation with 20 mM of LiCl	↓Vasopressin-stimulated cAMP formation	Goldberg et al., 1988
	Rat cerebral cortex	In vivo for 12–21 days at theraputic concentration of lithium	↓Noradrenergic and cholinergic agonist-induced increases in [³H]GTP binding	Avissar et al., 1988
	Rat hippocampus	In vivo for 4 weeks at therapeutic concentration of lithium	↓5-HT inhibition of cAMP	Mork and Giesler, 1989
	Rat cerebral cortex	In vivo for 4 weeks at therapeutic concentration of lithium	↓Isoprenaline-stimulated AC	Mork and Giesler, 1989
	Human platelets	Therapeutic concentration of lithium for >2 weeks	↑Basal, Gpp[NH]p and cesium fluoride–stimulated AC activity	Risby et al., 1991
	Rat cerebral cortex	In vivo for 4 weeks at therapeutic concentration of lithium	↑AC type I and type II mRNA/protein level; ↓$G_i\alpha_1$ and $G_i\alpha_2$ mRNA/protein level; no change in $G_o\alpha$, $G_s\alpha$, and $G\beta$	Colin et al., 1991
	Rat cerebral cortex	In vivo for 4 weeks at therapeutic concentration of lithium	↑Basal cAMP; ↓NE-stimulated cAMP formation	Masana et al., 1991
	Human platelets	Therapeutic concentration of lithium for 2 weeks	↑PTX-mediated ADP-ribosylation; no change in CTX-mediated ADP-ribosylation	Hsiao et al., 1992
	Rat frontal cortex	In vivo for 4 weeks at therapeutic concentration of lithium	↑DARPP-32 level	Guitart and Nestler, 1992
	Rat cerebral cortex	In vivo for 3 weeks at therapeutic concentration of lithium and carbamazepine	↓$G_s\alpha$, $G_i\alpha_1$, and $G_i\alpha_2$ mRNA	Li et al., 1993a

	Tissue/cells	Condition	Finding	Reference
	Rat neostriatum	In vivo for 4 weeks at therapeutic concentration of lithium	↓GTP-induced, DA-sensitive AC activity	Carli et al., 1994
	Rat frontal cortex	In vivo for 4 weeks at therapeutic concentration of lithium	↑Endogenous ADP-ribosylation	Nestler et al., 1995
	C6 glioma cells	Incubation with LiCl 1 mM, valproate 0.5 mM, and carbamazepine 0.05 mM for 1 week	↑Endogenous ADP-ribosylation after lithium, ↓by valproate, no change after carbamazepine	Young and Woods, 1996
Phosphoinositide generated second-messenger system	Rat hippocampus	In vivo for 5 weeks at therapeutic concentration of lithium	↓Membrane-associated PKC α isozyme	Manji et al., 1983
	Rat hippocampus	In vivo for 3 days at therapeutic concentration of lithium	↑PMA-induced 5-HT release	Anderson et al., 1988
	Mouse cerebral cortex	In vitro incubation with LiCl 5 mM for 10 min	↓Carbachol stimulation of IP_4	Whitworth and Kendall, 1988
	Rat cerebral cortex	In vitro incubation with LiCl 1 mM for 20–30 min	↓Carbachol stimulation of IP_3 and IP_4	Kennedy et al., 1989
	Rat brain	In vivo for 3 or 16 days at therapeutic concentration of lithium	↓Carbachol and NaF-stimulated inositol phosphate production	Godfrey et al., 1989
	Rat cortical tissue	In vivo for 3 weeks at therapeutic concentration of lithium	↓PMA-induced PKC translocation and 5-HT release	Wang and Friedman, 1989
	Rat hippocampus	In vivo for 3 weeks at therapeutic concentration of lithium	↓Phosphorylation and protein level of MARCKS	Lenox et al., 1992
	Rat cerebral cortex	In vivo 4 weeks at therapeutic concentration of lithium	↑GTPγS and NaF stimulation of [^{3}H]PI hydrolysis	Song and Jope, 1992
	Rat cortex	In vivo for 3 weeks at therapeutic concentration of lithium	↑Translocation and activation of PKC	Li et al., 1993b
	C6 glioma cells	In vitro incubation with valproate 0.6 mM for 6 to 7 days	↓Protein kinase C α and ε	Chen et al., 1994

mRNA or protein levels (Li et al., 1993a) and the effect of sodium valproate has not yet been determined. ADP-ribosylation of G-protein α subunits has been shown to be important in regulating their function and possibly turnover (Milligan et al., 1989; Milligan, 1993). An earlier study in platelets from healthy subjects treated chronically with lithium showed that the pertussis toxin–stimulated ADP-ribosylation of α_i was increased after chronic treatment, with no changes found in α_i, levels (Hsiao et al., 1992). Similar findings were also observed in platelets from lithium-treated subjects with BD (Manji et al., 1995a). More recently, Nestler et al. (1995) reported that lithium in vitro inhibits endogenous ADP-ribosylation of α_s in rat brain homogenates. They also found that chronic administration of lithium to rats in vivo, under conditions that result in therapeutically relevant serum levels, increases endogenous ADP-ribosylation activity. In our laboratory (Young and Woods, 1996), we also found that chronic treatment with lithium markedly increased endogenous ADP-ribosylation of both α_i and α_s in C6 glioma cells, whereas sodium valproate had an opposite effect and carbamazepine had little or no effect. Therefore, mood stabilizers may have different mechanisms of action with respect to G-protein regulation. Thus, to date, there is evidence that lithium may regulate G-proteins at both the transcriptional and the posttranslational levels. It is not yet clear how these actions account for its therapeutic effects.

Since lithium influences the activity of the cyclic AMP second-messenger system, protein phosphorylation mediated by the associated kinases might be expected to be altered by lithium administration. Indeed, chronic lithium treatment has been reported to alter the phosphorylation by cyclic AMP–dependent protein kinase of several proteins in vitro. For example, chronic lithium treatment increased the phosphoprotein DARPP-32, a major substrate for cyclic AMP–dependent protein kinase, by 30% in the rat frontal cortex (Guitart and Nestler, 1992). Chronic treatment with lithium also induced the translocation of cyclic AMP–dependent protein kinase from cytosol to the nucleus in the same tissue (Guitart and Nestler, 1992). Together, these findings further support an effect of lithium on the cAMP signaling pathway. Since specific transcriptional factors are targets of cyclic AMP–dependent protein kinases, it is not surprising that there has been much recent interest in whether lithium and other mood stabilizers regulate these downstream processes.

B. The PI-Generated Second-Messenger System

It has been clearly demonstrated that lithium affects phosphoinositide metabolism, apparently at multiple sites (Table 1). Lithium, at therapeutically relevant concentrations, is a noncompetitive inhibitor of the intracellular IMPase (Hallcher and Sherman, 1980), which is a key enzyme in the recycling of inositol phosphate (Naccarato et al., 1974; Atack et al., 1995a). As alluded to earlier, the ability of a neuron to maintain sufficient supplies of myo-inositol is critical for resynthesis of inositol phospholipids and the maintenance of PI-mediated signaling. It has been hypothesized that the therapeutic effect of lithium may derive from reduced agonist-induced PI hydrolysis consequent to inositol depletion by inhibition of IMPase and reduction in PI-generated second messengers. Belmaker and coworkers (Benjamin et al., 1995) have recently demonstrated that the addition of high concentrations of exogenous inositol can reduce but not completely reverse lithium's effects on the PI cycle. Furthermore, therapeutic concentrations of lithium only partially inhibited IMPase. The degree of IMPase inhibition needed to reduce symptoms in bipolar disorder is not known. Given this consistent effect of lithium in numerous studies, there has been much interest in the development of IMPase inhibitors that could potentially stabilize mood in patients with BD (Atack et al., 1994).

The hypothesis that lithium attenuates receptor-coupled phosphoinositide hydrolysis (Berridge et al., 1989a,b, 1992) is supported by findings from several groups showing that chronic lithium treatment attenuated agonist-stimulated phosphoinositide metabolism measured in rat brain. For example, lithium inhibited muscarinic agonist-stimulated $Ins(1,4,5)P_3$ and $Ins(1,3,4,5)P_4$ accumulation in rat and mouse cerebral cortical slices (Whitworth and Kendall, 1988; Kennedy et al., 1990). Godfrey et al. (1989) reported that the fluoride-stimulated PI response is reduced in cortical membranes of rats treated with lithium for 3 days. Since AlF_4^- is thought to directly activate G-proteins, these findings suggested that the lithium effect on PI signaling occurs at the G-protein level. This notion was further suggested by the findings that lithium administered chronically reduces both cholinergic- and GTPγS-stimulated [^{3}H]PI hydrolysis in rat cerebral cortex (Song and Jope, 1992).

As described earlier, PKC is a major signal mediator linked to PI-generated second messengers that influences many cell functions by protein phosphorylation (Nishizuka, 1984, 1986; Evans et al., 1990). Findings indicating that acute lithium administration increases PKC-mediated responses, whereas chronic treatment results in an attenuation of these responses, implicated this family of kinases in the action of this mood stabilizer. For example, in rat hippocampus, 3 days of lithium administration augments phorbol ester–induced 5-HT release, whereas 3 weeks of lithium administration at therapeutic levels attenuates both the phorbol ester–induced cytosol to membrane PKC translocation and 5-HT release (Anderson et al., 1988; Wang and Friedman, 1989). There are several reports of increased PKC translocation from cytosol to membrane after chronic lithium treatment based on phorbol ester binding (Bitran et al., 1989; Lenox and Watson, 1991; Li et al., 1993b). This is complemented by more recent studies that measured PKC isozymes by immunoblotting and also showed that lithium could selectively decrease membrane levels of the PKC α isozyme in hippocampus but not cortex or other brain regions (Manji et al., 1993). This effect also occurred after treatment with sodium valproate (Chen et al., 1994).

Such changes in cellular disposition and abundance of PKC subtypes may lead to further downstream effects and decreased PKC signaling since chronic lithium treatment reduced phosphorylation of the prominent PKC substrate, MARCKS in rat hippocampus, as well as that of a 45 kDa protein (Lenox et al., 1991, 1992). MARCKS protein was also reduced after chronic lithium treatment (Lenox et al., 1991, 1992). The ultimate effects of decreased PKC signaling may include the regulation of gene expression by changes in the levels or function of trancriptional factors linked to their specific signaling pathways.

C. Gene Expression

Mood stabilizers must be administered chronically to effectively treat BD. Long-term (i.e., several years or longer) treatment markedly improves the course of the illness, preventing relapses of either mania or depression. As long-term changes in neuronal synaptic function are thought to be related to changes of gene expression in brain that may underlie the effects of drugs such as the mood stabilizers, it is not surprising that there has been considerable interest in studying the effects of mood stabilizers on gene expression in brain (Post, 1992; Hyman and Nestler, 1996). Lithium-induced changes in expression of a number of genes including neuromodulators, enzymes, receptors, G-proteins, and other signal transduction molecules have been documented in studies of cultured cells and animal models (Kalasapudi et al., 1990; Williams and Jope, 1994; Manji et al., 1995b). Several studies have demonstrated that lithium alters the expression of the early response gene c-fos through a PKC-mediated mechanism (Divish et al., 1991; Manji et al., 1994). For example, incubation of PC12 cells for 16 hours with lithium significantly potentiates c-fos expression induced by the muscarinic agonist carbachol. Lithium pretreatment in these cells also potentiates c-fos expression in response to phorbol esters, which directly activate PKC (Divish et al., 1991). Acute lithium treatment also potentiates stimulation of AP-1 binding by the cholinergic agonist pilocarpine in rat cerebral cortex (Williams and Jope, 1995). As noted above, chronic lithium treatment reduces G-protein α subunit mRNA levels and increases expression of AC types I and II (Colin et al., 1991; Li et al., 1991, 1993a). It also alters the mRNA levels of a number of neuropeptides including neuropeptide Y in rat hippocampus (Weiner et al., 1992; Zachrisson et al., 1995) and prodynorphin mRNA abundance in the rat striatum (Sivram et al., 1988).

Differential display PCR has also been used to study the effects of mood stabilizers on gene expression. A recent study revealed four differentially expressed gene products after treatment with LiCl for 1 week at therapeutically relevant concentrations in C6 glioma cells (Wang and Young, 1996). Although the identity of three of these gene products is presently unknown, the expression of a cDNA with greater than 99% homology to the gene for the enzyme 2',3'-cyclic nucleotide 3'-phosphodiesterase type II (CNPaseII) was markedly increased after lithium treatment (Wang and Young, 1996). CNPaseII is a myelin-associated enzyme. Since CNPaseII is important in myelinogenesis, and possibly neuronal growth and repair, these findings suggest that lithium regulate these processes. This latter effect was not shared by either sodium valproate or carbamazepine.

In summary, although a number of effects on gene expression have been demonstrated following lithium treatment, the results are still very preliminary. Further gene-expression studies may help to place these effects in a larger context with respect to the mechanism of action of lithium which will probably include regulation of signal transduction pathways. In contrast, very little is known about the effects on gene expression of the other commonly prescribed mood stabilizers, carbamazepine and sodium valproate.

D. Summary

Considering the findings presented above, lithium, and possibly other mood stabilizers, have numerous effects on both the cyclic AMP and PI-generated second-messenger pathways in cultured cells, rat brain, and blood cells from patients after in vitro and vivo treatment (Table 1). A major body of evidence suggests that lithium attenuates G-protein function. Furthermore, treatment with this agent may decrease G-protein α subunit gene expression and increase pertussis toxin–catalyzed and endogenous ADP-ribosylation, which may inactive the α_i subunit or enhance α subunit protein turnover. There is, however, little evidence that lithium treatment alters cellular G-protein levels in animal models or in patients. Thus, the relevance of these changes to the clinical effects of this drug remains in question. Much less is known about the effects of either carbamazepine or sodium valproate treatment on G-protein or the cyclic AMP signaling pathways, but available evidence suggests these agents may act differently than lithium.

Substantial evidence also supports an effect of mood stabilizers on the PI-generated second-messenger pathway. Lithium inhibits IMPase and may lead to inositol depletion, in addition to decreased production of $Ins(1,4,5)P_3$ and/or $Ins(1,3,4,5)P_4$. The levels and activity of PKC (possibly limited to specific isozymes) in membrane appear to be reduced by chronic lithium treatment and possibly by sodium valproate. Attenuation of PKC signaling is also supported by downstream effects such as decreased MARCKS phosphorylation and decreased AP-1 binding after lithium treatment.

III. CLINICAL STUDIES IN BD

Findings from clinical studies complement the body of evidence on the effects of mood stabilizers on signal transduction pathways. Direct clinical evidence has been obtained in studies on postmortem brain and in peripheral blood cells (i.e., platelets, leukocytes) obtained from subjects with a diagnosis of BD. Although much less has been done in clinical investigations, the available findings, in general, support the conclusions drawn on the molecular pharmacology of mood-stabilizing medications (Table 2).

A. G-Protein-Coupled Cyclic AMP Signaling Pathway

Since lymphocytes have βAR coupled to AC through G_s, these cells have commonly been used as an analogous cellular model for clinical investigation of receptor sensitivity in BD (Landmann et al., 1983; Hudson et al., 1993). A number of groups found blunted norepinephrine (NE)- and isoproterenol-stimulated, but not PGE1-stimulated, cyclic AMP formation in mononuclear leukocytes (MNLs) from depressed patients compared with normal subjects (Pandey et al., 1979; Extein et al., 1979; Siever, 1984; Mann et al., 1985; Halper et al., 1988). This appears to be one of the few relatively consistent biochemical changes identified in depression. These changes have generally been been observed in unipolar patients but have also been reported in BD (see Hudson et al., 1993). Mann et al. (1985) also found that this change in receptor sensitivity was not accompanied by changes in βAR density and affinity. They concluded that the blunted β-adrenergic cyclic AMP response probably indicates a reduced responsiveness (desensitization)

Table 2 Clinical Studies in Patients with Bipolar Disorder

Intracellular messengers	Tissue	Techniques	Patient group	Physiological change	Ref.
G-protein-coupled cyclic AMP system	Platelets	Measurement of cAMP with RIA	Depressed	↓PGE$_1$-stimulated cAMP; ↓NE inhibition of PGE$_1$-stimulated cAMP production	Siever et al., 1984
	MNLs	Measurement of cAMP with RIA	Depressed	↓Isoproterenol-stimulated cAMP production	Mann et al., 1985; Halper et al., 1988
	MNLs	^{3}H-Gpp(NH)p Binding	BD (manic)	↑Isoproterenol and carbamylcholine-induced Gpp(NH)p binding	Schreiber et al., 1991
	Postmortem cerebral cortex	Western blot; measurement of cAMP with RIA	BD	↑G$_s$α; no change in G$_i$α, G$_o$α, and Gβ levels; ↑forskolin-simulated cAMP production	Young et al., 1991, 1993
	MNLs	Western blot	BD (depressed)	↑G$_s$α and G$_i$α levels	Young et al., 1994
	MNLs	Western blot	BD	↑G$_s$α levels	Manji et al., 1995
	Postmortem cerebral cortex	Semiquantitative RT-PCR	BD	No change in G$_s$α mRNA levels	Young et al., 1996
	Platelets	Protein phosphorylation	BD	↑cAMP-dependent endogenous phosphorylation	Perez et al., 1995
	Postmortem brain	^{3}H-cAMP Binding	BD	↓^{3}H-cAMP binding	Rahman et al., 1996
Phosphoinositide-generated second-messenger system	Platelets	Assay of PKC activity	BD (manic)	↑Membrane-bound/cytosolic PKC activity; ↑serotonin-elicited PKC translocation	Friedman et al., 1993
	Platelets	2-D and thin-layer chromatography	BD (manic)	↑PIP$_2$	Brown et al., 1993
	Occipital cortical membranes	Western blot	BD	↑G$_{q/11}$α and phospholipase C-β immunoreactivity	Matthews et al., 1996
	Occipital cortical membranes	[^{3}H]PI hydrolysis	BD	↓GTPγS and NaF-stimulated [^{3}H]PI hydrolysis	Jope et al., 1996

rather than a diminished number (down-regulation) of βAR sites in depressed subjects (Mann et al., 1985; Halper et al., 1988). This notion is supported by recent findings suggesting elevated NE turnover in cerebral cortical, but not subcortical, regions of BD postmortem brains (Young et al., 1994c) in the absence of changes in βAR densities (Young et al., 1994a) compared with controls. The lack of alterations in βAR number in transformed lymphocytes from BD subjects (Kay et al., 1993) and absence of linkage to chromosomal markers for βARs in either unipolar or BD (Berrettini et al., 1988) also support the dissociation of changes in post-βAR signaling and βAR density. This apparent densensitization was another of the findings that led a number of researchers to investigate possible alterations in postreceptor signaling in patients with BD.

Several studies have more directly examined G-protein function and levels in patients with BD (Table 2). Schreiber et al. (1991) reported increased agonist-stimulated [^{3}H]GppNHp binding in MNL membranes from manic patients compared with controls or euthymic lithium–treated BD subjects. Direct evidence indicating involvement of G-protein dysfunction in the pathophysiology of BD comes from findings of elevated $G\alpha_s$ immunoreactivity in postmortem brain from patients with an established lifetime diagnosis of BD (Young et al., 1991, 1993). Compared with controls matched on the basis of age, postmortem delay, and brain pH, $G\alpha_s$ immunoreactivity was significantly elevated in frontal, temporal, and occipital cortex but not in hippocampus, thalamus, or cerebellum. The lack of significant changes in $G\alpha_o$ or Gβ immunoreactivities, and the absence of evidence of G-protein abnormality in postmortem brain from patients with other psychiatric disorders including unipolar depression (Young et al, 1993; Ozawa et al., 1993; Cowburn et al., 1994), illustrate the specificity of changes to $G\alpha_s$ in this disorder. Preliminary efforts to determine the functional correlates of the elevated $G\alpha_s$ levels have revealed associated statistically significant increases in forskolin-stimulated AC activity in occipital and temporal cortical region (Young et al., 1993). These results suggest that increased amounts of $G\alpha_s$, and/or increased function of stimulatory G-protein, contribute to the pathophysiology of BD (Young et al., 1993).

It has also been reported that α_s and α_i immunoreactivity in MNL membranes was significantly increased in medication-free BD but not major depressive disorder (MDD) patients when compared with age- and sex-matched healthy controls (Young et al., 1994b). These findings suggest that similar disturbances occur in G-protein in peripheral MNLs, as in cerebral cortex of BD patients, and also raise the possibility that they are trait-related since the changes occurred in BD but not MDD patients (Young et al., 1994). Recently, Manji et al. (1995a) also reported elevated MNL α_s levels in drug-free and lithium-treated BD patients who were manic, depressed, or euthymic, which also supports the notion that these changes may be trait-related. These studies suggest that disordered signal transduction at the G-protein level, possibly linked to cortical noradrenergic postsynaptic receptors, is critical to the pathogenesis of BD.

A number of investigators have recently explored whether mutations might occur in the $G\alpha_s$ gene in BD patients and their family members since such mutations have been identified as critical to the pathophysiology of several medical conditions. No mutations have been identified, however, in either the 5' upstream or coding regions of the $G\alpha_s$ gene in several large pedigrees in both North America and Australia (Gejman et al., 1993; Le et al., 1994). Recent findings in our laboratory also show that $G\alpha_s$ mRNA levels are not altered in frontal, temporal, or occipital cortex from subjects with BD (Young et al., 1996). Considering these data together, it seems plausible that other unidentified mechanisms that regulate $G\alpha_s$ levels (for example, protein turnover or membrane attachment) may be important in the pathophysiology of BD. To date, however, there is no direct evidence to support this latter possibility.

There is also evidence of alterations in other components of the cyclic AMP signaling system in BD patients (Table 2). Ebstein et al. (1987a) found that basal and stimulated AC activity has decreased in platelets from euthymic lithium-treated patients with BD. Since they did not include drug-free BD subjects who were symptomatic, it was not possible in this study to attribute these findings either to the diagnosis of BD or to lithium treatment. Another study by this same group of investigators found that lithium inhibited basal AC activity when compared to pretreatment levels in eight subjects with BD (Ebstein et al., 1987b). This latter study did not include a comparison group of healthy subjects, limiting interpretation of the results. Along with the finding of increased forskolin-stimulated AC in BD cerebral cortex, the above findings in platelets suggest that in BD there may be increased AC activity (possibly due to hyperfunctional G-proteins), which is decreased by lithium treatment. The findings of increased cyclic AMP–stimulated phosphorylation of several protein substrates in platelets of untreated BD subjects (Perez et al., 1995) and of decreased ^{3}H-cyclic AMP binding (an index of cyclic AMP–dependent protein kinase regulatory subunit levels) in BD post-mortem brain (Rahman et al., 1996) provide further evidence of downstream effects suggestive of increased cyclic AMP signaling in BD.

B. The PI-Generated Second-Messenger Pathway

Despite the extensive body of evidence on lithium's effects on IMPase and the formation of $Ins(1,4,5)P_3$ and PKC activity, only a few studies have examined these second messengers directly in BD patients (Table 2). At least one study found that platelet PIP_2 levels were increased in untreated manic BD subjects (Brown, 1993). Since PIP_2 is the precursor of $Ins(1,4,5)P_3$ and DAG, this study was interpreted as evidence of increased PI signaling in mania. In support of this idea, Friedman et al. (1993) found that platelet membrane PKC activity was increased in manic patients and decreased after 1 to 2 weeks of lithium treatment. Furthermore, in an earlier study (Ebstein et al., 1987a), platelet PLC activity was found to be lower in lithium-treated BD subjects than in healthy subjects.

Several more recent findings have supported the notion that at least some of the PI abnormalities are due to a G-protein-mediated defect. Although $G_{q/11}$ levels were found to be increased in occipital cortex from subjects with BD (Mathews et al., 1996), GTPγS-stimulated [3H]PI hydrolysis, but not PLC activity, was decreased in this same region (Jope et al., 1996). The latter results were interpreted as evidence of an imbalance between the cyclic AMP (overactive) and PI (blunted) signaling systems, which may be important to the clinical symptoms of BD and may be regulated in part by G-proteins (Jope et al., 1996). Since lithium has numerous effects on PI-generated second messenger, it will be of interest to follow future work on this system in BD subjects to further clarify its relevance to pathophysiology of this disorder.

C. Calcium Studies

There are obvious links between the findings in cyclic AMP and PI signal transduction pathways described above and the calcium-mediated signaling disturbances implicated in BD. For instance, the major function of $Ins(1,4,5)P_3$ is to bind to a receptor that allows the ER Ca^{2+} to be released into the cytoplasm, so increased PI signaling might be expected to be accompanied by elevated intracellular Ca^{2+} levels. Additionally, since in some tissues $G_s\alpha$ couples to Ca^{2+} channels (Yatani et al., 1987, 1988), increased levels of this G-protein α subunit in BD might also lead to higher intracellular concentrations of this cation. Nonetheless, there has been a longstanding interest in calcium homeostasis in BD irrespective of the relevance to these second-messenger systems. Linnoila et al. (1983) reported that the activity of the red blood cell Ca^{2+}-ATPase was higher in manic and depressed BD subjects than in age-matched controls, and in another study there was a trend toward higher values in BD than in unipolar subjects. Bowden et al. (1988) also found increased levels of red cell Ca^{2+}-ATPase in both manic and depressed BD subjects but normal levels in unipolar depressed subjects. There are two possible explanations for the increment of Ca^{2+}-ATPase in BD. The first is that higher activity of Ca^{2+}-ATPase in BD is a secondary change that compensates for increased intracellular free Ca^{2+}. Alternatively, higher Ca^{2+}-ATPase activity may be a primary change leading to increased intracellular Ca^{2+} levels.

Direct measurement of intracellular free Ca^{2+} using the Ca^{2+} chelating fluorescent dyes Fura-2 and Quin-2 has demonstrated increased resting and agonist-stimulated intracellular free Ca^{2+} in platelets and resting Ca^{2+} lymphocyte levels in patients with BD compared with controls. Two independent laboratories (Dubovsky et al., 1989, 1992b; Tan et al., 1990) found that basal intracellular free Ca^{2+} concentrations were elevated in platelets and lymphocytes of patients with mania and bipolar depression. Simultaneous stimulation with platelet-activating factor and thrombin resulted in significantly higher intracellular free Ca^{2+} concentration in platelets of manic and bipolar depressed patients than in control subjects in another study by Dubovsky et al. (1989). However, other investigators (Bothwell et al., 1994; Eckert et al., 1994) did not find intracellular differences in resting Ca^{2+}, or in thrombin, platelet-activating factor, and serotonin-stimulated Ca^{2+} levels, between BD or unipolar patients and matched controls. Another question that has been partially studied is whether Ca^{2+} concentrations change after treatment of BD with mood stabilizers. Dubovsky et al. (1991) found that resting and stimulated intracellular free Ca^{2+} were significantly reduced in untreated BD patients' platelets incubated for 1 hour by treatment with a therapeutic concentration of lithium chloride, compared with those from control subjects. A therapeutic role for calcium channel blockers has also been described in this patient group (Dubovsky et al., 1986; Hoschl, 1989). Another possible mechanism leading to increased intracellular free Ca^{2+} in BD may be decreased in Na^+-K^+-ATPase activity, which regulates intracellular Na^+ and consequently Na^+-Ca^{2+} exchange. In this regard, some but not all groups have reported that red blood cell Na^+-K^+-ATPase activity in red blood cells is decreased in depressed patients with BD (Hokin-Neaverson et al., 1974; Johnston et al., 1980; Naylor, 1985).

D. Summary

Despite the limited number of direct clinical studies in subjects with BD and the limitations in extrapolating from findings from peripheral blood cells or postmortem brain (Table 2), a set of findings emerges from the research on signal transduction relevant to BD. To date, there is evidence of abnormalities in at least three signal transduction pathways that may be either independent or, more likely, interdependent, given the emerging complexity of crosstalk and regulation between signaling pathways in brain. First, based on findings from several independent laboratories, levels of the stimulatory G-protein α subunit appear to be increased in blood cells and postmortem brain from subjects with BD. Attempts to clarify the mechanism by which these abnormalities occur have been less conclusive. These findings are supported by downstream effects of increased cyclic AMP signaling in BD such as increased forskolin-stimulated AC activity and ^{3}H-cyclic AMP binding in postmortem brain, in addition to increased cyclic AMP–dependent protein phosphorylation in platelets from subjects with BD. The PI signal transduction pathway may also be altered in BD, with evidence of increased PIP_2 levels, increased PKC activity, and blunting of G-protein regulation of PLC activity. Finally, a series of studies has demonstrated increased basal intracellular Ca^{2+} and altered calcium homeostasis in blood cells from patients with BD. As yet there has been no attempt to show whether and how these signaling disturbances are linked and which might be the primary defect, if one indeed exists. Nonetheless, the findings of altered signal transduction in BD complement the growing body of evidence on the molecular pharmacology of mood stabilizers (especially lithium), demonstrating numerous effects of these agents on signal transduction pathways, often in opposing directions to those found in BD. Thus, in general it appears that increased signaling occurs through one or more of the transduction pathways considered here and that mood stabilizers may have the ability to dampen the activity of one or more of these systems.

IV. CONCLUSIONS

In summary, increasing evidence supports the hypothesis that abnormalities in signal transduction pathways are important in the pathophysiology of BD, and possibly in the response of this disorder to treatment with mood stabilizers. As described above, there is evidence of alterations in several second-messenger systems, possibly at multiple sites. It is not known whether the signal transduction abnormalities identified in BD are interrelated or independent. Given the complexities of cellular functioning and the multiple levels of cross-regulation between pathways, it would be hard to imagine that these findings were not related to one another. Some examples of possible interactions that might account for the identified findings in BD are: 1) increased PI hydrolysis leading to abnormally high production of DAG and IP_3 production, which may result in both increased PKC activity and intracellular calcium concentrations, 2) increased $G\alpha_s$ levels that couple to membrane channels, possibly resulting in increased intracellular calcium concentrations in addition to increased cAMP signaling, and 3) increased PKC and/or calcium levels that alter the degree of binding of specific transcription factors to AP-1, CRE, or SRE sites, which leads to increased expression of the genes for other signal transduction proteins (possibly including specific G-protein subunits).

Although it may be easier to conceptualize a single defect in the function of signal transduction pathways, there are a number of reasons to expect more than one biochemical abnormality resulting in BD. First, there are diverse clinical courses of BD with remarkable variability in symptomatic presentations, which may be due to different underlying abnormalities. Second, patients with BD respond differentially to medications. Third, as discussed in Chapter 10 there is mounting evidence of a number of susceptibility genes for this disorder on different chromosomes, and hypotheses about the inheritance of single mutations have been all but dismissed. Therefore, different genetic abnormalities could impinge on the normal functioning of components of one or more of these pathways, which could lead to phenotypic variability in the signal transduction abnormality noted. The agreement of several of these findings of signal transduction abnormalities in BD and on the effects of mood-stabilizing drugs in quite remarkable in the face of the lack of clear replicable findings in other fields of investigation on the neurobiology of BD.

REFERENCES

Anderson SMP, Godfrey PP, Grahame-Smith DG. The effects of phorbol esters and lithium on 5-HT release in rat hippocampal slices. Br J Pharmacol 1988; 93(suppl):96P.

Angel P, Imagawa M, Chiu R, Stein B, Imbra RJ, Rahmsdorf HJ, Jonat C, Herrlich P, Karin M. Phorbol ester-inducible genes contain a common cis element recognized by a TPA-modulated trans-acting factor. Cell 1987; 49:729–739.

Atack JR, Prior AM, Fletcher SR, Quirk K, McKernan R, Ragan CI. Effects of L-690,488, a prodrug of the bisphosphonate inositol monophosphatase inhibitor L-690,330, on phosphatidylinositol cycle markers. J Pharmacol Exp Ther 1994; 270:70–76.

Atack JR, Broughton HB, Pollack SJ. Inositol monophosphatase: a putative target for Li+ in the treatment of bipolar disorder. Trends Neurosci 1995a; 18:343–349.

Atack JR, Broughton HB, Pollack SJ. Structure and mechanism of inositol monophosphatase. FEBS 1995b; 361:1–7.

Avissar S, Schreiber G, Danon A, Balmaker RH. Lithium inhibits adrenergic and cholinergic increases in GTP binding in rat cortex. Nature 1988; 331:440–442.

Avissar S, Barki-Harrington L, Nechamkin Y, Roitman G, Schreiber G. Reduced β-adrenergic receptor-coupled Gs protein function and Gs immunoreactivity in mononuclear leukocytes of patients with depression. Biol Psychiatry 1996; 39:755–760.

Backlund PS Jr, Simonds WF, Spiegel AM. Carboxyl methylation and COOH-terminal processing of the brain G-protein gamma-subunit. J Biol Chem 1990; 265:15572–15576.

Beavo JA, Reifsnyder DH. Primary sequence of cyclic nucleotide phosphodiesterase isozymes and the design of selective inhibitors. Trends Pharmacol Sci 1990; 11:150–155.

Beavo JA, Bechtel PJ, Krebs EG. Activation of protein kinase by physiological concentrations of cyclic AMP. Proc Natl Acad Sci USA 1974; 71:3580–3583.

Beebe ST. The cAMP-dependent protein kinase and cAMP signal transduction. Sem Cancer Biol 1994; 5:285–94.

Benjamin J, Agam G, Levine J, Bersudsky Y, Kofman O, Belmaker RH. Inositol treament in psychiatry. Psychopharmacol Bull 1995; 31:167–175.

Berk AJ, Schmidt MC. How do transcription factors work? Genes Dev 1990; 4:151–155.

Berrettini WH, Hoehe M, Lentes KU. Molecular studies of beta-adrenergic receptors on lymphoblasts: a study of manic-depressive illness [abstr]. Presented at 43rd Annual Meeting of the Society of Biological Psychiatry, 1988.

Berridge MJ. Inositol triphosphate, calcium, lithium and cell signalling. JAMA 1989a; 262:1834–1841.

Berridge MJ, Irvine RF. Inositol phosphates and cell signalling. Nature 1989b; 341:197–205.

Berridge MJ, Downes CP, Hanley MR. Lithium amplifies the agonist dependent phosphatidylinositol responses in brain and salivary glands. Biochem J 1992; 206:587–595.

Birnbaumer L. Receptor-to-effector signaling through G proteins: roles for beta gamma dimers as well as alpha subunits. Cell 1993; 71:1069–1072.

Birnbaumer L, Abramowitz J, Brown AM. Receptor-effector coupling by G proteins. Biochem Biophys Acta 1990; 1031:163–224.

Bitran JA, Gusovsky F, Manji HK, Potter W. Effects of chronic lithium treatment on signal transduction mechanisms in HL60 cells. Biol Psychiatry 1989; 25:46A.

Blaustein M. Calcium transport and buffering in neurons. Trends Neurosci 1988; 11:438–443.

Bothwell RA, Eccleston D, Marshall E. Platelet intracellular calcium in patients with recurrent affective disorders. Psychopharmacology 1994; 114:375–381.

Bowden CL, Huang LG, Javors MA, Johnson JM, Seleshi E, McIntyre K, Contreras S, Maas JW. Calcium function in affective disorders and healthy controls. Biol Psychiatry 1988; 28:367–376.

Bray D. Intracellular signalling as a parallel distributed process. J Theor Biol 1990; 143:215–231.

Brown AS, Mallinger AG, Renbaum LC. Elevated platelet membrane phosphatidylinositol-4,5-bisphosphate in bipolar mania. Am J Psychiatry 1993; 150:1252–1254.

Buchner K. Protein kinase C in the transduction of signals toward and within the cell nucleus. Eur J Biochem 1995; 228:211–221.

Bunney WE Jr, Garland-Bunney BL. Mechanisms of action of lithium in affective illness: basic and clinical implications. In: Meltzer HY, ed. Psychopharmacology: The Third Generation of Progress. New York: Raven Press, 1987:553–565.

Burgess GM, Bird GSJ, Obie JF, Putney JW Jr. The mechanism for synergism between phospholipase C-and adenylyl cyclase-linked hormones in liver. Cyclic AMP-dependent kinase augments inositol trisphosphate-mediated Ca^{2+} mobilization without increasing the cellular levels of inositol polyphosphates. J Biol Chem 1991; 166:4772–4781.

Burgoyne RD, Geisow MJ. The annexin family of calcium-binding proteins. Cell Calcium 1989; 10:1–10.

Cali JJ, Zwaagstra JC, Mons N, Cooper DMF, Krupinski J. Type VIII adenylyl cyclase: a Ca^{2+}/calmodulin-stimulated enzyme expressed in discrete regions of rat brain. J Biol Chem 1994; 269:12190–12195.

Carafoli E. Intracellular calcium homeostasis. Annu Rev Biochem 1987; 56:395–433.

Carli M, Anand-Srivastava MB, Molina-Holgado E, Dewar KM, Reader TA. Effects of chronic lithium treatments on central dopaminergic receptor systems: G proteins as possible targets. Neurochem Int 1994; 24(1):13–22.

Casebolt TL, Jope RS. Effects of chronic lithium treatment on protein kinase C and cyclic AMP-dependent protein phosphorylation. Biol Psychiatry 1991; 29:233–243.

Chen G, Manji HK, Hawyer DB, Wright CB, Potter WZ. Chronic sodium valporate selectively decreases protein kinase C α and $\in$ in vitro. J Neurochem 1994; 63:2361–2364.

Clapham DE, Neer EJ. New roles for G protein $\beta\gamma$ dimers in transmembrane signaling. Nature 1993; 365:403–406.

Colin SF, Chang H-C, Mollner S, Pfeuffer T, Reed RR, Duman RS, Nestler EJ. Chronic lithium regulates the expression of adenylate cyclase and G_i-protein α subunit in rat cerebral cortex. Proc Natl Acad Sci USA 1991; 88:10634–10637.

Cooper DMF, Brooker G. Ca^2-inhibited adenylyl cyclase in cardiac tissue. Trends Pharmacol Sci 1993; 14:34–35.

Cowburn RF, Marcusson JO, Eriksson A, Wiehager B, O'Neill C. Adenylyl cyclase activity and G-protein subunit levels in postmortem frontal cortex of suicide victims. Brain Res 1994; 633:297–304.

Crespo P, Xu N, Simonds WF, Gutking JS. Ras-dependent activation of MAP kinase pathway mediated by G-protein $\beta\gamma$ subunits. Nature 1994; 369:418–420.

Curran T, Morgan JI. Fos: an immediate-early transcription factor in neurons. J Neurobio 1995; 26:403–412.

Curran T, Vogt PK. Dangerous liaisons: Fos and Jun, oncogenic transcription factors. In: McKnight SL, Yamamoto KR, eds. Transcriptional Regulation. Cold Spring Harbor, NY: Cold Spring Harbor Laboratory Press, 1992:797–831.

Defer N, Marinx O, Stengel D, Danisova A, Iourgenko V, Matsuoka I, Caput D, Hanoune J. Molecular cloning of the human type VIII adenylyl cyclase. FEBS Lett 1994; 351:109–113.

Dekker LV, Parker PJ. Protein kinase C—a question of specificity. Trends Biochem Sci 1994; 19:73–77.

Divish MM, Sheftel G, Boyle A, Kalasapudi VD, Papolos DF. Differential effect of lithium on fos protooncogene expression mediated by receptor and postreceptor activators of protein kinase C and cyclic adenosine monophosphate: model for its antimanic action. J Neurosci Res 1991; 28:40–48.

Dubovosky SL, Franks RD, Allen S. Calcium antagonists in mania: a double-blind study of verapamil. Psychiatry Res 1986; 18:309–320.

Dubovosky SL, Christiano J, Daniell LC, Franks RD, Murphy J, Adler L, Baker N, Harris RA. Increased platelet intracellular calcium concentration in patients with bipolar affective disorders. Arch Gen Psychiatry 1989; 46:632–638.

Dubovsky SL, Lee C, Christiano J. Lithium decreases platelet intracellular calcium ion concentrations in bipolar patients. Lithium 1991; 2:167–174.

Dubovsky SL, Murphy J, Christiano J, Lee C. The calcium second messenger system in bipolar disorders: data supporting new research directions. J Neuropsych Clin Neurosci 1992a; 4:3–14.

Dubovsky SL, Murphy J, Thomas M, Rademacher J. Abnormal intracellular calcium ion concentration in platelets and lymphocytes of bipolar patients. Am J Psychiatry 1992b; 149:118–120.

Dubovsky SL, Thomas M, Hijazi A, Murphy J. Intracellular calcium signalling in peripheral cells of patients with bipolar affective disorder. Eur Arch Psychiatry Clin Neurosci 1994; 243:229–234.

Ebstein RP, Lerer B, Bennett ER, Shapira B, Kindler S, Shemesh Z, Gerstenhaber N. Lithium modulation of second messenger signal amplification in man: inhibition of phosphatidylinositol-specific phospholipase C and adenylate cyclase activity. Psych Res 1987a; 24:45–52.

Ebstein RP, Moscovich D, Zeevi S, Amiri Z, Lerer B. Effect of lithium in vitro and after chronic treatment on human platelet adenylate cyclase activity: postreceptor modification of second messenger signal amplification. Psych Res 1987b; 24:221–228.

Eckert A, Gann H, Riemann D, Aldenhoff J, Muller WE. Platelet and lymphocyte free intracellular calcium in affective disorders. Eur Arch Psychiatry Clin Neurosci 1993; 243:235–239.

Evans MS, Zorumski CF, Clifford DB. Lithium enhances neuronal muscarinic excitation by presynaptic facilitation. Neurosci 1990; 38:457–468.

Extein I, Tallman J, Smith CC, Goodwin FK. Changes in lymphocyte beta-adrenergic receptors in depression and mania. Psychiatry Res 1979; 1:191–197.

Faure M, Voyno-Yasenetskaya A, Bourne HR. cAMP and βγ subunits of heterotrimeric G proteins stimulate the mitogen-activated protein kinase pathway in COS-7 cells. J Biol Chem 1994; 169:7851–7854.

Federman AD, Conklin BR, Schrader KA, Reed RR, Bourne HR. Hormonal stimulation of adenlyl cyclase through Gi-protein beta gamma subunits. Nature 1992; 356:159–161.

Fisch TM, Prywes R, Roeder RG. c-fos sequences required for basal expression and induction by epidermal growth factor, 12-O-tetradecanoyl phorbol-13-acetate, and the calcium ionophore. Mol Cell Biol 1987; 7:3490–3502.

Fish TM, Prywes R, Simon MC, Roeder RG. Multiple sequence elements in the c-fos promoter mediate induction by cyclic AMP. Genes Dev 1989; 3:98–211.

Forn J, Valdecasas FG. Effects of lithium on brain adenyl cyclase activity. Biochem Pharmaco 1971; 20:2773–2779.

Freissmuth M, Gilman AG. Mutations of $G_s\alpha$ designed to alter the reactivity of the protein with bacterial toxins: substitutions at ARG187 result in loss of GTPase activity. J Biol Chem 1989; 264:21907–21914.

Friedman E, Wang HY, Levinson D, Connell TA, Singh H. Altered platelet protein kinase C activity in bipolar affective disorder, manic episode. Biol Psychiatry 1993; 33:520–525.

Gejman PV, Martinez M, Cao QH, Friedman E, Berrettini WH, Goldin LR, Koroulakis P, Ames C, Lerman MA, Gershon ES. Linkage analysis of 57 microsatellite loci to bipolar disorder. Neuropsychopharmacology 1993; 9:31–40.

Gilman AG. G proteins: transducers of receptor-generated signals. Annu Rev Biochem 1987; 56:615–649.

Godfrey PP, McClue SJ, White AM, Wood AJ, Grahame-Smith DG. Subacute and chronic in vivo lithium treatment inhibits agonist- and sodium fluoride-stimulated inositol phosphate production in rat cortex. J Neurochem 1989; 52:498–506.

Goldberg H, Clayman P, Skorecki K. Mechanism of Li inhibition of vasopressin-sensitive adenylate cyclase in cultured renal epithelial cells. AM J Physiol 1988; 255:F995–F1002.

Gonzalez GA, Montiminy MR. Cyclic AMP stimulates somatostatin gene transcription by phosphorylation of CREB at serine 133. Cell 1989; 59:675–680.

Guitart X, Nestler EJ. Regulation of cylic AMP-dependent protein phosphorylation in rat frontal cortex by chronic lithium: identification of DARPP-32 and other lithium-regulated phosphoproteins. Soc Neurosci Abst 1992; 18:104.

Hallcher LM, Sherman WR. The effects of lithium ion and other agents on the activity of myo-inositol-1-phosphatase from bovine brain. J Biol Chem 1980; 255:10896–10901.

Halper JP, Brown RP, Sweeney JA, Kocsis JH, Peters A, Mann JJ. Blunted β-adrenergic responsivity of peripheral blood mononuclear cells in endogenous depression. Arch Gen Psychiatry 1988; 45:241–244.

Harvey B, Carstens M, Taljaard J. Absence of an effect of the lithium-induced increase in cyclic GMP on the cyclic GMP-stimulated phosphodiesterase (PDE II): evidence of cyclic AMP-specific hydrolysis. Neurochem Res 1993; 18:1095–1100.

Hepler JR, Gilman AG. G proteins. Trends Biochem Sci 1992; 17:383–387.

Hokin-Neaverson M, Spiegel DA, Lewis WC. Deficiency of erythrocyte sodium pump activity in bipolar manic depressive psychosis. Life Sciences 1974; 15:1739–1748.

Hope BT, Nye HE, Kelz MB, Self DW, Iadarola MJ, Nakabeppu Y, Duman RS, Nestler EJ. Induction of a long-lasting AP-1 complex composed of altered fos-like proteins in brain by chronic cocaine and other chronic treatments. Neuron 1994; 13:1235–1244.

Hoschl C, Kozeny J. Verapamil in affective disorders: a controlled double-blind study. Biol Psychiatry 1989; 25:128–140.

Hsiao JK, Manji HK, Chen G, Bitran JA, Risby ED, Potter WZ. Lithium administration modulates platelet G_i in humans. Life Sci 1992; 50:227–233.

Hudson CJ, Young LT, Li PP, Warsh JJ. CNS transmembrane signal transduction in the pathophysiology and pharmacology of affective disorders and schizophrenia. Synapse 1993; 13:278–293.

Hug H, Sarre TF. Protein kinase C isoenzymes: divergence in signal transduction? Biochem J 1993; 291:329–343.

Hyatt SL, Liao L, Aderem A., Nairn A, Jaken S. Correlation between protein kinase C binding proteins and substrates in REF52 cells. Cell Growth Differ 1994; 5:495–502.

Hyman SE, Nestler EJ. Initiation and adaptation: a paradigm for understanding psychotropic drug action. Am J Psychiatry 1996; 153:151–1626.

Irvine RF. Inositol phosphates and Ca^{2+} entry: toward a proliferation or a simplification? FASEB 1992; 6:3085–3091.

Iyengar R. Molecular and functional diversity of mammalian G_s-stimulated adenylyl cyclases. FASEB J 1993; 7:768–775.

Jacobowitz O, Chen J, Premont RJ, Iyengar R. Stimulation of specific types of G_s-stimulated adenylyl cyclase by phorbol ester treatment. J Biol Chem 1993; 268:3829–3832.

Jakobs KH, Watanabe Y, Bauer S. Interactions between the hormone-sensitive adenylate cyclase and the phosphoinositide-metabolizing pathway in human platelets. J Cardiovasc Pharmacol 1986; 8:S61–S64.

Janknecht R, Cahill MA, Nordheim A. Signal integration at the c-fos promoter. Carcinogenesis 1995; 16:443–450.

Johnston BB, Naylor GJ, Dick EG, Hopwood SE, Dick DA. Prediction of clinical course of bipolar manic depressive illness treated with lithium. Psychol Med 1980; 10:329–334.

Jope RS, Williams MB. Lithium and brain signal transduction systems. Biochem Pharmacol 1994; 47:429–441.

Jope RS, Song L, Li PP, Young LT, Kish SJ, Pacheco MA, Warsh JJ. The phosphoinositide signal transduction system is impaired in bipolar affective disorder brain. J Neurochem 1996; 66:2402–2409.

Kalasapudi VD, Sheftel G, Divish MM, Papolos DF, Lachman HM. Lithium augments fos protooncogene expression in PC12 pheochromocytoma cells: implications for therapeutic action of lithium. Brain Res 1990; 521:47–54.

Kay G, Sargeant M, McGuffin P, Whatley S, Marchbanks R, Baldwin D, Montgomery S, Elliott JM. The lymphoblast β-adrenergic receptor in bipolar depressed patients: characterization and down-regulation. J Affect Disord 1993; 27:163–172.

Kennedy MB. Second messengers and neuronal function. In: Hall ZW, ed. An Introduction to Molecular Neurobiology. Sunderland, MA: Sinauer Associates, 1993:207–246.

Kennedy MB, Bennett MK, Erondu NE, Miller SG. Calcium/calmodulin-dependent protein kinases. In: Cheung WY, ed. Calcium and Cell Function. Vol 7. New York: Academic Press, 1987:62–107.

Kennedy ED, Challiss RAJ, Nahorski SR. Lithium reduces the accumulation of inositol polyphosphate second messengers following cholinergic stimulation of cerebral corted slices. J Neurochem 1989; 53:1632–1635.

Krebs EG, Beavo JA. Phosphorylation and dephosphorylation of enzymes. Annu Rev Biochem 1980; 48:923–959.

Landmann R, Burgisser E, Buhler FR. Human lymphocytes as a model for beta-adrenergic receptors in clinical investigation. J Receptor Res 1983; 3:71–88.

Le F, Mitchell P, Vivero C, Waters B, Donald J, Selbie LA Shine J, Schofield P. Exclusion of close linkage of bipolar disorder to the G_s-α subunit gene in nine Australian pedigrees. J Affect Disord 1994; 32:187–195.

Lee KAW, Masson N. Transcriptional regulation by CREB and its relatives. Biochim Biophys Acta 1993; 1174:221–233.

Lee G, Yun Y, Hoeffler J, Habener J. Cyclic-AMP-responsive transcriptional activation of CREB-327 involves interdependent phosphorylated subdomains. EMBO J 1990; 13:4455–4465.

Lenox RH, Watson DG. Targets for lithium action in the brain: protein kinase C substrates and muscarinic receptor regulation. Clin Neuropharmacol 1991; 15(suppl):612A–613A.

Lenox RH, Watson DG, Patel J, Ellis J. Chronic lithium administration alters a prominent PKC substrate in rat hippocampus. Brain Res 1992; 570:333–340.

Lesch K. Aulakh C, Tolliver T, Hill J, Woldzin B. Differential effects of long-term lithium and carbamazepine administration of G_s and G_i protein in rat brain. J Pharmacol Mol Pharmacol 1991; 207:355–359.

Li X, Jope RS. Selective inhibition of the expression of signal transduction proteins by lithium in nerve growth factor-differentiated PC12 cells. J Neurochem 1995; 65:2500–2508.

Li PP, Young LT, Warsh JJ. Lithium decreased G_s, G_i-1 and G_i-2 α-subunit mRNA levels in rat cortex. Eur J Pharmacol Mol Pharmacol 1991; 206:165–166.

Li PP, Young LT, Tam YK, Sibony D, Warsh JJ. Effects of chronic lithium and carbamazepine treatment on G protein subunit expression in rat cerebral cortex. Biol Psych 1993a; 34:167–170.

Li PP, Sibony D, Green M, Warsh JJ. Lithium modulation of the phosphoinositide signalling system in rat cortex: selective effects on phorbol ester binding. J Neurochem 1993b; 61:1722–1730.

Linnoila M, MacDonald E, Rainila M, Leroy A, Rubinow DR, Goodwin FK. RBC membrane adenosine triphosphatase activities in patients with major affective disorders. Arch Gen Psychiatry 1983; 40:1021–1026.

Logothetis DE, Kurachi Y, Galper J, Neer EJ, Clapham DE. The βγ subunits of GTP-binding proteins activate the muscarinic K+ channel in heart. Nature 1987; 325:321.

Lustig KD, Conklin BR, Herzmark P, Taussig R, Bourne HR. Type II adenylylcyclase integrates coincident signals from G_s, G_i and G_q. J Biol Chem 1993; 268:13900–13905.

Manji HK, Lenox RH. Long-term action of lithium: a role for transcriptional and posttranscriptional factors regulated by protein kinase C. Synapse 1994; 16:11–28.

Manji HK, Etcheberrigaray R, Chen G, Olds JL. Lithium decreases membrane-associated protein kinase C in hippocampus: selectivity for the α isozyme. J Neurochem 1993; 61:2303–2310.

Manji HK, Chen G, Shimon H, Hsiao JK, Potter WZ, Belmaker RH. Guanine nucleotide-binding proteins in bipolar affective disorder. Arch Gen Psych 1995a; 52:135–144.

Manji H, Potter WA, Lenox RH. Molecular targets for lithium's actions. Arch Gen Psychiatry 1995b; 52:31–543.

Mann JJ, Brown RP, Halper JP, Sweeney JA, Kocsis JH, Stokes PE, Bilezikian JP. Reduced sensitivity of lymphocyte beta-adrenergic receptors in patients with endogenous depression and psychomotor agitation. N Engl J Med 1985; 313:715–720.

Masana MI, Bitran JA, Hsiao JK, Mefford IN, Potter WZ. Lithium effects on noradrenergic-linked adenylate cyclase activity in intact rat brain and in vivo microdialysis study. Brain Res 1991; 538:333–336.

Masana MI, Bitran JA, Hsiao JK, Potter WZ. In vivo evidence that lithium inactivates G_i modulation of adenylate cyclase in brain. J Neurochem 1992; 59:200–205.

Mathews R, Li PP, Young LT, Kish SJ, Warsh JJ. Increased Gq/11 immunoreactivity in postmortem occipital cortex from patients with bipolar affective disorder. Biol Psychiatry. 1997; 68:297–304.

Meyer TE, Habener JF. Cyclic adenosine 3',5'-monophasphate response element binding protein (CREB) and related transcription-activating deoxyribonucleic acid-binding proteins. Endocr Rev 1993; 14:269–290.

Milligan G. Agonist regulation of cellular G protein levels and distribution: mechanisms and functional implications. Trends Pharmacol Sci 1993; 14:413–416.

Milligan G, Unson GC, Wakelam MJO. Cholera toxin treatment produces down-regulation of the α-subunit of the stimulatory guanine-nucleotide-binding protein (Gs). Biochem J 1989; 262:643–647.

Mitchell PJ, Tjian R. Transcriptional regulation in mammalian cells by sequence-specific DNA binding proteins. Science 1989; 245:371–378.

Mork A, Geisler A. Effects of lithium ex vivo on the GTP-mediated inhibition of calcium-stimulated adenylate cyclase activity in rat brain. Eur J Pharmacol 1989a; 168:347–354.

Mork A, Geisler A. Effects of GTP on hormone-stimulated adenylate cyclase activity in cerebral cortex, striatum, and hippocampus from rats treated chronically with lithium. Biol Psych 1989b; 26:279–288.

Moss J, Vaughan M. ADP-ribosylation of guanyl mucleotide-binding regulatory proteins by bacterial toxins. Adv Enzymol 1988; 60:303–379.

Naccarato WF, Ray RE, Wells WW. Biosynthesis of myo-inositol in rat mammary gland: isolation and properties of the enzymes. Arch Biochem Biophys 1974; 164:194–201.

Nahorski SR, Jenkinson S, Challiss RA. Disruption of phosphoinositide signalling by lithium. Biochem Soc Trans 1992; 20:430–434.

Naylor GJ. Reversal of vanadate-induced inhibition of Na+, K+-ATPase: a possible explanation of the therapeutic effect of carbamazepine in affective illness. J Affective Illness 1985; 8:329–334.

Neer EJ. Heterotrimeric G proteins: organizers of transmembrane signals. Cell 1995; 80:249–257.

Nestler EJ, Terwilliger RZ, Duman RS. Regulation of endogenous ADP-ribosylation by acute and chronic lithium in rat brain. J Neurochem 1995; 64:2319–2324.

Newman ME, Drummer D, Lerer B. Single and combined effects of desimipramine and lithium on serotonergic receptor number and second messenger function in rat brain. J Pharmacol Exp Ther 1989; 252:826–831.

Newman ME, Ben-Zeev A, Lerer B. Chloramphetamine did not prevent the effects of chronic antidepressants on 5-hydroxytryptamine inhibition of forskolin-stimulated adenylate cyclase in rat hippocampus. Eur J Pharmacol 1991; 207:209–213.

Newton AC. Protein kinase C: structure, function and regulation. J Bio Chem 1995a; 270:28495–28498.

Newton AC. Protein kinase C: seeing two domains. Curr Biol 1995b; 5:973–976.

Nishizuka Y. The role of protein kinase C in cell surface signal transduction and tumour production. Nature 1984; 308:693–698.

Nishizuka Y. Studies and perspectives of protein kinase C. Science 1986; 233:305–312.

Nishizuka Y. The molecular heterogeneity of protein kinase C and its implications for cellular regulation. Nature 1988; 334:661–665.

Nye HE, Hope BT, Kelz MB, Iadarola M, Nestler EJ. Pharmacological studies of the regulation of chronic FOS-related antigen induction by cocaine in the striatum and nucleus accumbens. J Pharmacol Exp Ther 1995; 275:1671–1680.

Odagaki Y, Koyama Y, Yamashita I. Lithium and serotonergic neural transmission: a review of pharmacological and biochemical aspects in animal studies. Lithium 1992; 3:95–107.

Ozawa H, Gsell W, Frolich L, Zochling R, Pantucek F, Beckmann H, Riederer P. Imbalance of the G_s and $G_{i/o}$ function in postmortem human brain of depressed patients. J Neural Transm [Gen Sect] 1993; 94:63–69.

Palotta BS. Patch-clamp studies of ion channels. In: Meltzer HY, ed. Psychopharmacology: The Third Generation of Progress. New York: Raven Press, 1987:325–331.

Pandey GN, Dysken MW, Garver DL, Davis JM. Changes in lymphocyte beta-adrenergic receptor function in affective illness. Amer J Psychiatry 1979; 136:675–678.

Pennypacker KR, Hong J-S, McMillian MK. Implications of prolonged expression of fos-related antigens. TiPS 1995; 16:317–321.

Perez J, Zanardi R, Mori S, Gasperini M, Smeraldi E, Racagni G. Abnormalities of cAMP-dependent endogenous phosphorylation in platelets from patients with bipolar disorder. Am J Psychiatry 1995; 152:1204–1206.

Post RM. Transduction of psychosocial stress into the neurobiology of recurrent affective disorder. Am J Psychiatry 1992; 149:999–1010.

Premont RT, Matsuoka I, Mattei MG, Pouille Y, Defer N, Hanoune J. Identification and characterization of a widely expressed form of adenylyl cyclase. J Biol Chem 1996; 271:13900–13907.

Price LH, Charney DS, Delgado PL, Heninger DR. Lithium and serotonin function: implications for the serotonin hypothesis of depression. Psychopharmacology 1990; 100:3–12.

Rahman S, Li PP, Young LT, Kofman O, Kish SJ, Warsh JJ. Reduced ^{3}H cAMP binding in postmortem brain from subjects with bipolar affective disorder. J Neurochem 1997; 41:649–656.

Ramdas L, Disher RM, Wensel TG. Nucleotide exchange and cGMP phosphodiesterase activation by pertussis toxin inactivated transduction. Biochemistry 1991; 30:11637–11640.

Raymond JR. Multiple mechanisms of receptor-G protein signaling specificity. Am J Physiol 1995; 38:F141–F158.

Rens-Domiano S, Hamm H. Structural and functional relationships of heterotrimeric G-proteins. FASEB J 1995; 9:1059–1066.

Resnick T, Dimitrov D, Zschauer A. Platelet calcium-linked abnormalities in essential hypertension. Ann NY Acad Sci 1986; 488:252–265.

Reuter H. Calcium channel modulation by neurotransmitters, enzymes and drugs. Nature 1983; 301:569–574.

Reuveny E, Slesinger PA, Inglese J, Morales JM, Iniguez-Lluhi JA, Lefkowitz RJ, Bourne HR, Jan YN, Jan LY. Activation of the cloned muscarinic potassium channel by G protein $\beta\gamma$ subunits. Nature 1994; 370:143–146.

Rink TJ. A real receptor-operated calcium channel? Nature 1988; 334:649–659.

Risby ED, Hsiao JK, Manji HK. The mechanisms of action of lithium. II. Effects on adenylate cyclase activity and β-adrenergic receptor binding in normal subjects. Arch Gen Psychiatry 1991; 48:513–524.

Sachs G, Muallem S. Sites and mechanisms of Ca^{2+} movement in nonexcitable cells. Cell Calcium 1989; 10:265–273.

Schreiber G, Avissar S, Danon A, Belmaker RH. Hyperfunctional G proteins in mononuclear leukocytes of patients with mania. Biol Psychiatry 1991; 29:273–280.

Sharma RK. Signal Transduction: regulation of cAMP concentration in cardiac muscle by calmodulin-dependent cyclic nucleotide phosphodiesterase. Mol Cell Biochem 1995; 149(150):240–247.

Sheng M, Thompson MA, Greenberg ME. CREB: a Ca^{2+}-regulated transcription factor phosphorylated by calmodulin-dependent kinases. Science 1991; 252:1427–1430.

Siegfried A, Ziff EB. Transcriptional activation by serum, PDGF, and TPA through the c-fos DSE: cell type specific requirements for induction. Oncogene 1989; 4:3–11.

Siever LJ, Kafka MS, Targum S, Lake R. Platelet alpha-adrenergic binding and biochemical responsiveness in depressed patients and controls. Psych Res 1984; 11:287–302.

Sivram SP, Takeuchi K, Li S, Douglass J, Civelli O, Calvetta L, Herbert E, McGinty JF, Hong JS. Lithium increases dynornorphin A(1–8) and prodynorphin mRNA levels in the basal ganglia of rats. Mol Brain Res 1988; 3:155–163.

Smrcka AV, Sternweis PC. Regulation of purified subtypes of phosphatidylinositol-specific phospholipase Cβ by G protein α and βγ subunits. J Biol Chem 1994; 268:9667–9674.

Snyder SH, Supattapone S. Isolation and functional characterization of an inositol triphosphate receptor from brain. Cell Calcium 1989; 10:337–342.

Song L, Jope RS. Chronic lithium treatment impairs phosphatidylinositol hydrolysis in membranes from rat brain regions. J Neurochem 1992; 58:2200–2206.

Sonnenberg JL, Macgregor-Leon PF, Curran T, Morgan JI. Dynamic alterations occur in the levels and composition of transcription factor AP-1 complexes after seizure. Neuron 1989; 3:359–365.

Spiegel AM, Shenker A, Weinstein LS. Receptor-effector coupling by G proteins: implications for normal and abnormal signal transduction. Endo Rev 1992; 13:536–565.

Stabel S, Parker PJ. Protein kinase C. Pharmac Ther 1991; 51:71–95.

Strathman M, Simon MI. G protein diversity: a distinct class of α subunits is present in vertebrates and invertebrates. Proc Natl Acad Sci USA 1990; 86:9113–9117.

Strulovici B, Cerione RA, Kilpatrick BF. Direct demonstration of impaired functionality of a purified desensitized β-adrenergic receptor in a reconstituted system. Science 1984; 225:837–840.

Tamir A, Gill DM. ADP-ribosylation by chlera toxin of membranes derived from brain modifies the interaction of adenylate cyclase with guanine nucleotides and NaF. J Neurochem 1988; 50:1791–1797.

Tan CH, Javors MA, Seleshi E, Lowrimore PA, Bowden CL. Effects of lithium on platelet ionic intracellular calcium concentration in patients with bipolar (manic-depressive) disorder and healthy controls. Life Sci 1990; 46:1175–1180.

Tang WJ, Gilman AG. Type-specific regulation of adenylyl cyclase by G protein βγ subunits. Science 1991; 254:1500–1503.

Taussig R, Gilman AG. Mammalian membrane-bound adenylyl cyclases. J Bio Chem 1995; 270:1–4.

Taylor CW. The role of G proteins in transmembrane signalling. Biochem J 1990; 272:1–13.

Thiele EA, Eipper BA. Effect of secretogogues on components of the secretory system in AtT-20 cells. Endocrinology 1990; 126:809–817.

Thompson WJ, Appleman MM. Multiple cyclic nucleotide phosphodiesterase activities from rat brain. Biochemistry 1971; 10:311–316.

Tsien RW, Lipscombe D, Madison D, Bley K, Fox A. Multiple types of neuronal calcium channels and their selective modulation. Trends Neurosci 1988; 11:431–438.

Volonte C. Lithium stimulates the binding of GTP to the membranes of PC12 cells cultured with nerve growth factor. Neurosci Lett 1987; 87:127–132.

Wang H-Y, Friedman E. Lithium inhibition of protein kinase C activation-induced serotonin release. Psychopharmacology 1989; 99:213–218.

Wang J-F, Young LT. Differential display PCR reveals increased expression of 2',3'-cyclic nucleotide 3'-phosphodiesterase by lithium. FEBS Lett 1996; 386:225–229.

Warsh JJ, Matthews R, Young LT, Li PP. Brain $G\alpha q/11$ and phospholipase C-β_1 immunoreactivity in bipolar affective disorder (BD). Can J Physiol Pharmacol 1994; 72:545.

Weiner ED, Mallat AM, Papolos DF, Lachman HM. Acute lithium treatment enhances neuropeptide Y gene expression in rat hippocampus. Mol Brain Res 1992; 12:209–214.

Whitworth P, Kendall DA. Lithium selectively inhibits muscarinic receptor-stimulated inositol tetrakisphosphate accumulation in mouse cerebral cortex slices. J Neurochem 1988; 51:258–265.

Wickman KD, Iniguez-Lluhi JA, Davenport PA, Taussig R, Krapivinsky GB, Linder ME, Gilman AG, Clapham DE. Recombinant G-protein $\beta\gamma$ subunits activate the muscarinic-gated atrial potassium channel. Nature 1994; 368:255–257.

Williams MB, Jope RS. Distinctive rat brain immediate early gene responses to seizures induced by lithium plus pilocarpine. Mol Brain Res 1994; 25:80–89.

Williams MB, Jope RS. Circadian variation in rat brain AP-1 DNA binding activity after cholinergic stimulation: modulation by lithium. Psychopharmacology 1995; 122:363–368.

Wood AJ, Goodwin GM. A review of the biochemical and neuropharmacological actions of lithium. Psychol Med 1987; 17:579–600.

Yatani A, Codina J, Imoto Y. A G-protein directly regulates mamalian cardiac calcium channels. Science 1987; 238:1288–1291.

Yatani A, Imoto Y, Codina J, Hamilton SL. The stimulatory G-protein of adenylate cyclase, Gs, also stimulates dihydropyridine-sensitive Ca^{2+} channels. J Biol chem 1988; 263:9887–9895.

Young LT, Woods CM. Mood stabilizers have differential effects on endogenous ADP ribosylation in C6 glioma cells. Eur J Pharmacol 1996; 309:215–218.

Young LT, Li PP, Kish SJ, Siu LP, Kamble A, Hornykiewcz O, Warsh JJ. Cerebral cortex $G_s\alpha$ protein levels and forskolin-stimulated cyclic AMP formation are increased in bipolar affective disorder. J Neurochem 1991; 61:890–898.

Young LT, Li PP, Kish SJ, Siu LP, Warsh JJ. Postmortem cerebral cortex Gs alpha-subunit levels are elevated in bipolar affective disorder. Brain Res 1993; 551:323–326.

Young LT, Li PP, Kish SJ Warsh JJ. Cerebral cortex β-adrenoceptor binding in bipolar affective disorder. J Affect Disord 1994a; 30:89–92.

Young LT, Li PP, Kamble A, Siu KP, Warsh JJ. Mononuclear leukocyte levels of G-proteins in depressed patients with bipolar disorder or major depressive disorder. Amer J Psychiatry 1994b; 151(4):594–596.

Young LT, Warsh JJ, Kish SJ, Shannak K, Hornykeiwicz O. Reduced brain 5-HT and elevated NE turnover and metabolites in bipolar affective disorder. Biol Psychiatry 1994c; 35(2):121–127.

Young LT, Asghari V, Li PP, Kish SJ, Fahnestock M, Warsh JJ. Stimulatory G-protein α-subunit mRNA levels are not increased in autopsied cerebral cortex from patients with bipolar disorder. Mol Brain Res 1996. In press.

Zachrisson O, Mathe AA, Stenfors C, Lindefors N. Region-specific effects of chronic lithium administration on neuropeptide Y and somatostatin mRNA expression in the rat brain. Neurosci Lett 1995; 194:89–92.

3
Hormones and Bipolar Affective Disorder

Russell T. Joffe and Stephen T. H. Sokolov
McMaster University, Hamilton, Ontario, Canada

I. INTRODUCTION

There is a rich and extensive literature documenting a relationship between hormonal changes and mood disorders. However, by far the majority of studies have focused on hormonal changes in patients with major depressive disorder. As a result, abnormalities of the thyroid and adrenal axis, the pituitary hormones such as growth hormone and prolactin, and the pineal hormone melatonin have been well documented in unipolar major depression. Considerably less attention has been paid to the role of hormonal dysfunction in the biology of bipolar affective disorder, including acute mania. One of the obvious reasons for this is the methodological difficulties in obtaining reliable endocrine data in patients with acute manic syndromes. Therefore, most studies have examined milder forms of mania as well as possible trait hormonal changes in bipolar illness.

This chapter focuses on changes in the thyroid and adrenal axis in patients with bipolar affective disorder. In particular, the thyroid axis is comprehensively reviewed because of the potential therapeutic implications of thyroid abnormalities in bipolar illness, particularly the rapid-cycling subtype.

II. THE THYROID AXIS

Although the link between clinical thyroid disease, particularly hypothyroidism, and depression has been well established (1), the relationship

81

between manic symptoms and clinical thyroid disease is less clearly documented. However, it has been demonstrated that clinical hyperthyroidism can manifest with manic symptoms (2) and that mania may also be the consequence of rapid thyroid hormone–replacement treatment in patients with clinical hypothyroidism (3).

Consistent abnormalities of peripheral thyroid hormone levels have not been consistently documented in patients with bipolar affective disorder. However, the mood-stabilizing agents, particularly lithium and carbamazepine, have well-documented effects on the thyroid axis. In bipolar patients, both manic and depressed, carbamazepine treatment is associated with substantial decrements in measures of thyroxine (T4) with minimal alterations in thyrotropin (TSH) (4). These reductions, although substantial, are usually within the normal range of values reported for measures of T4 (4). Therefore, carbamazepine, unlike lithium, is not associated with the induction of clinical hypothyroidism. Although decreases in T4 are related to therapeutic response with carbamazepine treatment of depression, it is unclear to what extent this applies to the treatment of acute mania (4). The changes in T4 observed in patients with mood disorders are consistent with those observed in epileptic patients treated with carbamazepine (5–7). Lithium is known to have thyrostatic effects. It acts by having multiple effects on different stages in the production and release of thyroid hormones. Although lithium blocks thyroid hormone synthesis by reducing iodine uptake by the thyroid gland (8,9) and by inhibiting thyroid hormone production at various stages of synthesis (8,9), its major inhibitory effect is on the release of thyroid hormones from the thyroid gland (10). In addition to these direct effects on the thyroid gland, lithium also inhibits the conversion, by monodeiodination, of T4 to triiodothyronine (T3) (11,12). There is also suggestive evidence that lithium may have an inhibitory effect on the thyroid axis by acting proximal to the thyroid gland through an inhibitory effect on both TSH and thyrotropin-releasing hormone (TRH) levels (13,14).

The acute effects of lithium have been documented both in healthy volunteers (15–17) and in clinical populations (18–20). These studies (15–20) show that up to 6 weeks of lithium treatment leads to limited decreases in peripheral thyroid hormone levels, with increases in basal and TRH-stimulated TSH levels. However, if thyroid function tests are followed over a period of several months they tend to normalize, thereby correcting the initial acute changes observed (21). With long-term treatment, a substantial minority of patients will develop evidence of clinical hypothyroidism. Although there is wide variation in the prevalence rates reported for lithium-induced hypothyroidism (reviewed in Ref. 22), it is estimated that approximately 5–

10% of patients who receive long-term lithium will develop clinical evidence of hypothyroidism and require thyroid hormone–replacement therapy. It is possible that the inhibitory effect of lithium on the thyroid may be implicated in its therapeutic effect in bipolar disorder, although this requires further study (22).

A number of studies have investigated whether a higher prevalence of clinical and subclinical thyroid illness exists in patients with rapid-cycling bipolar illness (23–29) (see Table 1). Several studies have suggested a higher prevalence of subclinical and clinical hyperthyroidism in these patients (23,24,28,29). Cho et al. (23) found evidence of grade I clinical hypothy-roidism in one-third of rapid-cyclers versus approximately 2% of non-rapid-cycling women. Cowdry and collaborators (24) also reported a 3:1 preva-lence of grade I or II hypothyroidism in rapid-cycling versus non-rapid-cycling bipolar patients. Furthermore, Bauer et al. (28) found a higher prevalence of a variety of grades of hypothyroidism in their sample of rapid-cyclers compared to published prevalence rates in non-rapid-cycling bipolar illness. In a small series of 10 patients, Kusalic (29) reported that 50% of rapid-cyclers had grade II subclinical hypothyroidism and 10% had grade III subclinical hypothyroidism as compared to none of the non-rapid-cyclers.

However, there have to date been three negative studies (25–27) that have failed to replicate these findings. Wehr and collaborators (25) observed a high prevalence of hypothyroidism in both rapid- and non-rapid-cycling bipolar patients. Furthermore, Joffe and collaborators (26) evaluated 43 bipolar outpatients who had received at least 3 months of treatment with lithium. In 17 patients classified as rapid-cyclers and 25 classified as non-

Table 1 Hypothyroidism and Rapid-Cycling Bipolar Disorder

			Prevalence (%) of Hypothyroidism					
	Subjects (*n*)		Grade I		Grade II		Grade III	
Study	RC	NRC	RC	NRC	RC	NRC	RC	NRC
Cho et al., 1979 (23)	16	99	31.7	2.1	—	—	—	—
Cowdry et al., 1983 (24)	24	19	50.0	0	42.0	32.0	—	—
Wehr et al., 1988 (25)	51	19	47.0	39.0	—	—	—	—
Joffe et al., 1988 (26)	17	25	0	20.0	0	12.0	—	—
Bartalena et al., 1990 (27)	11	11	—	—	—	—	27.0	18.0
Bauer et al., 1990 (28)	30	—	23.0	—	27.0	—	10.0	—
Kusalic, 1992 (29)	10	10	0	0	50.0	0	10.0	0

RC = rapid-cycling; NRC= Non-rapid-cycling.

rapid-cyclers, course of illness was measured by detailed life charting and did not correlated with thyroid indices. Rather, it was a significantly longer mean duration of lithium treatment that correlated with the development of clinical hypothyroidism. Finally, Bartalena et al. (27) compared 11 rapid-cycling and 11 non-rapid-cycling women matched for age and mode of treatment and found a high prevalence of subclinical hyperthyroidism in both groups.

In summary, there is evidence from earlier studies of higher prevalence rates of different grades of thyroid dysfunction in bipolar patients overall, and rapid-cycling bipolars in particular (23,24,28,29). However, the three negative studies (25–27) found a higher than expected prevalence of hypothyroidism in both the rapid- and non-rapid-cycling groups but no significant difference in prevalence rates between them. This failure of consensus in the literature may be explained by some of the methodological differences in the studies to date. These include small sample sizes, the method of sample ascertainment, the gender ratio of the sample, and the types of treatment used in the different samples. Further large-scale studies are required to determine whether there is a particular association between thyroid dysfunction and the rapid-cycling subtype of bipolar illness.

Although no specific abnormalities of basal thyroid hormone levels have been demonstrated in bipolar affective disorder, two preliminary studies (30,31) suggest that higher T3 levels with lithium treatment are associated with a better long-term prognosis and a lower risk of relapse. Although this finding does not yet have clinical utility, if replicated in future studies, it may further elucidate the role of thyroid hormones in the propensity to cycling and in the biological basis for bipolar illness.

The TRH test is the measurement of serum TSH levels following the administration of a supramaximal dose of TRH. This standard endocrine test has been applied to a variety of psychiatric illnesses in a series of studies published largely in the early and late 1980s (reviewed in Refs. 32–34). Although the interpretation of this test has been quite variable in the psychiatric literature, the most useful approach appears to have been to define the frequency of blunting of the TSH response to TRH in a particular psychiatric diagnostic group. Using varying definitions of blunting, it has been suggested that about one-quarter to one-third of depressed patients have a blunted TSH response to TRH (32–34). The TRH stimulation test has been studied in acute mania. Patients with mania tend to have a higher frequency of blunted TSH responses to TRH than do healthy controls, comparable to that observed in major depression (35,36). As a result of these observations (35,36), it has been suggested that the TRH stimulation test may be useful in distinguishing patients with acute mania from those with schizophrenia, in which blunting of the TRH test is uncommon. However, because of the low sensitivity of this test, its clinical utility in separating mania from schizophrenia is limited, and a multidimensional hormonal profile, involving measurement of several hormonal systems, is required to improved sensitivity and thereby diagnostic utility (37).

III. THYROID HORMONE TREATMENT IN BIPOLAR DISORDER

A. Rapid Cyclers

Thyroxine has been used by several investigators to treat patients with bipolar affective illness, particularly the rapid-cycling form. These studies are reviewed in Table 2. Reports to date have utilized doses of T4 up to 500 μg/day, high enough to induce a hyperthyroid and consequently a hypermetabolic state (38–41). First, Stancer and Persad (38) openly treated with hypermetabolic thyroxine 10 rapid-cycling patients whose illness had been refractory to several conventional mood-stabilizing treatments including lithium, neuroleptics, and electroconvulsive therapy. Five of seven women treated with between 300 and 500 μg/day of T4 obtained complete remission of their illness with follow-up periods of 1.5–9 years. In addition, two women treated with between 240 and 400 μg/day of T3 had temporary or slight responses to treatment. Second, Leibow (39) reported a single case of rapid-cycling that responded to 400 μg/day of T4. More recently, Bauer and Whybrow (40) treated, in open fashion, 11 rapid-cycling patients with

Table 2 Thyroxine Treatment of Bipolar Disorder

Study	n	Design	Rapid-cycling	Thyroxine dose (μg/day)	Response
Stancer and Persad, 1982 (38)	10	Open	Yes	240–500	5—complete 2—slight
Cowdry et al., 1983 (24)	4	Open	Yes	Replacement	2—complete 1—partial
Leibow, 1983 (39)	1	Open	Yes	400	1—complete
Bauer and Whybrow, 1990 (40)	11	Open	Yes	150–400	10—marked
Kusalic, 1992 (29)	6	Open	Yes	75–125	Reduction in episodes
Baumgartner et al., 1994 (4)	6	Open	No	250–500	4—complete

150–400 μg/day of T4. Depressive symptoms improved in 10 of 11 patients and manic symptoms in five of seven patients who exhibited these symptoms at baseline. Three of four patients who were randomized in either single- or double-blind manner to discontinuation of T4 subsequently relapsed (40). Kusalic (29) and Cowdry and collaborators (24) also reported therapeutic effectiveness of T4 in rapid-cycling bipolar subjects.

B. Non-Rapid Cyclers

Recently, Baumgartner and collaborators (41) reported on the use of high-dose T4 in non-rapid-cycling treatment with refractory bipolar patients. Six patients were treated with between 250 and 500 μg/day of T4. Four of these patients obtained a significant response as measured by both the mean number of relapses and the mean length of hospitalization during the follow-up period of 12–46 months. However, four of six patients had evidence of subclinical hypothyroidism so it is unclear whether T4 was being used to provide thyroid hormone–replacement therapy.

In the reports to date, hypermetabolic T4 has been reported to be generally well tolerated since the treatment algorithms call for slow-dose titration, with the upper dose limit usually determined by the appearance of side effects. Because there is, nevertheless, a risk of iatrogenically inducing clinical hyperthyroidism, using this treatment technique requires caution. There is also a theoretical risk of osteoporosis; a high prevalence of this condition has been observed in untreated hyperthyroidism. To address this concern, Whybrow (42) followed up the original 11 patients previously studied (40) with serial bone densitometry. Rather than osteoporosis, a net increase in bone density was observed (42). However, all patients were treated with lithium in addition to the T4 and it is possible that lithium may have played a protective role against the development of osteoporosis.

With respect to thyroxine therapy in bipolar illness, there is limited controlled evidence for the efficacy of hypermetabolic T4 in the treatment of bipolar patients, rapid-cyclers or non-rapid-cyclers. Nonetheless, the dramatic nature of the responses obtained in the open trials to date (see Table 2) suggest that hypermetabolic T4 may be an important treatment for certain highly refractory patients, particularly rapid-cyclers. Further replication, utilizing larger patient numbers and a more rigorous study design, would clarify the clinical role of T4 in the treatment of bipolar illness.

It is of interest that Bauer and Whybrow (40) observed no relationship between baseline thyroid hormone levels and subsequent response to T4.

This suggests that the possible therapeutic effect of T4 in bipolar illness is not necessarily due to thyroid hormone–replacement treatment of clinical or subclinical hypothyroidism and that, regardless of whether clinical and subclinical hyperthyroidism are more common in rapid-cycling illness, T4 may prove to be an effective alternative therapy, particularly in refractory patients.

IV. THE ADRENAL AXIS

A concerted research effort over the last 30–40 years has documented consistent abnormalities of the adrenal axis in patients with unipolar major depressive disorder. Much less attention has been paid to the bipolar patient. However, abnormalities similar to those in major depression have been consistently observed in bipolar patients, including those with acute mania. These include elevations in both urinary free cortisol and cerebrospinal fluid cortisol levels (43); elevated circulating cortisol levels, particularly during the day (43,44); escape from dexamethasone suppression (45–49); and abnormal circadian rhythm of cortisol secretion, with an elevation of nocturnal cortisol levels and an early onset of the nadir of the circadian variation (50).

There is controversy in the literature over whether these changes suggestive of adrenal axis overactivity occur specifically in patients with mixed manic states and are less common or not observed in patients with pure mania. For example, Swann and collaborators (43) reported that measures of cortisol hypersecretion correlated significantly with measures of depressed mood in the mixed manic state. However, dexamethasone nonsuppression has been observed in both pure (45–47) and mixed manic (48,49) states, suggesting that adrenal axis hyperactivity occurs in all forms of mania but is less common in pure mania. In addition to the other abnormalities of the adrenal axis previously summarized, Gold et al. (51) noted that adrenocorticotropic hormone (ACTH) but not cortisol response to corticotropin-releasing factors (CRF) is lower in bipolar depressed patients and acute mania as compared with healthy controls.

Further studies are required to document the specific abnormalities of the adrenal axis common to patients with mania. Furthermore, documentation of adrenal axis abnormalities in pure as opposed to mixed manic states is required to determine whether the mania per se or the associated agitation and arousal, particularly with mixed manic states, may be responsible for the adrenal axis overactivity observed.

V. PITUITARY HORMONES

Consistent abnormalities of prolactin have not been observed in bipolar patients, including those with acute mania (52–54). Moreover, no abnormality of the circadian variation of prolactin has been observed in manic patients (50). Although one study (55) suggested that the prolactin response to TRH was increased in mania, this finding was not confirmed by Coppen and collaborators (56). Furthermore, any abnormalities of prolactin observed, particularly in response to TRH, may be a consequence of lithium treatment since hypothyroidism may be associated with elevated prolactin levels (57).

Consistent abnormalities in either basal or stimulated measures of growth hormone have not been reported in mania (44). Furthermore, Linkowski and collaborators (50) observed no abnormality in the circadian variation of growth hormone in manic patients.

VI. MELATONIN

The pineal hormone melatonin may be of interest in acute mania. This hormone has been shown to be reduced in cases of major depressive illness, and there are now two preliminary studies that suggest that nocturnal melatonin levels may be increased in mania (58,59). Moreover, in another preliminary study, Lewy and collaborators (60) showed that bipolar patients were more sensitive to the suppressive effects of bright light on melatonin than were healthy controls. Although the study was preliminary, involving only a small number of patients, the findings are provocative and call for replication. If this finding is confirmed, it may provide insight into the sensitivity of bipolar patients to changes in sleep–wake cycles as well as the seasonal variation in the onset of mania.

VII. CONCLUSIONS

With the exception of the thyroid, and perhaps the adrenal axis, there are very limited data on the neuroendocrinology of bipolar disorder, particularly acute mania. Further studies are required to determine whether specific abnormalities of prolactin and growth hormone can be documented in bipolar patients. Moreover, the specific abnormality of the adrenal axis and its clinical correlates requires further elucidation. The provocative findings related to changes in melatonin level in acute mania require further study because they may provide clues to the clinical and biological characteristics of the illness and possible factors influencing the long-term course of the illness. Although controversial, the thyroid abnormalities are of both theoretical and clinical interest, and further study is needed to determine whether T4 has a useful clinical role in the treatment of the refractory bipolar patient, particularly those with the rapid-cycling subtype of the illness.

REFERENCES

1. Reus VI. Psychiatric aspects of thyroid disease. In: Joffe RT, Levitt AJ, eds. The Thyroid Axis and Psychiatric Illness. Washington, DC: American Psychiatric Press 1993:171–194.
2. Corn TH, Checkley SA. A case of recurrent mania with recurrent hyperthyroidism. Br J Psychiatry 1983; 143:74–76.
3. Josephson AM, Mackenzie TB. Appearance of manic psychosis following rapid normalization of thyroid state. Am J Psychiatry 1979; 136:846–847.
4. Roy-Byrne PP, Joffe RT, Uhde TW, Post RM. Effects of carbamazepine on thyroid function in affectively ill patients: clinical and theoretical implications. Arch Gen Psychiatry 1984; 41:1150–1153.
5. Rootwelt K, Ganes T, Johannessen SI. Effects of carbamazepine, phenytoin and phenobarbitone on serum levels of thyroid hormones and thyrotropin in humans. Scand J Clin Lab Invest 1978; 38:731–736.
6. Leiwendahl K, Majuri H, Helenius T. Thyroid function tests in patients on long term treatment with various anticonvulsant drugs. Clin Endocrinol 1978; 8:185–191.
7. Bentsen KD, Gram L, Veje A. Serum thyroid hormones and blood folic acid during monotherapy with carbamazepine or valproate. ACTA Neurologica Scandinavica 1983; 67:235–241.
8. Burrow GN, Burke WR, Himmelhoch JM. Effect of lithium on thyroid function. J Clin Endocrinol Metab 1971; 32:647–652.
9. Mannisto PT. Thyroid iodine metabolism in vitro II. Effect of lithium ion. Ann Med Exp Biol 1973; 51:42–45.
10. Berens SC, Wolff J. The endocrine effects of lithium. In: Johnson FN, ed. Lithium Research and Therapy. New York: Academic Press, 1975:443–472.
11. Bagchi N, Brown TR, Mack RE. Effects of chronic lithium treatment on hypothalamic-pituitary regulation of thyroid function. Hormone Metabolic Res 1982; 14:92–93.
12. Voss C, Schober HC, Hartman N. Einfluss von lithium auf die invitro dejodierung von L-thyroxine in der rattenleber. ACTA Biologica Medica Germanica 1977; 36:1061–1065.
13. Bakker K. The influence of lithium carbonate on the hyperthalamic-pituitary-thyroid axis. Agressologie 1982; 23:89–93.
14. Halmi KA, Noyes R Jr. Effects of lithium on thyroid function. Biol psychiatry 1972; 5:211–215.
15. Kirkegaard C, Lauridsen UB, Nerup J. Lithium and the thyroid. Lancet 1973; ii:1210.

16. Lauridsen UB, Kirkegaard C, Nerup J. Lithium in the pituitary-thyroid axis in normal subjects. J Clin Endocrinol Metals 1974; 39:383–385.

17. Perrild H, Hegedus L, Arnung K. Sex related goiterogenic effect of lithium carbonate in healthy young subjects. ACTA Endocrinologica 1984; 106:203–208.

18. Sedvall G, Jonsson P, Pettersson U. Effects of lithium salts on plasma protein bound iodine and uptake of iodine in thyroid gland of man and rat. Life Sci 1968; 7:1257–1264.

19. Cooper TB, Simpson JM. Preliminary report of a longitudinal study on the effects of lithium on iodine metabolism. Curr Ther Res 1969; 11:603–608.

20. Fyr B, Pettersson U, Sedvall G. Time course for the effect of lithium on thyroid function in men and women. ACTA Psychiatrica Scandinavica 1973; 49:230–236.

21. Emerson CH, Dyson WL, Utiger RD. Serum thyrotropin and thyroxine concentrations in patients receiving lithium carbonate. J Clin Endocrinol Metab 1973; 36:338–346.

22. Joffe RT, Levitt AJ. The thyroid and depression. In: Joffe RT, Levitt AJ, eds. The Thyroid Axis in Psychiatric Illness. Washington, DC: American Psychiatric Press, 1993:195–253.

23. Cho JT, Bone S, Dunner DL, Colt E, Fieve RR. The effect of lithium treatment on thyroid function in patients with primary affective disorder. Am J Psychiatry 1979; 136:115–117.

24. Cowdry RW, Wehr TA, Zis AP, Goodwin SK. Thyroid abnormalities associated with rapid cycling bipolar illness. Arch Gen Psychiatry 1983; 40:414–420.

25. Wehr TA, Sack DA, Rosenthal NE, Cowdry RW. Rapid cycling affective disorder: contributing factors and treatment responses in 51 patients. Am J Psychiatry 1988; 145:179–184.

26. Joffe RT, Kutcher S, MacDonald C. The thyroid function in bipolar affective disorder. Psychiatry Res 1988; 25:117–121.

27. Bartalena L, Pallegrini L, Meschi M, Antonangeli L, Bogazzi F, Dell'Osso L, Pinchera A, Placidi GF. Evaluation of thyroid function in patients with rapid cycling and nonrapid cycling bipolar disorder. Psychiatry Res 1990; 34:13–17.

28. Bauer MS, Whybrow PC, Winokur A. Rapid cycling bipolar affective disorder. I. Association with grade I hypothyroidism. Arch Gen Psychiatry 1990; 47:427–432.

29. Kusalic M. Grade II and grade III hypothyroidism in rapid cycling bipolar patients. Neuropsychobiology 1992; 25:177–181.

30. Hatterer JA, Kocsis JH, Stokes PE. Thyroid function in patients maintained on lithium. Psychiatry Res 1988; 26:249–254.

31. Baumgartner A, Vonstuckrad M, MullerOerlinghauscen B, Graf KJ, Kurten I. The hypothalamic-pituitary-thyroid axis in patients maintained on lithium prophylaxis for years: high triiodothyronine serum concentrations are correlated to the prophylactic efficacy. J Affect Disord 1995; 34:211–218.

32. Sternbach H, Gerner RH, Gwirtsman HE. The thyrotropin releasing hormone simulation test: a review. J Clin Psychiatry 1982; 43:4–6.

33. Loosen PT, Prange AJ Jr. Serum thyrotropin response to thyrotropin-releasing hormone in psychiatric patients: a review. Am J Psychiatry 1982; 139:405–416.

34. Loosen PT. TRH-induced TSH response in psychiatric patients: a possible neuroendocrine marker. Psychoneuroendocrinology 1985; 10:237–260.

35. Extein I, Pottash ALC, Gold MS, Cowdry RW. Using the protirelin test to distinguish mania from schizophrenia. Arch Gen Psychiatry 1982; 39:77–81.

36. Kirike N, Izumiya Y, Nishiwaka S. TRH test and DST in schizoaffective mania, mania and schizophrenia. Biol Psychiatry 1988; 24:415–422.

37. Mason JW, Kosten TR, Giller EL. Multidimensional hormonal discrimination of paranoid schizophrenic from bipolar manic patients. Biol Psychiatry 1991; 29:457–466.

38. Stancer HC, Persad E. Treatment of intractable rapid cycling manic depressive disorder with levothyroxine. Arch Gen Psychiatry 1982; 49:311–312.

39. Leibow D. L-thyroxine for rapid cycling bipolar illness. Am J Psychiatry 1983; 140:1255.

40. Bauer MS, Whybrow PC. Rapid cycling in bipolar affective disorder. II. Treatment of refractory rapid cycling with high-dose levothyroxine: a preliminary study. Arch Gen Psychiatry 1990; 47:435–440.

41. Baumgartner A, Bauer MS, Hellweg R. Treatment of intractable non-rapid cycling bipolar affective disorder with a high-dose thyroxine: an open clinical trial. Neuropsychopharmacology 1994; 10:183–189.

42. Whybrow PC. The therapeutic use of triiodothyronine and high-dose thyroxine in psychiatric disorder. ACTA Medica Austriaca 1994; 21:47–52.

43. Swann AC, Stokes PE, Casper R, Secunda SK, Bowden CL, Berman N, Katz MM, Robins E. Hypothalamic-pituitary-adrenal cortical function in mixed and pure mania. ACTA Psychiatrica Scandinavica 1992; 85:270–274.

44. Cookson JC. The neuroendocrinology of mania. J Affect Disord 1985; 8:233–241.

45. Arana GW, Barreira PJ, Cohen BM, Lapinski JF, Fogelson D. The dexamethasone suppression test in psychotic disorders. Am J Psychiatry 1983; 140:1521–1523.

46. Goodwin CD, Greenberg LB, Shukla S. Predictive value of the dexamethasone suppression test in mania. Am J Psychiatry 1984; 141:1610–1612.

47. Graham PM, Booth J, Boranga G. The dexamethasone suppression test in mania. J Affect Disord 1982; 4:201–211.

48. Evans DA, Nemeroff CB. The dexamethasone suppression test in mixed bipolar disorder. Am J Psychiatry 1983; 140:615–617.

49. Krishnan RR, Maltbie AA, Davidson JRT. Abnormal cortisol suppression in bipolar patients with simultaneous manic and depressive symptoms. Am J Psychiatry 1998; 140:203–205.

50. Linkowski P, Kerkhofs M, VanOnderbergen A, Hubain P, Copinschi G, L'Hermit-Baleriaux M, Leclerc QR, Brasseur M, Mendlewicz J, VanCauter E. The 24-hour profiles of cortisol, prolactin and growth hormone secretion in mania. Arch Gen Psychiatry 1994; 51:616–624.

51. Gold PW, Chrousos G, Kellner C, Post R, Roy A, Avgerinos P, Schulte H, Oldfield E, Loriaux DL. Psychiatric implications of basic and clinical studies with corticotrophin-releasing factor. Am J Psychiatry 1984; 141:619–627.

52. Meltzer HY, Kolakowska T, Fang VS, Fogg L, Robertson A, Lewine R, Strahilevitz M, Busch D. Growth hormone and prolactin response to apomorphine in schizophrenia and the major affective disorders. Arch Gen Psychiatry 1984; 41:512–519.

53. Cookson JC, Silverstone T, Rees LH. Plasma, prolactin and growth hormone levels in manic patients treated with pimozide. Br J Psychiatry 1982; 140:274–279.

54. Joffe RT, Post RM, Ballenger JC, Rebar R, Gold PW. The effects of lithium on neuroendocrine function in affectively ill patients. ACTA Psychiatrica Scandinavica 1986; 73:524–528.

55. Tanimoto K, Maeda K, Yamaguchi N, Chihara K, Fujita T. Effect of lithium on prolactin response to thyrotropin releasing hormone in patients with manic state. Psychopharmacology 1981; 72:129–133.

56. Coppen A, Rao VAR, Bishop M, Aboue-Saleh MT, Wood K. Neuroendocrine studies in affective disorders. I. Plasma prolactin response to thyrotropin-releasing hormone in affective disorders: effects of ECT. J Affect Disord 1980; 2:311–315.

57. Yamaji T. Modulation of prolactin release by altered levels of thyroid hormones. Metabolism 1974; 23:745–749.

58. Lewy AJ, Whrt A, Gold PW, Goodwin FK. Plasma melatonin in manic depressive illness. In: Usdin E, Kopin IJ, Barchas J, eds. Catecholamines: Basic and Clinical Frontiers. Oxford: Pergamon Press, 1979:1173–1175.

59. Wirz-Justice A, Arendt J. Plasma melatonin and antidepressant drugs. Lancet 1980; i:425.

60. Lewy AJ, Wehr TA, Goodwin FK, Newsome DA, Rosenthal NE. Manic depressive patients may be supersensitive to light. Lancet 1981; i:383–384.

4

Kindling and Stress Sensitization

Robert M. Post and Susan R. B. Weiss
*National Institute of Mental Health, National Institutes of Health,
Bethesda, Maryland*

I. INTRODUCTION

Few animal models deal with recurrence and cyclicity in the affective disorders. In this chapter, we discuss two animal models—kindling and sensitization—that provide potential direction and insight into the phenomena of recurrence and cyclicity, and, are themselves models of long-term memory and synaptic plasticity in the central nervous system (CNS) (Table 1).

In the animal model of sensitization to the psychomotor stimulant cocaine, there are evident homologies between cocaine-induced behavioral syndromes and affective disorder syndromes of hypomania, dysphoric mania, full-blown psychotic mania, and paranoid psychoses (1–5). In the model of electrophysiological kindling, in which seizures are the endpoint, the analogies are indirect and behaviorally nonhomologous (6). Nevertheless, kindling provides an interesting model of increased responsivity over time, which may be pertinent to the development of progressively more severe and rapidly recurring affective episodes in the untreated or inadequately treated patient. The kindling model helps to consider the progression from minor to major episodes, which can eventually advance to a spontaneous state, such that episodes occur in the absence of exogenous stimulation (Figures 1a and b). This progression parallels a spontaneous state, such that aspects of the recurrences in affective illness in which initial episodes are triggered by psychosocial stresses but then begin to emerge autonomously (7).

Table 1 Phenomena in Course of Affective Disorders Modeled by Kindling and Behavioral Sensitization

Descriptors	Kindling (K)	Sensitization (S)	Phenomenon
Stressor vulnerability	++	++	Initial stressors early in development may be without effect but predispose to greater reactivity upon rechallenge.
Stressor precipitation	++	++	Later stress may precipitate full-blown episode.
Conditioning may be involved	—	++	Stressors may become more symbolic.
Episode autonomy	++	—	Initially precipitated episodes may occur spontaneously.
Cross-sensitization with stimulants	—	++	Comorbidity with drug abuse may work in both directions: affective illness ⇌ drug abuse.
Vulnerability to relapse	++	++	S and K demonstrate long-term increases in responsivity.
Episodes may:			
a. Become more severe	++	++	S and K both show behavioral evolution in severity or stages.
b. Show more rapid onsets		++	Hyperactivity and stereotypy show more rapid onsets.
Anatomical and biochemical substrates evolve	++	+	K memory-trace evolves from unilateral to bilateral; S evolves from midbrain to N. accumbens.
IEGs involved	++	++	Immediate early genes (IEGs) such as c-fos induced.
Alterations in gene expression occur	++	++	IEGs may change later gene expression, e.g. peptides over longer time domains.
Change in synaptic microstructure occurs	++	—	Neuronal sprouting and cell loss indicate structural changes.
Pharmacology differs as function or stage of evolution	++	++	K differs as a function of stage; S differs as a function of development versus expression.

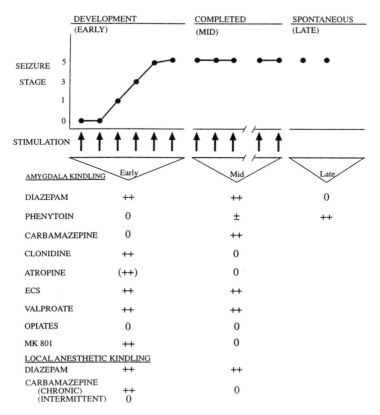

Figure 1a Pharmacological responsivity as a function of kindling stage. Early (developmental), mid (completed)-, and late (spontaneous) phases of amygdala (top) or local anesthetic (bottom) kindling evolution show differences in pharmacological responsivity (++ = very effective; 0 = not effective). The double dissociation in response to diazepam and phenytoin in the early versus the late phases, as described by Pinel, are particularly striking. Note also that carbamazepine is effective in inhibiting the developmental phase of local anesthetic but not amygdala kindling, whereas the converse is true for the mid (completed)-phase.

Finally, the kindling model is particularly useful for assessing various aspects of the molecular biology of tolerance development (8) and cyclic responsivity. For example, we have observed an episodic and cyclic pattern of tolerance development to the anticonvulsants carbamazepine and valproate when marginally effective doses or stimulation intensities are used (9). The cyclic pattern of seizure emergence, which also differs for individual

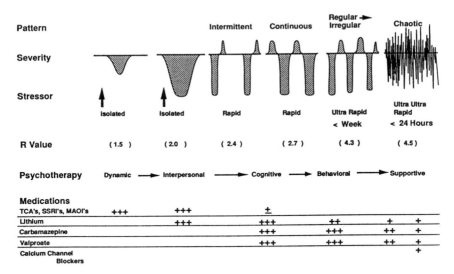

Figure 1b   Phases in evolution of mood cycling: potential relationship to treatment response. In an analogous fashion to kindling, episodes of affective illness may progress from triggered (arrows) to spontaneous and show different patterns and frequencies (top) as a function of stage of syndrome evolution. Just as different neural substrates are involved in different phases of kindling evolution, a similar principle is postulated in affective illness; these phases might also be responsive to different types of pharmacotherapies or psychotherapies. Although systematic and controlled studies have not examined the relationship of the illness phase to treatment response, anecdotal observations provide suggestive data that some treatments may be differentially highly effective (+++), moderately effective (++), or possibly effective (+) as a function of course of illness. Note that the pharmacological dissociations in the nonhomologous model of kindling are different from those postulated in mood disorders; nonetheless, the principle of differential response as a function of stage may be useful and deserves to be specifically examined and tested. The use of multiple agents in combination as a function of late or severe illness stage is standard in many medical illnesses and should be studied systematically in the refractory mood disorders.

animals, might provide insights into parallel mechanisms (in different neural systems) mediating cyclic recurrence of affective episodes in spite of long-term prophylactic treatment with lithium, carbamazepine, or valproate.

II.   KINDLING

The phenomenon of kindling, as first described by Goddard et al. (10), involves repeated intermittent stimulation of the brain that produces an

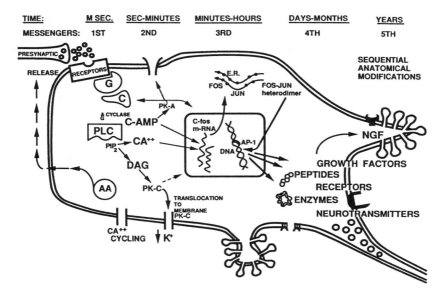

Figure 2 Neural mechanisms of synaptic plasticity, short- and long-term memory. This schematic of a cell illustrates how transient synaptic events induced by external stimuli can exert longer-lasting effects on neuronal excitability and the microstructure of the brain via a cascade of effects involving alterations in gene transcription. Neurotransmitters activate receptors and second-messenger systems, which then induce immediate early genes (IEGs) such as c-fos and c-jun. Fos and Jun proteins are synthesized on the endoplasmic reticulum (ER) and then bind to DNA to further alter transcription of late effector genes (LEGs) and other regulatory factors, the effects of which could last for months or years. PLC-phospholipase C; PIP_2-phosphatidyl inositol 4,5-biphosphate; AA = arachidonic acid; DAG = diacylglycerol; PK-C = protein kinase C; AP-1 = activator protein 1 (binding site on DNA); E.R. = endoplasmic reticulum; PK-A = protein kinase A; NGF = nerve growth factor.

increase in convulsive responsivity, resulting in the development of full-blown seizures in response to a previously subconvulsant stimulation. As kindling progresses, the threshold for afterdischarges in the amygdala decreases and afterdischarges spread to other areas of the brain (11).

Some of the key molecular aspects of kindling development include the induction of a sequential cascade of effects on immediate early genes (IEGs) and late effector genes (LEGs), as illustrated in Figure 2. In kindling evolution, transsynaptic activity resulting in depolarization of the cell activates second-messenger systems, which induce c-fos, zif268, and related transcription factors (12). These factors and an early wave of neurotrophic gene expression are followed by secondary effects on longer-term regulation of neuropeptide synthesis (Figure 3). For example, corticotropin-releasing hormone (CRH) is increased in the dentate hilus and is also observed in cells that do not normally express CRH mRNA (Figure 4) (13). The induction of c-fos is unilateral upon initial kindling stimulation, but becomes bilateral with additional stimulations as seizure generalization begins to occur (14). The mRNA for the peptide thyrotropin-releasing hormone (TRH) is expressed in the same areas as c-fos, e.g., the piriform cortex and dentate gyrus of the hippocampus, and in some cells, c-fos and TRH have been shown to coexist (15,16). Some peptides such as dynorphin are decreased rather than increased by amygdala-kindled seizures (Figure 4). The ultimate consequences for neuronal excitability of these peptide adaptations are not known, but recent observations of Weiss and associates (8) suggest that some adaptations may be anticonvulsant while others are likely related to the primary pathophysiology of the illness.

Weiss et al. (8) observed that seizures potentiate for the anticonvulsant efficacy of carbamazepine and diazepam. That is, animals given sufficient time off from the last seizure failed to respond to the anticonvulsant effects of these compounds when kindling stimulation was resumed. On the average, 4 days after the last kindled seizure, animals lost the anticonvulsant effects of carbamazepine reponsivity to (15 mg/kg), and 10 days after the last kindled seizure, animals lost their response to the anticonvulsant effects of diazepam (1–1.5 mg/kg). This disparity suggests that different and longer-lasting endogenous anticonvulsant mechanisms are needed for diazepam to work. These data suggest that some of the seizure-induced changes in IEG and LEG expression are adaptive, providing an endogenous anticonvulsant mechanism (8,17) that is sufficient to either prevent further seizures or supplement exogenous treatment.

Figure 3   Remodeling the central nervous system based on experience. This figure, an extension of Figure 2, portrays an evolving cascade of messenger systems, each with its own complex regulatory mechanisms and crosstalk with other systems (not illustrated). In addition to showing immediate early genes (IEGs) and late effector genes (LEGs) as illustrated in Figure 2, Figure 3 suggests that environmental stimulation can engage mechanisms that change the connectivity of the brain on a biochemical as well as microstructural basis, including cell sprouting, cell migration, or even cell death. These synaptic changes may ultimately be reflected in larger functional units (eighth and ninth messengers) that encode thoughts, memories, and preparation for action.

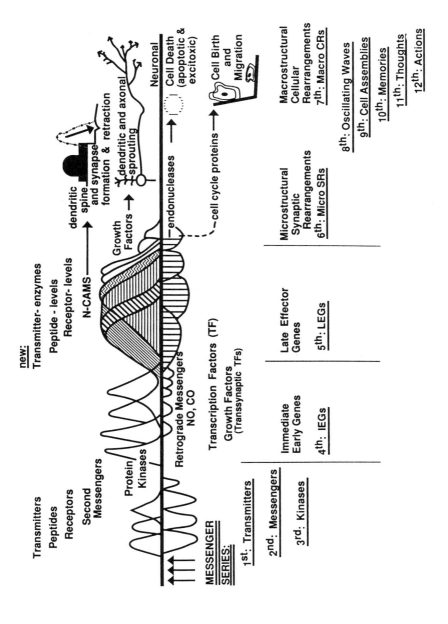

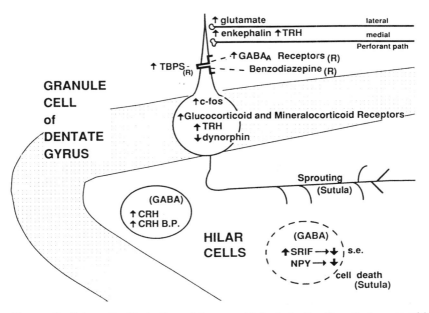

Figure 4 Schematic illustration of the neurobiological alterations that occur with amygdala kindling in the dentate gyrus of the hippocampus. Alterations in gene expression lead to transient to long-lasting changes in the biochemistry and neuroanatomy (sprouting and cell death) of the hippocampus. Some of these may account for the permanence of the kindled "memory trace." B.P. = binding protein; CRH = corticotropin-releasing hormone; GABA = gamma-aminobutyric acid; NPY = neuropeptide Y; s.e. = status epilepticus; SRIF = somatostatin; TBPS = t-butyl-bicyclophosphorothionate; TRH = thyrotropin-releasing hormone.

When these adaptations are lost (e.g., if enough time is allowed to elapse following the last seizure), the drugs are less effective. Since kindling produces enhanced mRNA expression for TRH, cholecystokinin (CCK), and enkephalin as well as increases in gamma-aminobutyric acid (GABA) and benzodiazepine receptor binding, these systems may be candidates for the endogenous compensatory mechanisms. TRH, CCK, and some opiate peptides have anticonvulsant effects in some seizure models and GABA is the major inhibitory neurotransmitter in the brain. Which of these is most important and in which areas of the brain is not yet known, but their physiological relevance is further suggested by the fact that there is a lowering of the seizure threshold in concert with this "time-off-seizure" effect on anticonvulsant drug efficacy (8).

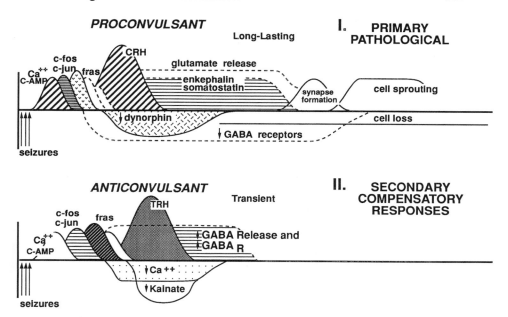

Figure 5 Competing pathological and adaptive endogenous responses to kindled seizures. C-AMP = cyclic adenosine monophosphate.

Other inductions of IEGs and LEGs appear to be part of the primary pathophysiological process of kindling and the mediator of the long-term "memory trace" (Figure 5). Sutula and colleagues (18) have demonstrated sprouting in the dentate granule cells as well as cell loss in the hilus area (Figure 4); the latter occurs in proportion to the number of kindled stimulations. Preliminary data in our laboratory suggest that this cell loss may be due to a preprogrammed or apoptotic cell death, as a number of the genes involved in such death programs are also induced by kindling (Zhang et al., unpublished observations). Since the neurotropic factors are involved in cell sprouting and, putatively, in cell death, there remains an intriguing possibility that they play a role in the anatomical rearrangement that occurs with kindling stimulation.

During kindling, brain-derived neurotropic factor (BDNF) is increased in the hippocampus while neurotropin-3 (NT-3) is decreased (Figure 6). These effects are opposite to what is observed following stress but are comparable to the effects of a variety of antidepressant compounds, as reported in the studies of Smith and colleagues (19,20). Thus, the biochemical alterations

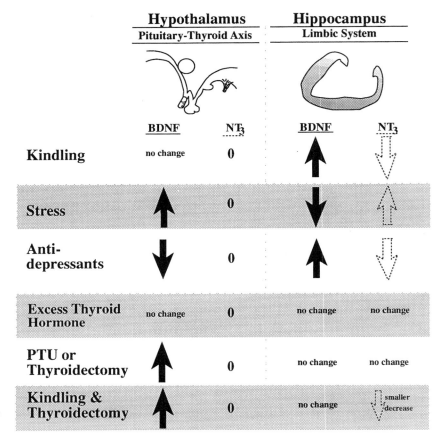

Figure 6 Differential regional regulation of neurotropins. (Data from 8; 20; Kim, Rosen, and Smith.)

leading to long-lasting changes in the anatomical circuitry of the hippo-campus and related areas of brain with kindling are likely related to the primary pathophysiology in kindled memory trace, while other more transient adaptations may be related to the secondary and compensatory anticonvulsant mechanisms.

This theme will be more systematically explored in considering the possible therapeutic use of TRH (21,22), a putative compensatory adaptive mechanism in depression (Figure 7). It is also possible that cyclic recurrence

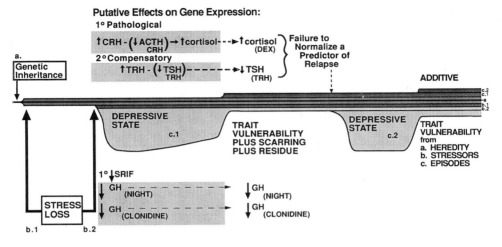

Figure 7 Accumulating experiential genetic vulnerability in recurrent affective illness. Initial stressors that might not be sufficient to trigger the full neurobiological concomitants of a depressive episode (STATE) may nonetheless leave behind biological (TRAIT) vulnerabilities (shaded center line) to further alterations. The state of depression with its associated peptide and hormonal increases (top) and decreases (bottom) may then leave behind additional trait vulnerabilities and residua. ACTH = adrenocorticotropic hormone; GH = growth hormone; TSH = thyroid-stimulating hormone.

of illness is related to the relative balance of primary pathological versus secondary adaptive mechanisms. When the adaptive changes predominate, there will be periods of relative wellness; when the pathological processes dominate, there will be periods of illness. However, the illness may be self-limiting with the generation of sufficient adaptive mechanisms (and the assistance of exogenous psychotropic agents) (Figure 8).

III. COCAINE SENSITIZATION

As illustrated in Figure 9, a related but differential unfolding cascade of IEG and LEG expression changes is programmed by chronic cocaine administration (23). The dosage, timing, and patterning of drug administration are also critical in the orchestration of this range of effects, as closely spaced, repeated administration of cocaine is associated with decreases in c-fos induction, while fos-related antigens (fras) are increased (15,24–26). How-

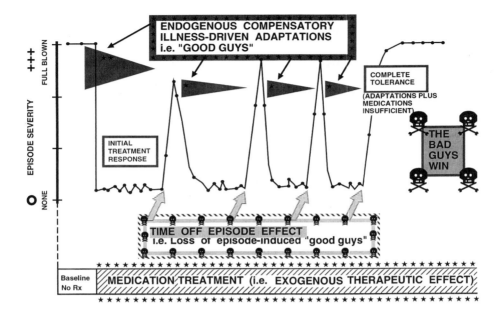

Figure 8 Hypothetical schema of the role of endogenous regulatory factors in the generation and progression of illness cyclicity. Following an illness episode, adaptive compensatory mechanisms are induced (i.e., "good guys"; large triangles), which, together with drug treatment, suppress the illness (initial treatment response; box). The "good guys" dissipate with time (i.e., the time-off-seizure effect), and episodes of illness re-emerge. While this re-elicits illness-related compensatory mechanisms, the concurrent drug treatment prevents some of the illness-induced adaptive responses from occurring (smaller triangles). As tolerance proceeds (associated with the loss of adaptive mechanisms), illness re-emergence occurs more rapidly. Thus, the drug is becoming less effective in the face of less robust compensatory adaptive mechanisms. The primary pathology is progressively re-emerging, driven both by additional stimulations and by episodes (i.e., the kindled memory trace of the "bad guys") along with a loss of illness-induced adaptations. Since this cyclic process is presumably driven by the ratio of bad to good guys at the level of changes in gene expression, we postulate that such fluctuations in the "battle of the oncogenes" arising out of illness- and treatment-related variables could account for individual patterns in illness cyclicity. An inherent abnormality in clock function is then not necessary to postulate. The illness is the clock and drives cyclicity.

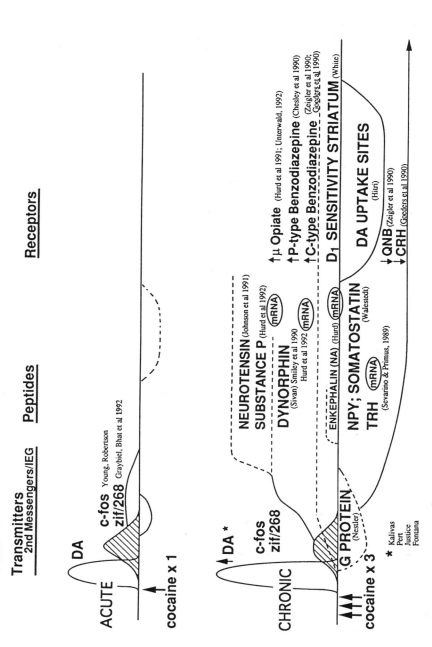

Figure 9 Evolution of biological changes associated with stimulant-induced behavioral sensitization. Acute cocaine administration (↑) induces IEGs such as c-fos and zif268 while chronic or repeated administration (↑↑↑) is associated with transient to long-lasting changes in LEGs, neuropeptides, and other adaptations that may provide the framework for longer-lasting changes in behavioral reactivity.

ever, more intermittent injections are associated with equal or greater increases in c-fos induction. The ultimate consequences for late effector changes are that some peptides are increased (such as dynorphin) (27–29) and others decreased (such as somatostatin and neuropeptide Y) (30). These potential long-term adaptations resulting from modification of in gene expression will come to play a crucial role in the interaction between stimulant abuse and affective disorders. Many of the alterations in the primary affective disorders are enhanced or exacerbated by the long-term changes produced by cocaine.

Since stresses are also capable of entering this same cascade (31) in a manner that closely overlaps with chronic cocaine, the potential for a destructive cycle exists, with stress sensitizing to cocaine abuse disorders or to primary affective disorders, and each predisposing to the other (Figure 10). This may account for the high incidence of comorbidity of bipolar illness and cocaine abuse disorders (32). Recent data of Kessler and collaborators (unpublished data) indicate an 8–10-fold greater potential of bipolar illness patients to have three or more comorbid psychiatric illnesses than patients with other primary psychiatric diagnoses. In addition, the substance abuse disorder rate in mania is double that of all other psychiatric illnesses (Kessler et al., unpublished observations; 33).

These clinical observations are supplemented by the preclinical observations that stress induction, particularly that of learned helplessness or unavoidable stress, predisposes to the acquisition of cocaine or amphetamine self-administration (34–36). At the same time, Wallace (37) and O'Brien and colleagues (38) have emphasized that dysphoric moods are one of the key elements, and can serve conditioned cues, that increase vulnerability to relapse in cocaine abusers. Thus, as schematized in Figure 10, stresses may be involved in the induction of either primary affective illness or the cocaine abuse disorders, but once they have been re-programmed through long-term changes in gene expression, they may become relatively autonomous of stresses, with dysphoric moods reinitiating substance abuse episodes and substance abuse exacerbating affective dysregulation.

Since dynorphin and related kappa opiate receptor ligands are dysphoric and psychotomimetic (39), it is possible that this long-term change is responsible for some of the increasing dysphoria observed in chronic cocaine abuse disorders. With increases in dynorphin as well as increases in kappa opiate receptors (39), substance abusers may never quite recapture their initial euphoric experiences of the first-time or early cocaine use. These data lead to the hypothesis that patients with primary dysphoric mania may also have increases in dynorphin and related kappa opiate activity, a

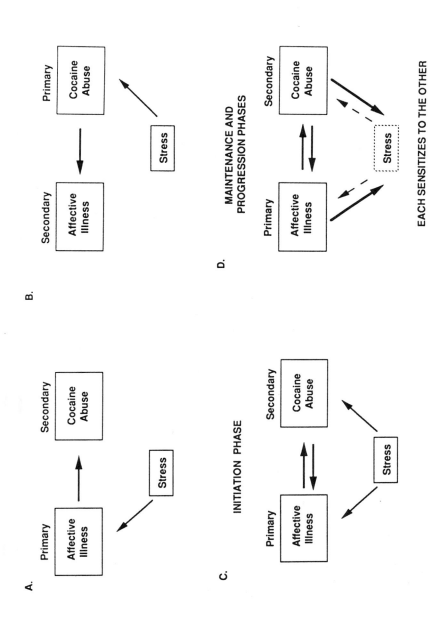

Figure 10 Diagram showing how stresses may be involved in the induction of either (A) primary affective illness or (B) cocaine abuse disorders, each possibly initiating the other (C), and then, in the maintenance and progression phases (D), each sensitizing to the other in the absence of stress.

postulate that could be studied directly by autopsy analyses comparing dysphoric and nondysphoric manic subjects.

IV. ILLNESS CYCLICITY

A. Primary Pathological Versus Secondary Compensatory Changes

As indicated above, we are postulating that TRH and $GABA_A$ receptors may be part of a compensatory response to the induction of kindled seizure episodes (Figure 5). Similarly, we asked whether excesses in TRH observed in patients in some studies of cerebrospinal fluid (CSF), and reflected in the increased blunting of thyrotropin-stimulating hormone (TSH) to TRH in depression, might be indicative of endogenous antidepressant alterations (40–42). If this is true, one would postulate that TRH injections during depression would evoke positive effects on mood, anxiety, and other symptoms of depression. A variety of early investigators observed this outcome, although findings were not always significantly different from those of placebo.

In an effort to circumvent the problem of TRH access to the brain, Marangell and collaborators (21) injected TRH intrathecally and found clinical improvement when compared to a sham procedure. Responders were further documented to have consistent response to active TRH administered parenterally as well as intrathecally in follow-up studies by Callahan and associates (22). These data support the view that TRH may be an endogenous adaptive substance, a postulate that is also consistent with the finding that TRH is substantially increased after electroconvulsive seizures (43–45). Interestingly, TRH is also increased in the CSF of patients treated with the mood-stabilizing anticonvulsant carbamazepine in one study but not another (46). It remains to be directly delineated whether TRH is directly related to or only one component of the mechanism of action of ECT or carbamazepine.

Given this perspective, one could envision that the induction of endogenous compensatory mechanisms, or their ascendency based on supplementation by exogenous agents such as ECT or carbamazepine, could be sufficient to successfully terminate an affective episode. However, with the dissipation of this active compensatory mechanism, or with the attenuation of the exogenous therapeutic regime—through dose reduction, medication discontinuation, or the development of tolerance—increased vulnerability to episode recurrence would resume (Figure 8).

B. Tolerance Development

When animals are treated once daily with an effective dose of carbamazepine (15 mg/kg i.p.), a marked anticonvulsant response is observed on fully developed amygdala-kindled seizures. However, after repeated stimulations, tolerance occurs and kindled seizures emerge through previously effective treatment (Figure 11) (47). This is not related to pharmacokinetic variables, since animals given equal doses of drug—but after the seizure has occurred—do not become tolerant. Moreover, a period of time off medication (i.e., with seizures occurring in the absence of drug) is sufficient to reinduce responsivity to the anticonvulsant (8).

The data of Weiss et al. (8) indicate that a variety of seizure-induced adaptations occur in response to amygdala-kindled seizures, and some of these fail to occur in animals that are tolerant to the anticonvulsant effects of carbamazepine or diazepam (Figure 12). In the case of tolerance to the anti-

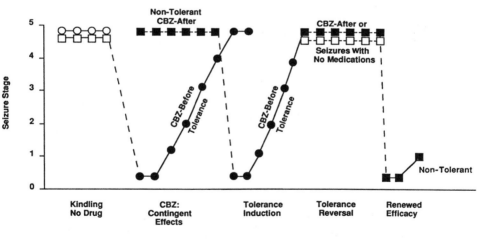

Figure 11 Schematic illustration of contingent tolerance development and reversal. In fully kindled animals (open symbols), carbamazepine treatment inhibits kindled seizures (filled circles). Repeated drug administration before (solid lines), but not after (dotted lines), kindling stimulation results in tolerance development. Tolerance induced in this manner can be reversed by a period of kindled seizures without drug administration (open squares; right) or even with continued drug administration but after each seizure (filled squares; right).

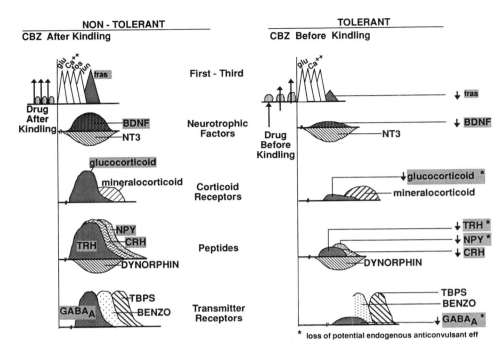

Figure 12 Neurochemistry of contingent tolerance to the anticonvulsant effects of carbamazepine (CBZ) on amygdala kindled seizures. Schematic illustration of seizure-induced changes in nontolerant animals (left) who receive CBZ after the seizure has occurred. These effects are the same as those observed in medication-free kindled animals. Although CBZ-tolerant animals (right) experience the same number of seizures and drug administrations, they fail to show the seizure-induced changes in TRH, CRH, GABA$_A$, and glucocorticoid receptors. *Putative endogenous anticonvulsant adaptations that may be lost with contingent tolerance.

convulsant effects of carbamazepine, seizures fail to increase TRH mRNA expression, or binding to GABA$_A$ receptors [at the α_4 subunit of the GABA$_A$ receptor (48)] as well as a variety of neurotropic factors (19). At the same time, seizures are able to induce other elements of the adaptive process, including increases in benzodiazepine receptors (Figure 12). While it has not been directly tested, we suggest that part of the pathophysiology of tolerance development is the failure of these endogenous adaptations to occur (8).

Consistent with this postulate is the observation described earlier that when sufficient time elapses, presumably associated with the dissipation of endogenous compensatory mechanisms, then carbamazepine and diazepam

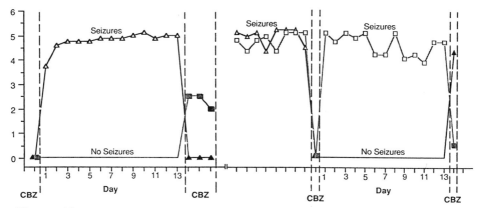

Figure 13   Seizures potentiate carbamazepine's anticonvulsant effect. In fully kindled animals, 15 mg/kg carbamazepine (CBZ) produced complete seizure suppression (CBZ, day 1). Animals were divided into two groups that received either 13 daily amygdala-kindled seizures (at 800 µA; open triangles) or no treatment. Both groups of animals then received 3 days of kindling stimulation preceded by CBZ administration on each day (15 mg/kg). The rats that did not experience seizures for the 13-day interval showed only a partial response to the CBZ (filled squares), whereas the rats that underwent seizures again showed complete seizure suppression by CBZ. Both groups were then given repeated seizures (open squares and triangles) to reinstate the original CBZ effect. A crossover design (right) was used to replicate the initial finding so that animals that had previously been given no treatment now received 13 days of seizures (open squares), and vice versa. Again, and even more robustly, the animals that did not experience seizures for 13 days showed no anticonvulsant response to CBZ administration (day 14; right), whereas the animals experiencing seizures showed almost complete seizure suppression.

become ineffective (Figure 13). We have also observed that under conditions of marginally effective drug treatment, tolerance can develop in an episodic and cyclic fashion which differs for individual animals (9) (Figure 14). Overall, there is a progression toward increasing numbers of seizures and complete drug tolerance over time. As illustrated in Figure 15, the intervals between successfully treated seizure episodes decrease as a function of the number of successive stimulations, just as the well intervals between successive episodes of untreated or treated affective illness on the average decrease over time. The striking similarities between the preclinical and clinical phenomenology suggest that this model may be useful for determining more optimal treatment stategies to prevent tolerance development as well as permitting the investigation of mechanisms involved in illness cyclicity (9).

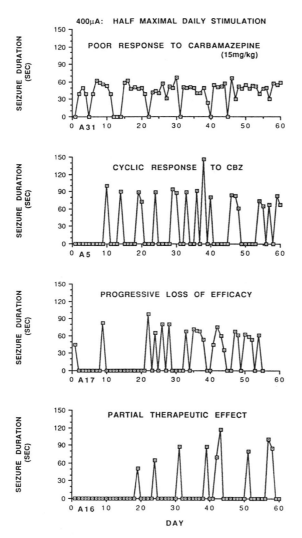

Figure 14 Individual patterns of loss of efficacy to the anticonvulsant effects of carbamazepine.

RECURRENT AFFECTIVE ILLNESS

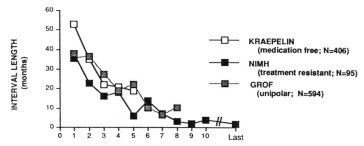

TOLERANCE TO VPA IN AFFECTIVE ILLNESS

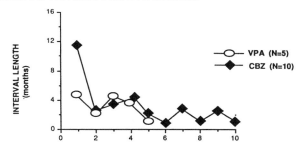

TOLERANCE TO VPA AND CBZ ON AMYGDALA-KINDLED SEIZURES

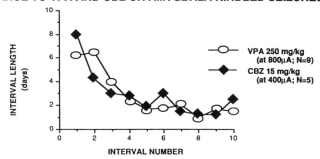

Figure 15 Decreasing well intervals between successive episodes in the emergence of recurrent affective illness (top). A similar progr ssive pattern (over different time frames) is observed during the development of tolerance to the psychotropic effects in patients with affective illness (center) and anticonvulsant effects in kindled animals (bottom) treated with carbamazepine and valproate. Following emergence of an illness episode, subsequent episodes occur more frequently, propelling the illness toward deterioration and loss of drug effect via tolerance.

C. Tolerance Reduction

A series of variables have been explored in an attempt to decrease the rate of tolerance development (Table 2). Weiss and associates (8) have found that lowering illness drive or increasing drug efficacy will slow tolerance development. Moreover, more chronic drug administration, compared to administration only immediately prior to amygdala-kindled stimulation, results in slower tolerance development (49). Kalynchuk et al. (50) have reported that ascending doses increase the rapidity of tolerance development; stable doses, or decreasing doses after initial high-dose treatment, may be relatively less likely to engender tolerance (Weiss et al., unpublished observations). Combination treatment with doses of two drugs such as carbamazepine and valproate, which individually cannot sustain a long period of anticonvulsant efficacy results in longer-term efficacy (Li et al., unpublished observations). Finally, treatment of seizures relatively early in the course of kindled stimulation is likely to result in better and more sustained therapeutic effects than treatment of seizures after many recurrences and later in the course of kindling (951).

Given this series of variables, one is now in a position to ask whether similar variables may also be pertinent to the long-term treatment of the affective disorders. For example, is early high-dose treatment with an effective mood stabilizer likely to be more efficacious than similar treatment later in the course of illness, after the occurrence of multiple episodes? It should be re-emphasized, however, that even if such a proposition is not yet proven,

Table 2 Other Predictions from Preclinical Model

Treatment resistance slowed by:	Future studies → predictive validity:
Higher doses	*Maximum tolerated doses*
Not escalating doses	*Stable dosing*
More efficacious drugs: VPA > CBZ	*Differential rate of treatment resistance?*
Treatments initiated early on illness	Gelenberg; O'Connell; Sarantidis; Denicoff
Combination treatment: CBZ plus VPA	*Combination > monotherapy?*
Reducing illness drive	*Treat comorbidities*
Response Restored by	
Period of drug discontinuation then re-exposure	*Randomized study of continuation vs. discontinuation*
Agents with different mechanisms of action: no cross-tolerance	*? Response to gaba pentin or lamotrigine*

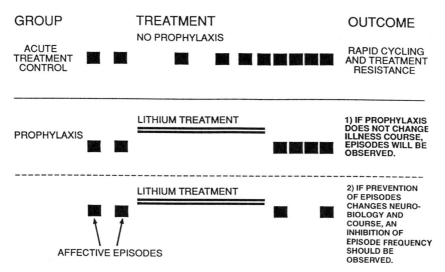

Figure 16 Postulated different outcomes of lithium prophylaxis on the course of illness. Squares represent affective episodes which, if untreated, may result in rapid cycling (top row). If prevention of episodes prevents sensitization (bottom), then patients who were randomized to lithium prophylaxis should show less rapid illness progression than those left untreated or only acutely dosed.

the clinical utility of such an approach would still be beneficial. The prevention of episodes at the earliest possible treatment point, and avoidance of the potential morbid and mortal consequences of affective episodes, would be inherently valuable, even if the subsequent course of illness was not affected.

The preliminary, uncontrolled data are nonetheless consistent with the formulation that early treatment may be advantageous to the long-term course of illness and ultimate pharmacological response (Figure 16). Gelenberg (52), O'Connell (53), Sarantadis (54), Denicoff (55), and their colleagues, and a variety of other investigators, have observed that patients with greater numbers of affective episodes prior to initiating long-term treatment with lithium are less likely to respond than are those with three or fewer episodes prior to initiation of treatment. Similarly, the data are overwhelming that rapid-cycling patients are less likely to respond to lithium than non-rapid-cycling patients (56). There is the issue of whether rapid cycling is a marker for more malignant forms of the illness from the onset, or whether it occurs relatively later in illness evolution and could have been prevented with early institution of treatment. In either instance, rapid cyclers appear to be less responsive to lithium and carbamazepine (55,57), suggesting the importance of early treatment to avoid rapid cycling and its accompanying risk of lower pharmacoresponsivity.

Similarly, in our initial observations with open treatment in a naturalistic follow-up study, we observed the greatest incidence of tolerance to the anticonvulsant effects of carbamazepine in those patients with the most rapidly progressive course of illness prior to institution of treatment (58). Thus, as in the amygdala-kindling paradigm, a rapidly progressive or rapidly cycling course may suggest the utility of initiating combination treatment from the outset. This view would be consistent with the empirical data of Denicoff and collaborators (55), who found that the combination of carbamazepine and lithium was more effective in the treatment of rapid cyclers than either monotherapy alone, even though the year on combination treatment was always at the end of the clinical trial and, theoretically, the least likely to evoke response based on the temporal course of illness evolution. A Clinical Global Impressions (CGI) response of moderate to marked improvement was achieved in 53% of rapid cyclers on combination treatment in the third year, compared with 19% on carbamazepine and 28% on lithium in the first or second years of the study.

Combination of lithium and valproate is also highly efficacious for many rapid-cycling patients, as is valproate alone in some instances (59–62). Optimal dosing strategies for valproate and carbamazepine in the treatment of bipolar illness are not known. However, the preclinical data noted above would suggest that maximizing the dose from the outset might ultimately be more effective than attempting to use minimally effective doses and escalating doses in the face of tolerance development.

In the prophylactic study of Kupfer and associates (63) in unipolar depression, effectiveness was achieved using full-dose antidepressant therapy (with imipramine 200 mg/day). When the dose was halved, a substantial percentage of patients relapsed. Related observations have been made with lithium dose reductions. In the study of Gelenberg et al. (52), reanalysis of the data (64) suggests that most of the relapses in the low-dose group were in those patients who were switched from the higher to the lower dose ranges. Other authorities, however, including Coppen et al. (65), have suggested that some patients may be able to tolerate such dose reductions without relapses. The area remains highly controversial, and given a side-effects rate three times greater in the high-dose group of Gelenberg et al. (52), and a very high noncompliance rate with lithium in general (mediated in part by its side-effects profile), optimal dosing strategies are far from well delineated.

Table 3 Rationales for Combination Therapy

Stage: with illness progression, *multiple systems* involved, e.g., in cancer, TB, congestive heart failure
Mechanisms of action
    Target "good guys" for augmentation
    Target "bad guys" for suppression
    Drugs without cross-tolerance
Avoidance of side effects
Need: if patient remains ill on monotherapy

D. Complex Combination Therapy

Again, the preclinical data, supported by uncontrolled clinical observations, suggest the potential utility of combinations of agents, particularly in rapid cycling. It is possible that different agents with different mechanisms of action may be more effective in preventing tolerance than maximizing the dose of a single agent, although this remains to be demonstrated. Such a strategy is nevertheless utilized in a variety of other areas of medicine, including the treatment of tuberculosis, most cancer chemotherapies involving complex multimodal regimens, and the treatment of congestive heart failure. Possibly, side effects could be minimized and efficacy maximized by judicious use of combination therapy (Table 3). In some instances, it may also be possible to utilize the side-effects profile of a given agent in a propitious fashion (Table 4). Thus, in a patient with comorbid migraines, valproate or the calcium channel blockers (CCBs) may be useful monotherapies or adjuncts, because clinical trials have shown them to be effective in migraines (66). Similarly, the anticonvulsant carbamazepine with valproate may be

Table 4 Possible Benefits of Combination Therapy: Side Effects Countered

Drug	Effect	Counter-Action	Drug
Li	↑ Diarrhea	↓	Calcium channel blockers
	↑ Polyuria	↓	Inositol
CBZ	↓ WBC	↑	Lithium
	↓ Sodium	↑	Lithium
	↓ Calcium	↓	Lithium
Li/VPA	↑ Weight	? ↓	Bupropion/T_3
Venlafaxine	↑ BP	↓	Calcium channel blockers

better tolerated by patients with head injuries and other medical or neurological conditions such as multiple sclerosis, in whom lithium is often poorly
tolerated (67,68).

Mechanistic diversity may also be specifically utilized. The CCBs have
been reported to be effective in some patients with bipolar illness, but previous research suggests that lithium and verapamil share similar spectra of
action and lithium nonresponders are not highly responsive to verapamil
(69). In contrast, the dihydropyridine L-type CCBs nimodipine and isradipine
appear to be effective in some patients who are not responsive to lithium, and
in some patients with ultra-rapid and ultra-ultra-rapid (ultradian) cycling
(70,71). These data suggest that there is heterogeneity of clinical response
even within the class of L-type CCBs. This suggestion is further supported by
the observations that nimodipine responders with bipolar illness failed to
respond to verapamil but did respond to isradipine in three double-blind,
crossover trials (Pazzaglia et al., unpublished observations, 1996).

While some patients responded to nimodipine alone, others required
combination treatment with nimodipine and carbamazepine (70). These
observations are of interest from the perspective that different types of
effects on calcium metabolism may interact in a cumulative fashion to
produce a more optimal therapeutic result. Recent data suggest that
carbamazepine, among a panoply of other actions (72–74), also blocks
calcium influx through the NMDA receptor (75). The different types of
calcium channel influx have different effects on the transcription of
immediate early genes, and thus it is possible that two types of calcium
blockade could affect calcium dysregulation to a greater degree than either
one alone. These data are also of interest in relationship to observations that
patients with unipolar and bipolar affective disorders have increased
accumulation of calcium in platelets, lymphocytes, and other blood elements
(76), further suggesting that increased calcium influx could be related to part
of the pathophysiology of the illness.

Whether carbamazepine's combination effects with nimodipine are due
to its effects on NMDA channels or some other mechanism of action remains
to be delineated. Moreover, Manna et al. (77) found that lithium in combination with nimodipine is more effective than monotherapy with either agent
alone, again suggesting that utilization of two drugs with different mechanisms of action may be an effective approach to the refractory bipolar
patient, and a useful way of preventing breakthrough episodes and the
ultimate manifestation of complete loss of efficacy through tolerance.

In cancer chemotherapy, systematic clinical trials exist to demonstrate
that four drugs are better in combination than three, or a given three are more

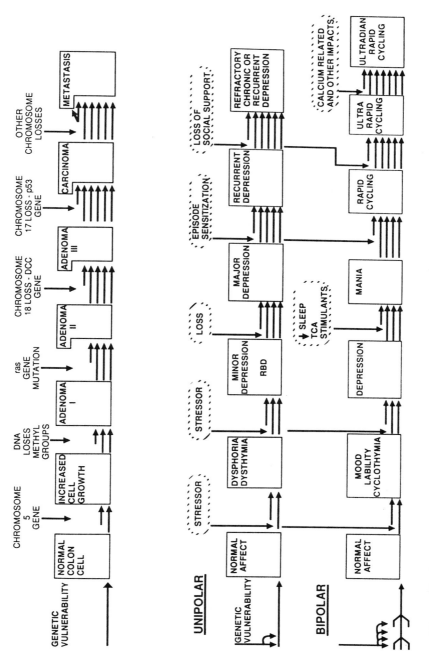

Figure 17 Similarities between somatic mutations in gene expression underlying carcinogenesis and experiential modulation of gene expression observed in unipolar affective disorder. RBD = recurrent brief depression; TCA = tricyclic antidepressant.

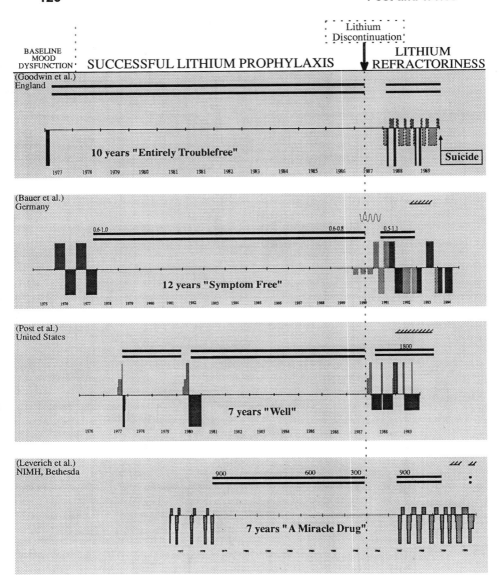

Figure 18 Life charts from four patients showing previous successful lithium prophylaxis, lithium discontinuation, and subsequent lithium discontinuation–induced refractoriness.

effective than a different regimen. In bipolar illness, the patient and treating psychopharmacologist are faced with an almost complete lack of a systematic database to guide clinical decision-making, and only the barest framework of preclinical principles and empirical databases. Thus, the clinician must titrate doses against clinical response and use systematic clinical trials and add-on therapies to achieve optimal clinical results. This method is precarious, and could entail an inordinate amount of time, money, and pain and suffering, if initial treatment options prove to be ineffective.

Preliminary data of Ketter et al. (78) have identified possible differential cerebral topographies of glucose metabolism related to treatment and response. Depressed patients with temporal lobe hypermetabolism were among those who responded to carbamazepine whereas those with a profile of frontal hypometabolism responded to nimodipine. Perhaps a combination of clinical, familial, and biological markers of response to different therapeutic agents and their combinations will ultimately be developed to more optimally guide therapeutics of bipolar illness from the outset.

V. CONCLUSION

The perspective of the stress sensitization and kindling models suggests that, as in the cancer chemotherapies, early aggressive and preventive treatment may help prevent the build-up of progressive vulnerabilities (Figure 17) to more severe and recurrent illness. These formulations also offer one potential explanation for the small percentage of patients who fail to re-respond to lithium once they have discontinued the drug and experienced new episodes (79,80) (Figure 18). It is possible that a new episode (like alterations in progression of metastatic cancer) can engender a new set of biological processes that are no longer amenable to treatment. Treatment of bipolar illness should focus on the likelihood of recurrences and ways of minimizing the risk not only of new episodes but also of treatment resistance in the form of either tolerance or refractoriness.

REFERENCES

1. Post RM. Cocaine psychoses: a continuum model. Am J Psychiatry 1975; 132:225–231.
2. Post RM. Clinical aspects of cocaine: assessment of acute and chronic effects in animals and man. In: Mule S, ed. Cocaine: Chemical, Biological, Clinical, Social, and Treatment Aspects. Cleveland: CRC Press, 1976:203–215.

3. Satel SL, Edell WS. Cocaine-induced paranoia and psychosis proneness. Am J Psychiatry 1991; 148:1708–1711.
4. Satel SL, Southwick SM, Gawin FH. Clinical features of cocaine-induced paranoia. Am J Psychiatry 1991; 148:495–498.
5. Brady KT, Lydiard RB, Malcolm R, Ballenger JC. Cocaine-induced psychosis. J Clin Psychiatry 1991; 52:509–512.
6. Weiss SRB, Post RM. Caveats in the use of the kindling model of affective disorders. J Toxicol Industr Health 1995; 10:421–447.
7. Post RM. Transduction of psychosocial stress into the neurobiology of recurrent affective disorder. Am J Psychiatry 1992; 149:999–1010.
8. Weiss SRB, Clark M, Rosen JB, Smith MA, Post RM. Contingent tolerance to the anticonvulsant effects of carbamazepine: relationship to loss of endogenous adaptive mechanisms. Brain Res Rev 1995; 20:305–325.
9. Post RM, Weiss SRB. A speculative model of affective illness cyclicity based on patterns of drug tolerance observed in amygdala-kindled seizures. Mol Neurobiol 1996; 13:33–60.
10. Goddard GV, McIntyre DC, Leech CK. A permanent change in brain function resulting from daily electrical stimulation. Exp Neurol 1969; 25:295–330.
11. Racine R. Kindling: the first decade. Neurosurgery 1978; 3:234–252.
12. Morgan JI, Curran T. Inducible proto-oncogenes of the nervous system: their contribution to transcription factors and neuroplasticity. Prog Brain Res 1990; 86:287–294.
13. Smith M, Weiss SRB, Abedin T, Post RM, Gold P. Effects of amygdala-kindling and electroconvulsive seizures on the expression of corticotropin releasing hormone (CRH) mRNA in the rat brain. Mol Cell Neurosci 1991; 2:103–116.
14. Clark M, Post RM, Weiss SRB, Cain CJ, Nakajima T. Regional expression of c-fos mRNA in rat brain during the evolution of amygdala-kindled seizures. Mol Brain Res 1991; 11:55–64.
15. Rosen JB, Cain CJ, Weiss SRB, Post RM. Alterations in mRNA of enkephalin, dynorphin and thyrotropin releasing hormone during amygdala kindling: an in situ hybridization study. Mol Brain Res 1992; 15:247–255.
16. Rosen JB, Abramowitz J, Post RM. Co-localization of TRH mRNA and Fos-like immunoreactivity in limbic structures following amygdala kindling. Mol Cell Neurosci 1993; 4:335–342.
17. Post RM, Weiss SRB. Endogenous biochemical abnormalities in affective illness: therapeutic vs. pathogenic. Biol Psychiatry 1992; 32:469–484.
18. Sutula TP, Cavazos JE, Woodard AR. Long-term structural and functional alterations induced in the hippocampus by kindling: implications for memory dysfunction and the development of epilepsy. Hippocampus 1994; 4:254–258.
19. Smith MA, Makino S, Kvetnansky R, Post RM. Stress and glucocorticoids affect the expression of brain-derived neurotropic factor and neurotrophin-3 mRNAs in the hippocampus. J Neurosci 1995; 15:1768–1777.
20. Smith MA, Makino S, Altemus M, Michelson D, Hong SK, Kvetnansky R, et al. Stress and antidepressants differentially regulate neurotrophin 3 mRNA expression in the locus coeruleus. Proc Natl Acad Sci USA 1995; 92:8788–8792.

21. Marangell LB, George MS, Callahan AM, Ketter TA, Pazzaglia PJ, L'Herrou TA, et al. Effects of intrathecal protirelin (thyrotropin-releasing hormone) in refractory depressed patients. Arch Gen Psychiatry 1997; 54:214–222.

22. Callahan AM, Frye MA, Marangell LB, George MS, Ketter TA, L'Herrou T, et al. Comparative antidepressant effects of intravenous and intrathecal thyrotropin-releasing hormone: Confounding effects of tolerance and implications for therapeutics. Biol Psychiatry 1997; 41:264–272.

23. Post RM, Weiss SRB, Smith M. Sensitization and kindling: implications for the evolving neural substrate of PTSD. In: Friedman MJ, Charney DS, Deutch AY, eds. Neurobiology and Clinical Consequences of Stress: From Normal Adaptation to PTSD. Philadelphia: Lippincott-Raven Publishers 1995:203–224.

24. Hope B, Kosofsky B, Hyman SE, Nestler EJ. Regulation of immediate early gene expression and AP-1 binding in the rat nucleus accumbens by chronic cocaine. Proc Natl Acad Sci USA 1992; 89:5764–5768.

25. Iadarola MJ, Chuang EJ, Yeung CL, Hoo Y, Silverthorn M, Gu J, et al. Induction and suppression of proto-oncogenes in rat striatum after single or multiple treatments with cocaine or GBR-12909. NIDA Res Monogr 1993; 125:181–211.

26. Bhat RV, Worley PF, Cole AJ, Baraban JM. Activation of the zinc finger encoding gene krox-20 in adult rat brain: comparison with zif268. Mol Brain Res 1992; 13:263–266.

27. Smiley PL, Johnson M, Bush L, Gibb JW, Hanson GR. Effects of cocaine on extrapyramidal and limbic dynorphin systems. J Pharmacol Exp Ther 1990; 253:938–943.

28. Sivam SP. Cocaine selectively increases striatonigral dynorphin levels by a dopaminergic mechanism. J Pharmacol Exp Ther 1989; 250:818–824.

29. Hurd YL, Brown EE, Finlay JM, Fibiger HC, Gerfen CR. Cocaine self-administration differentially alters mRNA expression of striatal peptides. Brain Res Mol Brain Res 1992; 13:165–170.

30. Wahlestedt C, Karoum F, Jaskiw G, Wyatt RJ, Larhammar D, Ekman R, et al. Cocaine-induced reduction of brain neuropeptide Y synthesis dependent on medial prefrontal cortex. Proc Natl Acad Sci USA 1991; 88:2078–2082.

31. Smith MA, Banerjee S, Gold PW, Glowa J. Induction of c-fos mRNA in rat brain by conditioned and unconditioned stressors. Brain Res 1992; 578:135–141.

32. Post RM, Weiss SRB, Rosen J, Smith M, Thomas N, Pert A. Co-morbidity of cocaine abuse and affective disorders. Am J Psychiatry 1995. Unpublished manuscript.

33. Brady KT, Sonne SC. The relationship between substance abuse and bipolar disorder. J Clin Psychiatry 1995; 56 (suppl 3):19–24.

34. Antelman SM. Stressor-induced sensitization to subsequent stress: implications for the development and treatment of clinical disorders. In: Kalivas PW, Barnes CD, eds. Sensitization in the Nervous System. Caldwell, NJ: Telford Press, 1988:227–254.

35. Kalivas PW, Stewart J. Dopamine transmission in the initiation and expression of drug- and stress-induced sensitization of motor activity. Brain Res Rev 1991; 16:223–244.

36. Piazza PV, Deminiere JM, Le Moal M, Simon H. Stress- and pharmacologically-induced behavioral sensitization increases vulnerability to acquisition of amphetamine self-administration. Brain Res 1990; 514:22–26.

37. Wallace BC. Psychological and environmental determinants of relapse in crack cocaine smokers. J Subst Abuse Treat 1989; 6:95–106.

38. O'Brien C, Childress AR, Ehrman R, Robbins S, McLellan AT. Persistent conditioned responses in former cocaine addicts. ACNP Abstracts 1991; 54.

39. Pfeiffer A, Brantl V, Herz A, Emrich HM. Psychotomimesis mediated by kappa opiate receptors. Science 1986; 233:774–776.

40. Loosen PT. The TRH-induced TSH response in psychiatric patients: a possible neuroendocrine marker. Psychoneuroendocrinology 1985; 10:237–260.

41. Kirkegaard C, Faber J, Hummer L, Rogowski P. Increased level of TRH in cerebrospinal fluid from patients with endogenous depression. Psychoneuroendocrinology 1979; 4:227–235.

42. Banki CM, Bissette G, Arato M, Nemeroff CB. Elevation of immunoreactive CSF TRH in depressed patients. Am J Psychiatry 1988; 145:1526–1531.

43. Kubek MJ, Meyerhoff JL, Hill TG, Norton JA, Sattin A. Effects of subconvulsive and repeated electroconvulsive shock on thyrotropin-releasing hormone in rat brain. Life Sci 1985; 36:315–320.

44. Kubek MJ, Sattin A. Effect of electroconvulsive shock on the content of thyrotropin-releasing hormone in rat brain. Life Sci 1984; 34:1149–1152.

45. Sattin A, Hill TG, Meyerhoff JL, Norton JA, Kubek MJ. The prolonged increase in thyrotropin-releasing hormone in rat limbic forebrain regions following electroconvulsive shock. Regul Pept 1987; 19:13–22.

46. Marangell L, George MS, Bissette G, Pazzaglia P, Huggins T, Post RM. Carbamazepine increases CSF thyrotropin-releasing hormone in affectively ill patients. Arch Gen Psychiatry 1994; 51(8):625–628.

47. Weiss SRB, Post RM. Development and reversal of conditioned inefficacy and tolerance to the anticonvulsant effects of carbamazepine. Epilepsia 1991; 32:140–145.

48. Clark M, Massenburg GS, Weiss SRB, Post RM. Analysis of the hippocampal GABA A receptor system in kindled rats by autoradiographic and in situ hybridization techniques: contingent tolerance to carbamazepine. Mol Brain Res 1994; 26:309–319.

49. Weiss SRB, Post RM. Contingent tolerance to the anticonvulsant effects of carbamazepine: implications for neurology and psychiatry. In: Canger R, Sacchetti E, Perini GI, Canevini MP, eds. Carbamazepine: A Bridge Between Epilepsy and Psychiatric Disorders. Origgio, Italy: Ciba-Geigy Edizioni, 1990:7–32.

50. Kalynchuk LE, Kim CK, Pinel JPJ, Kippin TE. Effect of an ascending dose regimen on the development of tolerance to the anticonvulsant effect of diazepam. Behav Neurosci 1994; 108:213–216.

51. Weiss SRB, Heynen T, Noguera CC, Li X, Post RM. Oscillating patterns of anticonvulsant responsivity: putative model of affective illness cyclicity. ACNP Abstracts 1994; 210.

52. Gelenberg AJ, Kane JM, Keller MB, Lavori P, Rosenbaum JF, Cole K, et al. Comparison of standard and low serum levels of lithium for maintenance treatment of bipolar disorder. N Engl J Med 1989; 321:1489–1493.

53. O'Connell RA, Mayo JA, Flatow L, Cuthbertson B, O'Brien BE. Outcome of bipolar disorder on long-term treatment with lithium. Br J Psychiatry 1991; 159:123–129.

54. Sarantidis D, Waters B. Predictors of lithium prophylaxis effectiveness. Prog Neuropsychopharmacol 1981; 5:507–510.

55. Denicoff KD, Smith-Jackson EE, Disney ER, Ali SO, Leverich GS, Post RM. Comparative prophylactic efficacy of lithium, carbamazepine, and the combination in the treatment of bipolar affective illness. J Clin Psychiatry 1997; in press.

56. Post RM, Kramlinger KG, Altshuler LL, Ketter TA, Denicoff K. Treatment of rapid cycling bipolar illness. Psychopharmacol Bull 1990; 26:37–47.

57. Okuma T. Effects of carbamazepine and lithium on affective disorders. Neuropsychobiology 1993; 27:138–145.

58. Post RM, Leverich GS, Rosoff AS, Altshuler LL. Carbamazepine prophylaxis in refractory affective disorders: a focus on long-term follow-up. J Clin Psychopharmacol 1990; 10:318–327.

59. Calabrese JR, Markovitz PJ, Kimmel SE, Wagner SC. Spectrum of efficacy of valproate in 78 rapid-cycling bipolar patients. J Clin Psychopharmacol 1992; 12:53S–56S.

60. McElroy SL, Keck PE Jr, Pope HG Jr, Hudson JI. Valproate in the treatment of rapid-cycling bipolar disorder. J Clin Psychopharmacol 1988; 8:275–279.

61. Kravitz HM, Fawcett J. Efficacy of divalproex vs lithium and placebo in mania. JAMA 1994; 272:1005–1006.

62. Emrich HM, Dose M, Von Zerssen D. Action of sodium-valproate and of oxcarbazepine in patients with affective disorders. In: Emrich HM, Okuma T, Muller AA, eds. Anticonvulsants in Affective Disorders. Amsterdam: Excerpta Medica, 1984:45–55.

63. Kupfer DJ, Frank E, Perel JM, Cornes C, Mallinger AG, Thase ME, et al. Five-year outcome for maintenance therapies in recurrent depression. Arch Gen Psychiatry 1992; 49:769–773.

64. Keller MB, Lavori PW, Kane JM, Gelenberg AJ, Rosenbaum JF, Walzer EA, et al. Subsyndromal symptoms in bipolar disorder: a comparison of standard and low serum levels of lithium. Arch Gen Psychiatry 1992; 49:371–376.

65. Coppen A, Ghose K, Montgomery S, Rama Rao VA, Bailey J, Jorgensen A. Continuation therapy with amitriptyline in depression. Br J Psychiatry 1978; 133:28–33.

66. Freedman DD, Waters DD. "Second generation" dihydropyridine calcium antagonists: greater vascular selectivity and some unique applications. Drugs 1987; 34:578–598.

67. Bouvy PF, van de Wetering BJM, Meerwaldt JD, Bruijn JB. A case of organic brain syndrome following head injury successfully treated with carbamazepine. Acta Psychiatr Scand 1993; 77:363.
68. Sechi GP, Piras MR, Demurtas A, Tanca S, Rosati G. Dexamethasone-induced schizoaffective-like state in multiple sclerosis: prophylaxis and treatment with carbamazepine. Clin Neuropharmacol 1987; 10:453–457.
69. Dubovsky SL, Franks RD. Verapamil: a new antimanic drug with potential interactions with lithium. J Clin Psychiatry 1987; 48:371–372.
70. Pazzaglia PJ, Post RM, Ketter TA, George MS, Marangell LB. Preliminary controlled trial of nimodipine in ultra-rapid cycling affective dysregulation. Psychiatry Res 1993; 49:257–272.
71. McDermut W, Pazzaglia PJ, Huggins T, Mikalauskas K, Leverich GS, Ketter TA, et al. Use of single case analyses in off-on–off-on trials in affective illness: a demonstration of the efficacy of nimodipine. Depression 1995; 2:259–271.
72. Post RM, Weiss SRB, Chuang D-M. Mechanisms of action of anticonvulsants in affective disorders: comparisons with lithium. J Clin Psychopharmacol 1992; 12:23S–35S.
73. Post RM, Weiss SRB, Chuang D, Ketter TA. Mechanisms of action of carbamazepine in seizure and affective disorders. In: Joffe RT, Calabrese JR, eds. Anticonvulsants in Mood Disorders. New York: Marcel Dekker, 1994:43–92.
74. Post RM, Chuang D-M. Mechanism of action of lithium: comparison and contrast with carbamazepine. In: Birch NJ, ed. Lithium and the Cell: Pharmacology and Biochemistry. London: Academic Press, 1991:199–241.
75. Hough CJ, Irwin RP, Gao X-M, Rogawski MA, Chuang D-M. Carbamazepine inhibition of N-methyl-D-aspartate-evoked calcium influx in rat cerebellar granule cells. J Pharmacol Exp Ther 1996; 276:143–149.
76. Dubovsky SL, Thomas M, Hijazi A, Murphy J. Intracellular calcium signalling in peripheral cells of patients with bipolar affective disorder. Eur Arch Psychiatry Clin Neurosci 1994; 243:229–234.
77. Manna V. [Bipolar affective disorders and role of intraneuronal calcium: therapeutic effects of the treatment with lithium salts and/or calcium antagonist in patients with rapid polar inversion] Article translation from French. Minerva Med 1991; 82:757–763.
78. Ketter TA, Kimbrell TA, George MS, Stein RM, Willis MW, Benson BE, et al. Baseline hypermetabolism may predict carbamazepine response, and hypometabolism nimodipine response in mood disorders [abstr]. Abstracts of the XXth CINP Congress, 1996; (abstract 0-5-6):10.
79. Post RM, Leverich GS, Altshuler L, Mikalauskas K. Lithium discontinuation–induced refractoriness: preliminary observations. Am J Psychiatry 1992; 149:1727–1729.
80. Post RM, Leverich GS, Pazzaglia PJ, Mikalauskas K, Denicoff K. Lithium tolerance and discontinuation as pathways to refractoriness. In: Birch NJ, Padgham C, Hughes MS, eds. Lithium in Medicine and Biology. Lancashire, England: Marius Press, 1993:71–84.

5
The Chronobiology of Mood-Related Disorders

Meir Steiner and Diana Ingram
McMaster University,
Hamilton, Ontario, Canada

I. INTRODUCTION

Chronobiology is the study of the rhythmic changes in living organisms that govern homeostasis and synchrony of the internal milieu. Rhythms may have short periods—oscillating with high frequency, such as the heartbeat—or longer periods—such as 24-hour (circadian), monthly (circalunar, menstrual), or yearly (circannual) cycles. These rhythmic variations in the body's physiology have implications for the clinician and are relevant not only in diagnosis but also in implementing effective treatments and in designing preventive measures. Current research in chronobiology has already established that some diseases are associated with malfunction of rhythms and others are more likely to occur at certain times during a cycle period. Clinical signs and symptoms may vary in a cyclical manner. Results of biochemical and physiological measurements and tests may be subject to circadian, circalunar, and circannual variations. Appropriate treatment can thus be targeted and timed to have maximal action during a specific phase of a cycle, but particular attention must also be given to potential interaction and synergy between interventions and rhythms that may affect side effects as well as efficacy. Specific treatments may also be aimed at correcting desynchronization of rhythms.

In general medicine, the importance of chronobiology is well recognized (Hrushesky, 1994). Myocardial infarction and cerebrovascular accidents tend to have a peak incidence in the early morning, when pulse and blood pressure, which have dropped overnight, rise sharply, together with an increase in catecholamine levels and platelet aggregation. Airway resistance increases at night, when cortisol levels drop and bronchial reactivity to allergens is maximal; the majority of asthma attacks occur between 2 and 6 A.M. Rheumatoid arthritis is symptomatically worse early in the day following nocturnal low cortisol levels and rhythmic variation of the immune system.

Another new and intriguing area of research, chronopharmacology, deals with the impact of biological rhythms on the efficacy as well as the toxicity of medication. Time- and phase-specific interventions have been established for anticancer drugs (Hrushesky, 1985), drugs given to alleviate the symptoms of asthma (Smolensky et al., 1987), and anti-inflammatory agents (Clench et al., 1981), to name a few. For example, anticancer agents such as doxorubicin are known to be most cytotoxic when cells are moving into DNA synthesis. These drugs are toxic not only to tumor cells but also to host cells. When doxorubicin is given in the late afternoon or evening, white-cell recovery is affected for more than 28 days. When given in the morning, white cells are less affected and recovery to normal levels occurs within 21 days (Hrushesky, 1994). Such basic concepts as chronotoxicity, chronotolerance, and chronoefficiency, and the temporal relationship between these effects, have greatly advanced the management of cancer patients (Focan, 1995). Similarly, in asthmatics, inhaled steroids have been found to be more effective when given in morning and afternoon doses, mimicking the endogenous cortisol rhythms. This type of dosing has also been found to be less toxic than evening dosing of steroids, which is more likely to lead to adrenal suppression (Minors, 1985). Circadian differences in analgesic efficacy have been observed, confirming a circadian rhythm of pain as well as circadian variations in the desired chronoeffectiveness and undesired chronotoxicity of opioids (Labrecque and Vanier, 1995) and nonsteroidal anti-inflammatory drugs (Labrecque et al., 1995). A recently documented circadian pattern of acute, neuroleptic-induced dystonic reactions suggests that the efficacy of neuroleptics might also vary over the course of the day (Mazurek and Rosebush, 1996).

Abnormal biological rhythms have long been associated with affective disorders, and the ever-expanding knowledge base regarding mechanisms involved in desynchronized rhythmicity is clearly relevant to understanding these disorders and their treatments.

II. CIRCADIAN RHYTHMS

A. Normal Physiology and "Minor" Disruptions

In humans, 24-hour physiological and biological rhythms are endogenously sustained by a circadian pacemaker or clock. In the absence of light or of day–night cycles, these rhythms "free-run" with a 25-hour period. This has been observed in the blind and in some conditions of stringent isolation from external cues (Lewy and Sack, 1988). The visual system has a unique role in the temporal organization of physiological and neuroendocrine rhythms as well as behavior. This synchronization is not just a passive response to the light–dark cycle, but rather a complex interaction among the endogenous circadian pacemaker or clock, the suprachiasmatic nucleus (SCN) of the hypothalamus, and the environment. It has been generally assumed that intact vision is a prerequisite for circadian synchrony, but a recent study has shown that ocular light exposure caused a robust neuroendocrine response (melatonin suppression) in some blind patients, challenging the presumption that the loss of conscious perception of light also indicates a loss of function of the retinohypothalamic tract (Czeisler et al., 1995; Moore, 1995). In some blind individuals, it appears that a 24-hour period may also become entrained by social routines and other environmental cues. Thus, it is apparent that the central circadian pacemaker has an afferent pathway that is light-sensitive and that may also be influenced by other exogenous time-givers, or *Zeitgebers* (Aschoft et al., 1975; Wever, 1986).

The purpose of the circadian clock is to recognize local time and mark passage of time, ensuring that bodily activities are appropriately integrated for sleep–wake cycles at local time. Efferent outputs from the pacemaker modulate not only the sleep–wake cycle but also temperature and endocrine rhythms. To date, the results of most human experiments on circadian rhythmicity confirm the existence of more than one internal clock, pacemaker, or oscillator. This dual- or even multioscillatory concept of the human circadian system explains how different oscillators contribute to the control of different rhythms (Wever, 1986). Thus, the endogenous circadian components of both melatonin and body-temperature rhythms are believed to be generated by a single central circadian pacemaker (Shanahan and Czeisler, 1991), whereas the relationship between sleep and the circadian secretory profile along the hypothalamic-pituitary-adrenal (HPA) axis of cortisol continues to be controversial (Weibel et al. 1995). Light exposure early in the dark period will reset the pacemaker by delaying it, whereas light exposure late in the dark period advances it. Defects in rhythmicity may occur from central pacemaker malfunction or if a biological rhythm comes uncoupled from the pacemaker. Rhythms may also be affected by influences that did not originate in the pacemaker. Thus, while body temperature and plasma cortisol levels are partly under the control of the same pacemaker, they are also lowered by sleep alone (Schwartz, 1993).

Sleep and wakefulness are under predominant circadian control. Nocturnal sleep is accompanied by a drop in body temperature and a rise in light-sensitive melatonin. Sleep at other times of the day becomes uncoupled from body-temperature rhythmicity and shows a change in sleep architecture, with changes in the duration of total sleep and onset and amount of rapid eye movement (REM) sleep (Schwartz, 1993).

The psychiatric implications of disrupted circadian rhythms become evident when one considers the consequences of disturbed sleep–wake cycles in non-psychiatrically-ill populations. Examples of such "minor" disruption include shift work, jet lag, and insomnia.

Shift workers with shifts that violate circadian sleep–wake cycle physiology report chronic fatigue, difficulty concentrating, irritability, impaired performance, difficulty sleeping, and a variety of gastrointestinal disturbances as well as an increased risk of cardiovascular disease. Shift work has been noted to be associated with heavier use of caffeine and alcohol and an increase in divorce (Schwartz, 1993; Healy and Waterhouse, 1995). Many of these medical and psychosocial problems associated with rotating shift work can be prevented by introducing schedules designed to incorporate circadian principles (Czeisler et al., 1982, 1990; Campbell, 1995; Eastman et al., 1995a, 1995b; Dawson et al., 1995).

Jet lag is a phenomenon well known to long-distance travelers and especially to flight crews on transmeridian long hauls (Dodge et al., 1982). Typical symptoms include fatigue, temporal disorientation with difficulty sleeping at the destination's nighttime, impairment in concentration and performance, loss of appetite, and even impaired mood (Comperatore and Krueger, 1990). The longer the journey and the more time zones crossed, the worse are the symptoms. These symptoms are the result of a temporary and abrupt loss of synchrony between the sleep–wake cycle and the day–night cycle in the new time zone. Travel eastward (phase advance) is more disruptive than travel westward (phase delay) since re-entrainment following westward travel is faster. Jet lag seems to affect middle-aged and older people more than younger ones. Older subjects show more sleep disruption, greater deficits in daytime alertness, and greater increase in sleepiness (Moline et al., 1992). Measures useful for adjusting circadian time to the new time zone include exposure to bright light, regular meals and activity during daytime in the new zone, and short-acting hypnotics or melatonin capsules at night (Boulos et al., 1995).

Sleep disorders are currently classified as either sleep-phase or duration disturbances. Sleep-phase disorders include delayed and advanced sleep-phase syndromes, whereas duration disorders primarily include insomnia and hypersomnia (Terman et al., 1995).

Shiftwork, jet lag, and sleep disorders are all conditions associated with disrupted circadian rhythmicity similar to disturbances observed in mood disorders.

B. Circadian Dysfunction and Mood Disorders

Many of the clinical characteristics of mood disorders are indicative of an association with disrupted circadian rhythms. These include abnormal sleep–wake cycles with insomnia or hypersomnia, early morning awakening, shortened REM latency, and other changes in sleep architecture. Diurnal variations in mood occur with symptoms of depression being at their worst in the morning whereas manic symptoms mostly peak in the early evening hours. In addition, bipolar patients, especially rapid cyclers who experience the "switch" phenomenon, will switch from depression into mania at night (Bunney et al., 1972). A similar switch may also be induced by any of the antidepressive treatments (Altshuler et al., 1995).

A number of chronobiological hypotheses have been proposed to explain the pathophysiology of mood disorders.

1. Internal Desynchronization

In 1968 Halberg proposed that two or more circadian rhythms might not be entrained to the 24-hour cycle and might free-run, falling out of phase with any rhythms that remained entrained to the normal cycle. According to this hypothesis, the temporary coincidence between the maxima of two independent rhythms generates a "beat" phenomenon that triggers an episode of depression or mania. In support of this theory were some preliminary observations in rapid cyclers kept in temporal isolation who switched each time the sleep–wake cycle coincided with the cortisol and temperature rhythms (Kripke, 1983). However, more recently, Checkley (1989) has concluded that desynchronized circadian cycles do not fully account for the length of psychiatric symptoms. This hypothesis has fallen out of favor.

2. Phase Advance

This hypothesis is based on the observation that some depressed patients experience a shortened REM latency as well as early morning awakening. Their rhythms are partially desynchronized and resynchronize each night. It appears that these patients sleep earlier than biologically expected, leading to a depressogenic effect similar to that found in shift workers or long-distance travelers. The biological etiology of this abnormality is unclear. Early work suggested that serum cortisol might be involved, in that the nadir of cortisol secretion is advanced by several hours whereas peak secretion, which is invariably increased, occurs at normal times (for review, see Sack et al., 1987). Additional support for the phase-advance hypothesis comes from several clinical observations: in some patients a phase advance of the sleep–wake cycle can improve depressive symptoms (Wehr, 1990), but when the sleep period of some subjects has been delayed (artificially advancing their circadian rhythm), shortened REM latency, early morning wakenings, and depressed mood have been reported (David et al., 1991).

3. Blunted Amplitude

It has been suggested that blunted amplitude of normal rhythmic circadian fluctuations in the body, such as temperature, melatonin, TSH, heart rate, and other rhythms, may be the primary chronobiological abnormality in depression, resulting in shortened REM latency and early morning wakenings. Nevertheless, research in this area is difficult to interpret because measurements of diminished core temperature, heart rate, and other variables may reflect consequences of disturbed sleep–wake cycles and not disturbed circadian central function. Similarly diminished melatonin secretion may reflect response to external factors such as light exposure rather than providing a valid measure of central production deficit. Studies to date have failed to validate measured variables as appropriate markers of circadian amplitude (Checkley, 1989; Souêtre et al., 1989; Wirz-Justice, 1995).

4. Deficient Process S

This hypothesis is based on the two-process model of sleep regulation (Borbély, 1988). Process C—the central circadian oscillator responsible for the circadian rhythmicity of physiological variables, including REM sleep—is unaffected. Process S, which generates slow-wave sleep, is a homeostatic process that builds up during wakefulness and dissipates during slow-wave sleep. Process C also drives the endogenous rhythms of body temperature, melatonin, and cortisol. Process C drive is highest in the early morning and low during the day. It has been proposed that the sleep disturbance in depression is due to a deficient accumulation of Process S. Such a deficiency would explain prolonged sleep latency, increased waking through the night, and an overall reduction in time spent in slow-wave sleep, which could also explain changes in REM sleep in depressed patients (Borbély et al., 1989).

5. Kindling

The kindling hypothesis is a conceptual framework that attempts to describe neurobiological processes that explain the spatial and temporal evolution of mood disorders. Thus, mood episodes are thought of as seizure-like episodes in the brain. These episodes are conceived of as manifesting themselves with increased responsivity to similar stimuli over time, and as progressing to spontaneous recurrence. At the cellular level, memory of a kindled episode appears to be gene-encoded with messenger RNA inducing spontaneous repetitive events. Synaptic and neural remodeling is thought to occur during kindling, resulting in permanent alteration in neurons and behaviors. Hypothetically recurrent stressors in genetically prone individuals may result in subclinical episodes of kindling that, with repeated episodes of stress or stimulation, lead to full-blown affective episodes with a recurrent pattern (Post et al., 1995; Wirz-Justice, 1995).

6. Exogenous Zeitgebers

Ehlers and her colleagues (1988, 1993) have proposed that psychosocial and external events can be important in the maintenance or disruption of biological rhythms. They suggest that social rhythms help to act as *Zeitgebers* ("time-givers") to entrain biological rhythms. It has now been established that bright light and social cues may have differential effects on the re-entrainment of human circadian rhythms (Honma et al., 1995). These rhythms may be disrupted by travel, shift work, or loss of regular social routine following the death or loss of a partner. They have coined the term *Zeitstörer* ("time-disrupter") for physical, chemical, or psychosocial events resulting in disruption of circadian rhythms. In the healthy individual, central rhythm disruption with disturbed sleep and mood is transient. The biologically vulnerable individual develops a pathological dysrhythmia of endogenous rhythms, resulting in manic or depressive episodes.

C. Circadian Rhythms: Summary

These chronobiological hypotheses are not mutually exclusive; most can be subsumed under the dysregulation hypothesis of the central clock. Accordingly, during an episode of dysrhythmia some rhythms may phase-advance, some will lose amplitude, and others may entrain inappropriately (Healy, 1987). In humans, such dysrhythmia introduces unpredictability and uncertainty into the most vital areas of personal functioning (sleep, appetite, motivation, libido, interest, concentration, etc.), eventually leading to a clinical presentation more typical of a mood disorder (Healy and Waterhouse, 1991).

Circadian rhythms seem also to have the capacity to entrain to nonphotic stimuli. Experiments with animals have shown that it is possible to influence the clock through behavior and that behavioral events (such as social interactions or vigorous activities) can shift rhythms by several hours (Mrosovsky et al., 1989, 1992). Similar data are now also available for humans (Piercy and Lack, 1988; Wirz-Justice, 1995). This new evidence for the existence of a nonphotic phase response curve may help us in further understanding the circadian system and its disruption, especially in situations in which the photic stimuli are inadequate.

Most mammalian circadian rhythms are regulated by neural mechanisms centered on the SCN—the endogenous generator of most circadian rhythms as well as the synchronizer of these rhythms to local time cues (light–dark). Light is communicated to the circadian system via the retina by photoreceptors with connections that terminate in the SCN (the retinohypothalamic tract). Light seems to entrain circadian rhythms by altering activity of cells in the SCN. There is evidence to suggest that these cells undergo alterations in gene expression in response to retinal illumination, but only at times in the circadian rhythm when light is capable of influencing entrainment (Rusak et al., 1990).

Several neurotransmitters and neuromodulators have been suggested as playing a role in the generation and entrainment of rhythms by the SCN. These include serotonin, acetylcholine, glutamate, GABA, a large number of peptides, enzymes, and hormones. These neurotransmitters and neuromodulators are of particular relevance and interest to the study of the chronobiology of mood disorders because they are also thought to be involved in the pathophysiology and pharmacotherapy of these disorders. Unfortunately, evidence of their direct regulation of the SCN is still very inconclusive. Nevertheless, several pharmacological studies have demonstrated that chemical agents can phase-shift circadian rhythms similar to those induced in response to brief light pulses, although the receptor mechanisms underlying these effects are still uncertain (for review, see Rusak and Bina, 1990). A cholinergic pathway projecting from the forebrain and brainstem to the SCN has been localized in the rat (Bina et al., 1993), but the functional significance of these pathways is still unknown. More recently, it has been suggested that in the rat the SCN circadian rhythm is under cholinergic regulation via a muscarinic mechanism that operates only during the dark phase (Liu and Gillette, 1996). The involvement of other neurotransmitters is even less clear. The SCN also receives a major input from the raphe nuclei. Studies suggest that serotonergic agonists can produce circadian time-dependent phase shifts in rhythms of neuronal activity in vitro (Prosser et al., 1993) as well as in behavioral rhythms in vivo (Edgar et al., 1993).

The SCN is further connected to the pineal gland, thereby forming the retinohypothalamic-pineal (RHP) axis. Melatonin is the primary indoleamine hormone produced by the pineal gland. It is synthesized and secreted into the bloodstream during the dark period only and is activated by the noradrenergic system. The pineal gland translates light–dark information (received via the RHP axis) into a chemical messenger (Reiter, 1991). In humans, daytime levels of this messenger, melatonin, are barely detectable with nocturnal peaks at the early part of the night (the "chemical expression of darkness"). These circulating levels of melatonin convey information about the light–dark cycle to the rest of the organism. Melatonin is unique among the neurotransmitter and neuromodulators involved in chronobiology in that it seems to have both a regulatory and a modulatory role. In most mammals, which are seasonal breeders, reproductive potential is linked to photoperiodic information and this information (both absolute and relative) is provided by the nightly changes in circulating melatonin levels (Kennaway and Rowe, 1995). In humans, the role of the pineal is less defined but it seems that melatonin plays a role in the organization of circadian rhythms, and that appropriately timed administration of melatonin can be utilized to phase-shift these rhythms (Attenburrow et al., 1995; Lewy et al., 1996). Furthermore, a functional relationship between the pineal gland and the HPA axis has been suggested in mood disorders. Low nocturnal melatonin secretion and hypercortisolemia were found in acutely depressed inpatients who were also nonsuppressive on the dexamethasone suppression test (Steiner et al., 1990). Thus, changes in availability of melatonin along the RHP axis and dysregulation along the HPA axis may interact in the genesis of mood disorders (Steiner et al., 1987). It is conceivable that in patients with recurrent unipolar depression, changes in central monoamines and in circadian rhythms are secondary to the stress-induced activation of the HPA axis (Dinan, 1994) whereas the trigger for an episode in bipolar mood disorder may be primarily along the RHP axis, i.e., dysrhythmia.

It is hypothesized that bipolar patients have increased sensitivity to light in the morning, and that they have a phase advance of some cycles during the depressed state and a phase delay during mania (Lewy et al., 1985;

Sack et al., 1987). It is also suggested that the amplitude of melatonin secretion is state-dependent in bipolar patients (for review, see Mayeda and Nurnberger, 1990).

Some of the characteristics of circadian rhythms are sex-dependent. In experiments in which external stimuli are excluded, i.e., under constant conditions and in temporal isolation from all time cues, rhythms will free-run according to internal synchrony. Under such conditions the period in women of reproductive age is shorter than in men (on the average by 28 minutes), and the ratio of sleep within the sleep–wake cycle is significantly greater (by ~18% or by 1.46 hours in a 24-hour day). The rhythm of deep body temperature is also different in women: the amplitude is smaller (by ~41%), the value higher (by ~0.15°C), and the fluctuations (the range) of all rhythm parameters are larger in women (Wever, 1986). Significant differences also exist between the sexes in other sleep parameters: women have an earlier onset of sleep, a longer sleep period, and a greater tendency to have disturbed sleep than men (Reyner and Horne, 1995). These sex differences in rhythms seem to disappear in postmenopausal women. It is likely that these differences in circadian rhythmicity may put women of reproductive age at a higher risk for dysrhythmia, especially that due to phase advancement, but possibly also due to greater vulnerability of the shorter cycle to *Zeitstörers*. Such a hypothesis would be in line with the epidemiological data showing a higher incidence of mood disorders in women during their reproductive years (Weissmann and Olfson, 1995).

Age-related changes in the circadian system have been well documented in animals and humans (Touitou and Haus, 1995). The most marked change is an attenuation of amplitude, but an advance in phase and a shortening of period are also observed. The exact physiological mechanisms underlying these age-related deteriorations are still unknown, but changes along the RHP tract seem to play a role. Reduction in the sensitivity to photic stimulation as well as reduction in physical activity may cause dysrhythmia, with potential disruption of sleep and diminished daytime alertness and performance (Myers and Badia, 1995). Studies in hamsters have shown that aging alters monoaminergic inputs to the clock, and that some of the age-related changes in the response of the clock can be reversed by implanting old animals with fetal SCN tissue (Turek et al., 1995). Recent data provide strong evidence that significant alterations occur in gene regulation in the SCN of the aged hamster. The concomitant age-related decreases observed in behavioral phase-shifting and in the expression of c-fos in the SCN support the hypothesis that transcription factors and their target genes are important for photic phase-shifting of circadian rhythms (Zhang et al., 1996).

Taken together, the hypotheses of desynchronization of circadian rhythms and the periodicity of mood disorders can be explained mostly by the temporary coincidence between the maxima of two independent rhythms, generating a "beat" phenomenon that triggers an episode. Thus, rapid cyclers in temporal isolation will "switch" each time the sleep–wake cycle and the cortisol-temperature rhythms concide. The hypotheses also predict shortening of cortisol-temperature rhythms, directly affected by sleep that in itself is disturbed (mostly insomnia but also hypersomnia, reduction in total sleep time, delayed onset and interrupted sleep with early wakening, and shortened REM latency). Ultimately, clinical tests, which can establish whether circadian rhythms are phase-advanced or -delayed, may indicate in individual patients the type of treatment they require and predict response.

III.   MENSTRUAL, MONTHLY CYCLES (CIRCALUNAR)

A. Normal Physiology

From puberty to menopause, women are subject to monthly menstrual cycles. At puberty, the hypothalamic-pituitary-gonadal (HPG) axis begins to function in a cyclical, regulated manner, which persists in terms of fluctuating steroid hormone levels until menopause. The hallmark of puberty is the positive estrogen feedback to the hypothalamus and pituitary. The nature of the "clock" governing the inherent timing of the ontogeny of the HPG system and the control of the onset of puberty remains a mystery (Bettendorf and Bettendorf, 1993). It is probably internally regulated by genetic coding, as well as externally influenced by exteroceptive factors such as light exposure, geographic location, general health, and nutrition. Menarche is reasonably well correlated between mothers, daughters, and sisters. Children who live close to the equator, at low latitudes, and are mildly obese have been found to experience menarche earlier than those who live in northern latitudes, at higher altitudes, or who are of normal weight (Tanner, 1962). Blindness has also been reported to be associated with an earlier menarche (Zacharias and Wurtman, 1964).

From the time of menarche, menstrual function is initiated by the release of gonadotropin-releasing hormone (GnRH) from the hypothalamus. Normal menstrual function requires pulsatile GnRH discharge within a critical range of frequency and amplitude. Pulses of GnRH are influenced by a dual catecholamine system: norepinephrine-facilitatory, dopamine-inhibitory. Endogenous opioids modulate the catecholamine pathway. Gonadal steroids feed back to influence neurotransmitters directly, and possibly interact at the hypothalamus directly as catecholsteroids (Speroff et al., 1994). Following menstruation, in response to low levels of estrogen, GnRH action results in the synthesis and release of follicle-stimulating hormone (FSH) from the anterior pituitary. FSH acts on a group of growing follicles in the ovary, promoting their growth and the elaboration of estrogen. At mid-cycle, a critical estradiol level triggers a surge of luteinizing hormone (LH) from the anterior pituitary, which affects the dominant follicle, causing ovulation—the formation of a corpus luteum and elaboration of proges-terone. While fertile, women's monthly cycles are traditionally described in terms of their overt manifestation—menstruation—and further described in terms of the related gonadal hormone fluctuations: follicular phase, ovula-tion, luteal phase, and menstruation. These cycles persist as long as func-tional ovarian follicles produce estrogen. Menopause occurs when the ovary no longer contains functional follicles.

Most of the physiological parameters that follow a circadian pattern also have, in women of reproductive age, a superimposed circalunar rhythm (for review, see Leibenluft et al., 1994). Sleep varies through the cycle, with total sleep probably being greater in the luteal than in the follicular phase. 24-hour temperature mean, minimum, and maximum are all greater in the luteal phase of the cycle. Studies of melatonin are inconclusive with regard to variations in secretion throughout the cycle. However, levels of melatonin, which has been shown to inhibit ovulation, have been found to be elevated in amenorrheic women (generally anovular) and those receiving oral contra-ceptives. Plasma monoamines seem to fluctuate through the menstrual cycle; in particular, plasma levels of serotonin have been found to be lowest in the ovulatory phase (Blum et al., 1992). It is unclear whether these fluctuations parallel events in the central nervous system. Studies on prolactin secretion are inconclusive, with many studies not evaluating levels during sleep when prolaction secretion is maximal. Basal cortisol levels do not appear to fluctu-ate through the menstrual cycle.

Since the effects of the fluctuations in gonadal steroids on circadian rhythms have been studied primarily in animals, the effects in humans are still mostly unknown (Leibenluft, 1993). Estrogen has been shown to shorten the period of free-running circadian rhythms in ovariectomized rats, and to advance entrained circadian rhythms. In menopausal women, estrogen has also been demonstrated to decrease sleep latency and advance the onset of sleep. It is hypothesized that gonadal steroids may be implicated in disorders that disturb circadian rhythms that are more prevalent in women (rapid-cycling and seasonal affective disorders) and disorders that show atypical symptoms of depression such as hypersomnia, which may also be more prevalent in women.

B. Mood-Related Disorders in Women

The two-females-to-one-male prevalence in unipolar depression is well documented in the epidemiological psychiatric literature (Weissman and Olfson, 1995). Of note is the fact that this sex difference is not present in children but is present by early adolescence (Offord et al., 1987; Radloff, 1991). While gender difference in developmental experience and socialization may account for this sex-ratio difference, it is also possible that sex-steroid changes initiated at menarche may play a role. The NIMH Epidemiologic Catchment Area (ECA) Study found that women aged 18–44 have the greatest risk for depression in 1-year prevalence (Wolk and Weissman, 1995). There is no increased risk for development of depression at menopause, or evidence for specific symptom development in menopausal years (Hallstrom and Samuelsson, 1985; McKinlay et al., 1987; Weissman, 1979).

Unlike unipolar depression, in which there is a 2:1 prevalence of women to men, the rate of bipolar affective disorders is equal in men and women (Weissman et al., 1993). However, extreme rhythmic or cyclical patterns of bipolar disorder occur in women more commonly than men, including rapid-cycling disorders (Coryell et al., 1992; Wehr et al., 1988; Alarcon, 1985) as well as the seasonal form of the disorder (Wehr and Rosenthal, 1989). Bipolar women are also likely to suffer from other cyclical disturbances of mood such as severe premenstrual dysphoria (Price and DiMarzio, 1986; Endicott et al., 1985) and postpartum disturbances (Leibenluft, 1996).

Hormones are only partial determinants of gender-specific behaviors, interacting with other physiological, environmental, and psychosocial factors. In most women of reproductive age and beyond, the hormonal fluctuations are not associated with major physical discomfort or mental distress. But in some women changes in mood, levels of anxiety and irritability, sleep, eating habits, and levels of energy as well as physical symptoms appear to be linked temporally to these hormonal fluctuations. In these women, a cascade of events triggered originally along the HPG axis brings about the shift from an existing vulnerability to the actual manifestations of the various female-specific mood disorders. The degree of vulnerability becomes apparent at puberty, when women are exposed to increasing estrogenic influences.

Particularly vulnerable times are the periods that mark shifts in the reproductive stages: menarche, the premenstruum, puerperium, and menopause, all associated with major hormonal turmoil as well as with psychosocial stresses (Steiner and Dunn, 1996).

Minor physical and emotional changes (premenstrual molimina) precede menstruation in the ovulatory cycles of 60–70% of women. A small percentage of women, 3–8%, suffer from severe mood changes in the luteal phase of the cycle that are sufficient to interfere with their work, activities, or relationships (Andersch et al., 1986; Johnson et al., 1988; Rivera-Tovar and Frank, 1990; Ramcharan et al., 1992; Merikangas et al., 1993). This syndrome, categorized as premenstrual dysphoric disorder (PMDD) in the DSM-IV, occurs regularly in the week before menstruation and disappears within a few days of menstrual bleeding (APA, 1994). A number of investigators have reported an increased incidence of major depression in women who suffer from severe PMDD (Endicott, 1993). Others have noted prior episodes of postpartum depression or bipolar affective disorder in these women (Pearlstein et al., 1990; Endicott et al., 1985). It seems that there is often a "magnification" of affective symptoms in the luteal phase of the cycle (Steiner, 1996). Women with "treated" depression have been noted to report premenstrual exacerbations of mood symptoms when carefully evaluated throughout their cycle (Yonkers and White, 1992). In some studies, one-quarter to one-third of women presenting with complaints of severe premenstrual symptoms are found to have ongoing major depression (Stout and Steege, 1985; McMillan and Pihl, 1987). Women with affective disorders are more likely to have a psychiatric admission in the luteal phase (Janowsky et al., 1969; Targum et al., 1991), although studies attempting to relate suicide in women to phases of the menstrual cycle remain inconclusive at this time (MacKinnon and MacKinnon, 1959; Lester, 1990; Vanezis, 1990).

Gonadal hormones appear to modify psychosis. Female schizophrenic patients have a later onset schizophrenia and better outcome than males. Prior to menopause they require smaller neuroleptic doses for both acute and maintenance treatment, whereas following menopause they need higher doses than men (for review, see Seeman and Lang, 1990). It is speculated that estrogen is protective by down-regulating dopamine D_2-receptor sensitivity. Hallonquist et al. (1993) reported that symptom severity changed over the course of the menstrual cycle in a small number of treated schizophrenics, with worsening of symptoms in the luteal (hypoestrogenic) phase. Brockington et al. (1988) reported on eight patients with puerperal psychosis who recovered, and then suffered premenstrual relapses. Five suffered recurrent premenstrual relapses. Sothern et al. (1993) documented the case of a woman with schizoaffective disorder who had recurrent "manic" bouts of psychosis with onset perimenstrually and the predominance of affected days in the follicular phase of her cycles.

It is now being acknowledged that the complexity of gender-specific biological rhythms is also extremely relevant to treatment. The enzymes responsible for the oxidative metabolism of drugs—including many of the psychotropic medications and, in particular, tricyclic antidepressants as well as selective serotonin-reuptake inhibitors (SSRIs)—include the cytochromes P450-2D6 and the P450-3A family (Moltke et al., 1994; Preskorn et al., 1994). These are the same enzymes that are involved in metabolizing not only many other medications but also, more importantly, gonadal steroids (Kato, 1974), and the expression of these enzymes is subject to genetic polymorphism (Coutts, 1994). Sex-specific cytochrome P450 has also been identified as the cause for gender- and species-related differences in drug toxicity (Kato and Yamazoe, 1992). Rhythms in efficacy as well as side effects of psychotropic drugs may be due to rhythms in the brain's susceptibility, which reflects shifting relationships among the drug, the receptor sybtype it affects, and the surrounding neuroendocrine environment (Nagayama, 1993).

Future research will have to establish whether the genetic expression and function of 5-HT receptor subtypes are influenced by gonadal and adrenal steroid hormones, and whether an inbalance in the interaction of these two systems may contribute to the vulnerability of women to mood disorders.

C. Mood Disorders and the HPG Axis

Bipolar affective disorder may be considered a primary rhythm or chronobiological disturbance. The presence of yet one more rhythm—the menstrual cycle—puts women at risk for dysregulation in more rhythm systems than men. It is interesting that in a disorder with equal prevalence between the sexes women suffer from the highly rhythmic form of the disorder, rapid cycling, more frequently than men do.

Rapid cycling is defined as more than four episodes of mood disturbance in a 12-month period (Dunner and Fieve, 1974; APA, 1994). Most studies indicate the presence of three women to one man in reviews of patient populations of rapid cyclers (Dunner et al., 1977; Kukopulos et al., 1980; Wehr et al., 1988; Coryell et al., 1992). Furthermore, among patients who have 12 or more episodes of affective disturbance occur per year, the ratio of women to men is even greater (Bauer and Whybrow, 1991). Female rapid cyclers in their reproductive years are more likely to complain of severe premenstrual changes than controls, and those complaining of severe premenstrual changes have a tendency to have more affective episodes per year than those with mild premenstrual symptoms (Price and DeMarzio, 1986). Previous studies have related rapid cycling to hypothyroidism (Cowdry et al., 1983). However, more recent studies have suggested the hypothyroidism is no more associated with rapid-cycling illness than non-rapid-cycling disorder, but rather has a high prevalence in women who are treated with lithium (Wehr et al., 1988; Joffe et al., 1988).

At least one case report exists of a women in her 80s, not reported to be on hormone-replacement therapy, who has well-documented regular 3–4-week episodes of affective disorder (either mania or depression) that started postmenopausally (Mizukawa et al., 1991). Such episodes obviously do not result from the flux of gonadal hormones, but rather may reflect a persistent central *Zeitgeber* or kindling phenomenon in the brain triggered by previous menstruation-related changes. A recent report on five females with ultra-rapid and ultradian cycling of bipolar affective illness further confirms the notion that women may have faster patterns of mood oscillation (Kramlinger and Post, 1996). Wehr and coworkers (1988) have also reported on rapid cycling beginning at or persisting into menopause.

Pregnancy results in a significant disruption of the cyclical activity of the HPG axis. While pregnancy itself seems protective against serious psychiatric illness (Paffenbarger, 1982), the postpartum period is associated with an increased risk of psychiatric admission (Kendell et al., 1987). A number of studies have indicated that affective disorders account for 75–80% of severe postpartum disorders, whereas schizophrenia accounts for only 2–3% (Dean and Kendell, 1981; Kendell et al. 1987). Bipolar women and women with schizoaffective disorder are found more frequently than expected in most studies of severe puerperal disorder (Brockington et al., 1981; Kendell et al. 1987; Platz and Kendell, 1988; Wisner et al., 1995). In the largest study available, Kendell et al. (1987) linked a psychiatric registry with an obstetrical registry, and were able to estimate the risk of needing psychiatric hospitalization within 90 days of childbirth in women who had previous psychiatric diagnoses. They found that the risk of admission post-partum was highest in women with a lifetime diagnosis of manic-depressive illness. Researchers have also looked at the difference between bipolar patients with de novo onset of episodes postpartum and those with a diagnosis preceding pregnancy. Puerperal-onset bipolar patients have been found to have fewer recurrences and a better prognosis than non-puerperal-onset patients (Kadrmas et al., 1979; Dean et al., 1989). Others have indicated a better long-term outcome in women with first onset of a postpartum disorder other than bipolars (Platz and Kendell, 1988; Bell et al., 1994; Cooper and Murray, 1995). This heterogeneity in outcomes is thought to reflect two groups of patients, with women suffering from puerperal-only forms of the illness being seen to have less vulnerability to the illness unless exposed to a significant biological challenge such as pregnancy and parturition.

As previously noted, there is no documented evidence that there is an increase in unipolar depression or a unique depressive syndrome in monopausal women (Wolk and Weissman, 1995; Weissman, 1979), or that perimenopausal mood disorders should be classified as a separate entity (Youngs, 1990). However, methodological problems exist with previous studies (Schmidt and Rubinow, 1991), while experimental work shows that estrogen enhances mood, sexual desire, and memory in postmenopausal women, especially those who have undergone surgical menopause (Sherwin et al., 1985; Sherwin, 1988, 1991). It remains to be seen whether women who are susceptible to puerperal-related episodes of mood disorder, perhaps hormonally triggered, are also susceptible to menopausally triggered bouts.

IV. CIRCANNUAL SEASONAL RHYTHMS

A. Normal Physiology

For most mammalian species, especially in middle and high latitudes, physiological adaptation to the extreme conditions of winter is a matter of survival. Some animals adapt to extremely low temperatures and scarce food supplies by hibernating. Hibernation is a circannual rhythm in which a warm-blooded animal can control and regulate a reduction in body temperature, respiration, heart rate, metabolic rate, and food consumption. Many of the neurophysiological and biochemical aspects of hibernation remain unexplained (Lyman, 1984). The annual timing of hibernation is synchronized with the seasons and is dependent on the gradual shortening of the photoperiod. The message of changes in photoperiodicity is conveyed along the RHP axis and further transduced to the rest of the organism by melatonin. The message to the hypothalamus (the locus of the "thermostat") is to reset at a lower level. Melatonin is also implicated in the regulation of reproduction: extended melatonin production during longer prehibernation dark periods results in suppression of gonadal activity, which in turn facilitates entry into hibernation. There is an inverse relationship between the annual gonadal and hibernation cycles (Pevet el al., 1989). During hibernation, levels of both temperature and melatonin drop sharply and the circadian pacemaker in the

SCN loses its rhythmicity (Jansky et al., 1989). The hypothalamic thermostat is also responsible for a similar but lesser downward resetting of nighttime body temperature during slow-wave sleep; indeed, animals seem to enter hibernation during slow-wave sleep, perhaps indicating that both sleep–wakefulness and hibernation–euthermia cycles are regulated by the same neural circuit (Heller, 1979) and that slow-wave sleep and hibernation are homologous states (Walker and Berger, 1980; Kilduff et al., 1993).

Seasonal fluctuations in a number of body functions have also been observed in humans. Seasonal rhythms may be dependent on either photoperiodic regulation or a circannual clock (Pittendrigh, 1988). Seasonal variations in healthy adults have so far been observed in the timing of sleep, mean body temperature, phases of circadian temperature, and the phase relationship between sleep and rectal-temperature rhythm (Honma et al., 1992). These findings indicate that not only the external (local time) but also the internal (between circadian rhythms) phase relationships of the human circadian rhythms depend on season. Seasonal variations have also been observed in total sleep duration and body weight (Terman, 1988) and in the circadian rhythms of melatonin (Illnerova et al., 1985; Kennaway and Royles, 1986). Research into the relationship of circadian and seasonal rhythms continues to support the notion that melatonin's main function is to coordinate biological rhythms. Melatonin rhythms are normally slightly delayed and its secretion increased in winter, and it has been suggested that hibernation is analogous to seasonal depression in humans (Pohl and Giedke, 1987; Mrosovsky, 1988).

B. Seasonality of Mood Disorders

Seasonal rhythms in mood and behavior in humans have been known to occur for centuries. It is only in more recent years that seasonal disturbances in mood have been delineated and categorized as syndromes, including seasonal affective disorder (SAD) (Rosenthal et al., 1984) or recurrent winter depression and summer depression (Wehr et al., 1991). It has been suggested that SAD runs in families and that this is largely due to a biological predisposition, thus emphasizing the role of genetic factors in this disorder (Madden et al., 1996).

In addition, any recurrent mood disorder with a regular seasonal cyclicity can now be identified by the qualifier "with seasonal pattern" (APA, 1994). Winter depression seems to be induced in vulnerable individuals by the decreased ambient light during the winter, and summer depression seems to be associated more with high temperatures (Wehr, 1992).

Contemporary research into the epidemiology of mood disorders seems to confirm a strong seasonal pattern. Suicides as well as hospital admissions for depressive illness peak in spring and autumn (Eastwood and Peter, 1988). Similar patterns have also been established for onset of episodes, first prescription of antidepressants, and ECT (for review, see Wehr and Rosenthal, 1989).

Seasonal influences on the onset of episodes of depression and mania are thus relevant to the treatment and crucial in the prevention of these episodes. In 15% of patients with recurrent depression, episodes will recur almost exclusively in one of the two seasonal risk periods, suggesting that they may be influenced by environmental changes. Two major seasonal patterns have been described: 1) autumn–winter depression with or without spring–winter mania or hypomania and 2) spring–summer depression with or without autumn–winter mania or hypomania (Faedda et al., 1993). These patterns seem to apply to both unipolar and bipolar disorders, although the onset of depression episodes seems to be determined in part more by seasonality than mania (Silverstone et al., 1995). Winter depressives are more likely to have atypical vegetative symptoms such as increased appetite, carbohydrate craving, weight gain, and hypersomnia, whereas summer depressives are more likely to have endogenous vegetative symptoms, with decreased appetite and insomnia (Wehr et al., 1991). The question of whether patients with pure SAD (winter depression) are different from patients with nonseasonal episodes seems to be as yet unresolved (Lewy et al., 1981; Reme et al., 1991; Cummings et al., 1989). It has been suggested that there is an abnormal seasonal variation in the suppression of melatonin by light in SAD with a supersensitivity during the winter and possibly subsensitivity during summer (Thompson et al., 1990).

Others have shown no significant differences in melatonin rhythms in SAD (Checkley et al., 1993). However, differences have been documented in the HPA axis profiles in SAD when compared to melancholics, with SAD patients having a deficient, attenuated ACTH and cortisol response to CRH (Joseph-Vanderpool et al., 1991).

V. TREATMENT

The impact of recent developments in the studies of biological rhythms is very much in evidence, especially in the area of chronopharmacology (Nagayama, 1993). General new principles of chronotherapeutics are being introduced, and topics such as chronopharmacokinetics and chronopharmacodynamics can no longer be ignored. Biological rhythms affect absorbtion, metabolism, and excretion of drugs and their metabolites, resulting in different concentrations of a drug at different times of the day, month, or year.

Rhythmic changes also occur in the susceptibility of a system to a fixed dose of a drug at different times of the circadian or other relevant cycle (e.g., menstrual cycle). This phenomenon, known as chronesthesy, can result from changes in membrane permeability or in receptor sensitivity.

Drugs that specifically shift rhythms are known as chronobiotics; these are chemical substances capable of therapeutically re-entraining short-term dissociated or long-term desynchronized rhythms, or prophylactically prevent such disruptions (Dawson and Armstrong, 1996).

The mechanism of action of many, if not most, of the modern therapeutic interventions geared toward helping patients with mood disorders involves shifting of biological rhythms. These interventions include mood stabilizers and/or antidepressants, sleep induction, sleep deprivation, and phototherapy. Thus, the overall aim of these treatments is, at least in part, to shift and correct desynchronized rhythms.

In support of this hypothesis is the fact that most antidepressants, despite the lack in specificity of their chemical or therapeutic properties, are consistent in their effect on the clock. Antidepressants slow the pacemaker and lengthen the circadian cycle period, thereby resynchronizing the intrinsic rhythms to the light–dark cycle. Lithium, which until recently was—and in many cases still is—the treatment of choice for bipolar mood disorder, has no generalized behavioral effects; i.e., it is not a sedative, depressant, or euphoriant but rather seems to stabilize mood by slowing circadian rhythms. Lithium lengthens the intrinsic period of free-running rhythms. In hamsters, lithium was found to delay or suppress natural hibernation, again suggesting the involvement of circadian rhythms in its mechanism of action (Pohl and Giedke, 1987). In depressed patients, it is believed that these interventions resynchronize a phase-advanced cycle (Goodwin et al., 1982; Wirz-Justice and Campbell, 1982; Kripke et al., 1985; Klemfuss, 1992; Healy and Waterhouse, 1995; Dawson and Armstrong, 1996).

Benzodiazepines such as triazolam, which are commonly used in the treatment of insomnia, are also capable of phase-advancing the circadian clock, and this effect seems to be partially but not completely additive to the effect of bright light (Joy and Turek, 1992).

Total sleep deprivation (TSD) has been found to improve depression in about 50–60% of unipolar and bipolar depressed patients (Wehr, 1990; Wu and Bunney, 1990). However, a total relapse into depression may occur following recovery sleep, and TSD in bipolar patients may precipitate mania (Wehr, 1990, 1991). Partial sleep deprivation (PSD) has also been associated with clinical improvement in depressed patients (Sack et al., 1988; Elsenga et al., 1990; Giedke et al., 1992; Leibenluft et al., 1993). A recent review suggests that timing of sleep is less important than its duration (Van den Hoffdakker, 1994), but the timing of sleep following successful TSD may be crucial for stabilization of its antidepressant effect (Rieman et al., 1996). Advancing the sleep cycle by 6 hours has also been found to have a beneficial effect on mood (Sack et al., 1985; Vollman and Berger, 1993).

To restore rhythm disorders generated by the lack of *Zeitgeber* effectiveness, one must intensify the *two* effective *Zeitgeber* modes: social contacts and intensity of daytime illumination.

It is not known how much daily illumination is required in humans for optimal physical and mental health. Exposure to 1000–10,000 lux illumination for up to several hours each day might be required to produce maximal changes in human circadian rhythms (Wever, 1985) and melatonin secretion (Bojkowski et al., 1987) as well as to maintain optimal euthymia (Terman et al., 1989), although dim light also seems to have substantial effects (Bojkowiski et al., 1987; Brainard et al., 1988; Avery et al., 1993). Both season and geographic location (latitude) strongly influence human illumination exposure (Cole et al., 1995). Recent results from a study of adults in San Diego who experienced daily exposure to only low illumination suggest that many Americans may be receiving insufficient light exposure to maintain optimal mood (Espiritu et al., 1994).

Bright light has been shown to be able to reset the human circadian pacemaker independent of the timing of the sleep–wake cycle (Czeisler et al., 1986), and the sensitivity (phase-response curve) of the human circadian pacemaker to light has been characterized (Czeisler et al., 1989). These findings have major implications for the treatment of circadian sleep disorders as well as SAD.

Phototherapy with bright artificial light (BAL) has been accepted by most clinicians as an effective treatment for SAD. It seems to be independent of time of day, suppression of melatonin, or circadian phase (Wehr et al., 1986; Wirz-Justice et al., 1993; Tam et al., 1995). However, SAD patients also seem to respond to "natural" light (Wirz-Justice et al., 1986, 1996). The therapeutic effects of BAL in SAD are believed to involve a serotonergic mechanism (Lam et al., 1996) and a specific serotonin-reuptake inhibitor was also found to be effective in this disorder (Lam et al., 1995). BAL is now also utilized in the treatment of sleep disorders associated with shift work (Eastman et al., 1995a,b) and jet lag (Boulos et al., 1995).

Based on the sleep-inducing properties of melatonin, and the fact that BAL suppresses nighttime melatonin secretion (Lewy, 1983), it has been suggested that the effects of BAL are mediated through the action of melatonin. Moreover, administration of melatonin, which is believed to have chronobiotic effects (Dawson and Armstrong, 1996), counteracts the effects of BAL on body temperature and alertness (Badia et al., 1991; Sack et al., 1992). BAL may also cause hypomanic irritability and hyperactivity in SAD patients (Rosenthal et al., 1984; Levitt et al., 1993), and hypomania and mania were also reported in nonseasonal depressives treated with BAL (Schwitzer et al., 1990).

VI. FUTURE DIRECTIONS

Solving the underlying genetic and molecular mechanisms of biological clocks has become an important goal with the growing realization that intracellular tiny biochemical clocks maintain, at least in the fruitfly, the daily rhythms in physiology, biochemistry, and behavior (Hall, 1995). Not only does light—i.e., environmental input—regulate IEG expression (Rusak et al., 1990), but there are clock-controlled target genes, and more recently several clock genes have also been isolated in *Drosophila* (for review, see Takahashi, 1995). Two genes in particular, *period* (PER) and *timeless* (TIM), are required for production of circadian rhythms in *Drosophila*, and the phase of these rhythms can be differentially advanced or delayed by light pulses (Myers et al., 1996). Newly discovered four *clock* mutant genes in the nematode suggest that bodily functions such as metabolic rate are also controlled and paced by genetic clocks, thus determining the lifespan of the worm (Lakowski and Hekimi, 1996).

Biological rhythms are ubiquitous, and seem to be governed by clocks that respond to similar stimuli in species as varied as prokaryotes, aplysia, *Drosophila*, and mammals. The most recent genetic studies seem to indicate that the clock genes have not changed in evolution. The hope is therefore that learning more about the system in one or more species may also teach us about the implications these rhythms have in humans.

More advanced strategies for studying the biological clock and the role of melatonin in entrainment in mammals will also become available now that the melatonin receptor gene has been cloned (Ebisawa et al., 1994). A recently discovered second 24-hour circadian clock in the mammalian retina seems to regulate the synthesis of melatonin in the retina and is entrained by light cycles. This oscillator, which is genetically programmed, is essential for normal photoreceptor function (Tosini and Menaker, 1996). The implications of these findings for the chronobiology of mood disorders are yet to be determined.

Future research should focus on the phase relationship among physiological rhythms, clock and sleep time, and onset of episodes of mood disorders. Animal models of mood disorders, with particular emphasis on models of circadian dysregulation, continue to be extremely valuable to these studies. It is also important to remember that not all clinical features of the mood disorders are related to biological rhythms, and that the chronobiological approach has to be reconciled with other theoretical concepts of mood disorders.

REFERENCES

Alarcon RD. Rapid cycling affective disorders: a clinical review. Compr Psychiatry 1985; 26:522–540.

Altshuler LL, Post RM, Leverich GS, et al. Antidepressant-induced mania and cycle acceleration: a controversy revisited. Am J Psychiatry 1995; 152:1130–1138.

Andersch B, Wendestam C, Hahn L, et al. Premenstrual complaints. I. Prevalence of premenstrual symptoms in a Swedish urban population. J Psychosom Obstet Gynaecol 1986; 5:39–49.

APA. Diagnostic and Statistical Manual of Mental Disorders. 4th ed. Washington, DC: American Psychiatric Association, 1994.

Aschoff J, Hoffman K, Pohl H, et al. Re-entrainment of circadian rhythms after phase shifts of the Zeitgeber. Chronobiologia 1975; 2:23–78.

Attenburrow ME, Dowling BA, Sargent PA, et al. Melatonin phase advances circadian rhythm. Psychopharmacology 1995; 121:503–505.

Avery DH, Bolte MA, Dager SR, et al. Dawn simulation treatment of winter depression: a controlled study. Am J Psychiatry 1993; 150:113–117.

Badia P, Myers B, Boecker M, et al. Bright light effects on body temperature, alertness, EEG and behavior. Physiol Behav 1991; 50:583–588.

Bauer MS, Whybrow PC. Rapid cycling bipolar disorder: clinical features, treatment and etiology. In: Amsterdam JD, ed. Advances in Neuropsychiatry and Psychopharmacology. Vol 2. Refractory Depression. New York: Raven Press, 1991:191–208.

Bell AJ, Land NM, Milne S, et al. Long-term outcome of postpartum psychiatric illness requiring admission. J Affective Disord 1994; 31:67–70.

Bettendorf M, Bettendorf G. Search for a biological clock in the ontogeny of puberty. Human Reprod 1993; 8:791–792.

Bina KG, Rusak B, Semba K. Localization of cholinergic neurons in the forebrain and brainstem that project to the suprachiasmatic nucleus of the hypothalamus in rats. J Comp Neurol 1993; 335:295–307.

Blum I, Nessiel L, David A, et al. Plasma neurotransmitter profile during different phases of the ovulatory cycle. J Clin Endocrin Metab 1992; 75:924–929.

Bojkowski CJ, Aldhous ME, English J, et al. Suppression of nocturnal plasma melatonin and 6-sulphatoxymelatonin by bright and dim light in man. Horm Metab Res 1987; 19:437–440.

Borbély AA. The two-process model of sleep regulation. In: Kupfer DJ, Monk TH, Barchas JD, eds. Biological Rhythms and Mental Disorders. New York: Guilford Press, 1988:55–81.

Borbély AA, Achermann P, Trachsel L, et al. Sleep initiation and initial sleep intensity: interactions of homeostatic and circadian mechanisms. J Biol Rhythms 1989; 4:149–160.

Boulos Z, Campbell SS, Lewy AJ, et al. Light treatment for sleep disorders: consensus report. VII. Jet lag. J Biol Rhythms 1995; 10:167–176.

Brainard GC, Lewy AJ, Menaker M, Fredrickson RH, Miller LS, Weleber RG, Cassone V, Hudson D. Dose-response relationship between light irradiance and the suppression of plasma melatonin in human volunteers. Brain Res 1988; 454:212–218.

Brockington IF, Cernik KF, Schofield EM, et al. Puerperal psychosis. Arch Gen Psychiatry 1981; 38:829–833.

Brockington IF, Kelly A, Hall P, et al. Premenstrual relapse of puerperal psychosis. J Affective Disord 1988; 14:287–292.

Bunney WE Jr, Goodwin FK, Murphy DL. The "switch process" in manic-depressive illness. III. Theoretical implications. Arch Gen Psychiatry 1972; 27:312–317.

Campbell SS. Effects of timed bright-light exposure on shift-work adaptation in middle-aged subjects. Sleep 1995; 18:408–416.

Checkley S. The relationship between biological rhythms and the affective disorders. In: Arendt J, Minors DS, Waterhouse JM, eds. Biological Rhythms in Clinical Practice. London: Wright, 1989:160–183.

Checkley SA, Murphy DG, Abbas M, et al. Melatonin rhythms in seasonal affective disorder. Br J Psychiatry 1993; 163:332–337.

Clench J, Reinberg A, Dziewanowska Z, et al. Circadian changes in the bioavailability and effects of indomethacin in healthy subjects. Eur J Clin Pharmacol 1981; 20:359–369.

Cole RJ, Kripke DF, Wisbey J, et al. Seasonal variation in human illumination exposure at two different latitudes. J Biol Rhythms 1995; 10:324–334.

Comperatore CA, Krueger GP. Circadian rhythm desynchronosis, jet lag, shift lag and coping strategies. Occup Med 1990; 5:323–341.

Cooper PJ, Murray L. Course and recurrence of postnatal depression: evidence for the specificity of the diagnostic concept. Br J Psychiatry 1995; 166:191–195.

Coryell W, Endicott J, Keller M. Rapidly cycling affective disorder: demographics, diagnosis, family history and course. Arch Gen Psychiatry 1992; 49:126–131.

Coutts RT. Polymorphism in the metabolism of drugs, including antidepressant drugs: comments on phenotyping. J Psychiatr Neurosci 1994; 19:30–44.

Cowdry RW, Wehr TA, Zis AP, et al. Thyroid abnormalities associated with rapid-cycling bipolar illness. Arch Gen Psychiatry 1983; 40:414–420.

Cummings MA, Berga SL, Cummings KL, et al. Light suppression of melatonin in unipolar depressed patients. Psychiatr Res 1989; 27:351–355.

Czeisler CA, Moore-Ede MC, Coleman RH. Rotating shift work schedules that disrupt sleep are improved by applying circadian principles. Science 1982; 217:460–463.

Czeisler CA, Allan SJ, Strogatz SH, et al. Bright light resets the human circadian pacemaker independent of the timing of the sleep-wake cycle. Science 1986; 233:667–671.

Czeisler CA, Kronauer RE, Allan JS, et al. Bright light induction of strong (type O) resetting of the human circadian pacemaker. Science 1989; 244:1328–1333.

Czeisler CA, Johnson MP, Duffy JF, et al. Exposure to bright light and darkness to treat physiologic maladaptation to night work. N Engl J Med 1990; 322:1253–1259.

Czeisler CA, Shanahan TL, Klerman EB, et al. Suppression of melatonin secretion in some blind patients by exposure to bright light. N Engl J Med 1995; 332:6–11.

David MM, MacLean AW, Knowles JB, et al. Rapid eye movement latency and mood following a delay of bedtime in healthy subjects: do the effects mimic changes in depressive illness? Acta Psychiatr Scand 1991; 84:33–39.

Dawson D, Armstrong SM. Chronobiotics—drugs that shift rhythms. Pharmacol Ther 1996; 69:15–36.

Dawson D, Encel N, Lushington K. Improving adaptation to simulated night shift: timed exposure to bright light versus daytime melatonin administration. Sleep 1995; 18:11–21.

Dean C, Kendell RE. The symptomatology of puerperal illnesses. Br J Psychiatr 1981; 139:128–133.

Dean C, Williams RJ, Brockington IF. Is puerperal psychosis the same as bipolar manic-depressive disorder? A family study. Psychol Med 1989; 19:637–647.

Dinan TG. Glucocorticoids and the genesis of depressive illness: a psychobiological model. Br J Psychiatry 1994; 164:365–371.

Dodge R. Circadian rhythms and fatigue: a discrimination of their effects on performance. Aviat Space Environ Med 1982; 53:1131–1137.

Dunner DL, Fieve RR. Clinical factors in lithium carbonate prophylaxis failure. Arch Gen Psychiatry 1974; 30:229–233.

Dunner DL, Patrick V, Fieve RR. Rapid-cycling manic-depressive patients. Compr Psychiatry 1977; 18:561–566.

Eastman CI, Boulos Z, Terman M, et al. Light treatment for sleep disorders: consensus report. VI. Shift work. J Biol Rhythms 1995a; 10:157–164.

Eastman CI, Liu L, Fogg LF. Circadian rhythm adaptation to simulated night shift work: effect of nocturnal bright-light duration. Sleep 1995b; 18:399–407.

Eastwood MR, Peter AM. Epidemiology and seasonal affective disorder. Psychol Med 1988; 18:799–806.

Ebisawa T, Karne S, Lerner MR, et al. Expression cloning of a high-affinity melatonin receptor from Xenopus dermal melanophores. Proc Natl Acad Sci 1994; 91:6133–6137.

Edgar DM, Miller JD, Prosser RA, et al. Serotonin and the mammalian circadian system. II. Phase-shifting rat behavioral rhythms with serotonergic agonists. J Biol Rhythms 1993; 8:17–31.

Ehlers CL, Frank E, Kupfer DJ. Social Zeitgebers and biological rhythms: a unified approach to understanding the etiology of depression. Arch Gen Psychiatry 1988; 45:948–952.

Ehlers CL, Kupfer DJ, Frank E, et al. Biological rhythms and depression: the role of Zeitgebers and Zeitstorers. Depression 1993; 1:285–293.

Elsenga S, Van den Hoofdakker RH, Dols LCS. Early and late partial sleep deprivation in psychiatry. In: Stefanis C, Soldatos C, Rabavilas A, eds. Psychiatry: A World Perspective. Vol 2. Amsterdam: Excerpta Medica, 1990:374–379.

Endicott J. Differential diagnosis and comorbidity. In: Gold JH, Severino SK, eds. Premenstrual Dysphoria: Women's Reality. Washington, DC: APA Press, 1993:3–17.

Endicott J, Halbreich U, Schacht S, et al. Affective disorder and premenstrual depression. In: Osofsky HJ, Blumenthal SJ, eds. Premenstrual Syndrome: Current Findings and Future Directions. Washington, DC: APA Press, 1985:3–11.

Espiritu RC, Kripke DF, Ancoli-Israel S, et al. Low illumination experienced by San Diego adults: association with atypical depressive symptoms. Biol Psychiatry 1994; 35:403–407.

Faedda GL, Tondo L, Teicher MH, et al. Seasonal mood disorders: patterns of seasonal recurrence in mania and depression. Arch Gen Psychiatry 1993; 50:17–23.

Focan C. Circadian rhythms and cancer chemotherapy. Pharm Ther 1995; 67:1–52.

Giedke H, Geilenkirchen R, Hauser M. The timing of partial sleep deprivation in depression. J Affective Disord 1992; 25:117–128.

Goodwin FK, Wirz-Justice A, Wehr TA. Evidence that the pathophysiology of depression and the mechanism of action of antidepressant drugs both involve alterations in circadian rhythms. Adv Biochem Psychopharmacol 1982; 32:1–11.

Halberg F. Physiologic considerations underlying rhythmometry with special reference to emotional illness. In: de Ajuriaguerra J, ed. Symposium Bel-Air III. Cycle Biologiques et Psychiatrie, Masson et Cie, Paris, 1967:73–126.

Hall JC. Tripping along the trail to the molecular mechanisms of biological clocks. TINS 1995; 18:230–240.

Hallonquist JD, Seeman MV, Lang M, et al. Variation in symptom severity over the menstrual cycle of schizophrenics. Biol Psychiatry 1993; 33:207–209.

Hallstrom T, Samuelsson S. Mental health in the climacteric: the longitudinal study of women in Gothenburg. Acta Obstet Gynecol Scand Suppl 1985; 130:13–18.

Healy D. Rhythm and blues: neurochemical, neuropharmacological and neuropsychological implications of a hypothesis of circadian rhythm dysfunction in the affective disorders. Psychopharmacology 1987; 93:271–285.

Healy D, Waterhouse JM. Reactive rhythms and endogenous clocks. Psychol Med 1991; 21:557–564.

Healy D, Waterhouse JM. The circadian system and the therapeutics of the affective disorders. Pharm Ther 1995; 65:241–263.

Heller HC. Hibernation: neural aspects. Annu Rev Physiol 1979; 41:305–321.

Honma K, Honma S, Kohsaka M, et al. Seasonal variation in the human circadian rhythm: dissociation between sleep and temperature rhythm. Am J Physiol 1992; 262:R885–R891.

Honma K, Honma S, Nakamura K, et al. Differential effects of bright light and social cues on reentrainment of human circadian rhythms. Am J Physiol 1995; 268:R528–R535.

Hrushesky WJ. Circadian timing of cancer chemotherapy. Science 1985; 228:73–75.

Hrushesky WJ. Timing is everything. Sciences 1994; July/August:32–37.

Illnerova H, Zvolsky P, Vanecek J. The circadian rhythm in plasma melatonin concentration of the urbanized man: the effect of summer and winter time. Brain Res 1985; 328:186–189.

Janowsky DS, Gorney R, Castelnuovo-Tedesco P, et al. Premenstrual-menstrual increases in psychiatric hospital admission rates. Am J Obstet Gynecol 1969; 103:189–191.

Jansky L, Vaneck J, Hanzal V. Absence of circadian rhythmicity during hibernation. In: Malan A, Canguilhem B, eds. Living in the Cold. II. John Libbey Eurotext, London. 1989:33–39.

Joffe RT, Kutcher S, MacDonald C. Thyroid function and bipolar affective disorder. Psychiatry Res 1988; 25:117–121.

Johnson SR, McChesney C, Bean JA. Epidemiology of premenstrual symptoms in a nonclinical sample. I. Prevalence, natural history and help-seeking behavior. J Reprod Med 1988; 33:340–346.

Joseph-Vanderpool JR, Rosenthal NE, Chrousos GP, et al. Abnormal pituitary-adrenal responses to corticotropin-releasing hormone in patients with seasonal affective disorder: clinical and pathophysiological implications. J Clin Endocrinol Metab 1991; 72:1382–1387.

Joy JE, Turek FW. Combined effects of the circadian clock of agents with different phase response curves: phase-shifting effects of triazolam and light. J Biol Rhythms 1992; 7:51–63.

Kadrmas A, Winokur G, Crowe R. Postpartum mania. Br J Psychiatry 1979; 135:551–554.

Kato R. Sex related differences in drug metabolism. Drug Metab Rev 1974; 3:1–32.

Kato R, Yamazoe Y. Sex-specific cytrochrome P450 as a cause of sex-related and species-related differences in drug toxicity. Toxicol Lett 1992; 64/65:661–667.

Kendell RE, Chalmers JC, Platz C. Epidemiology of puerperal psychosis. Br J Psychiatry 1987; 150:662–673.

Kennaway DJ, Rowe SA. Melatonin binding sites and their role in seasonal reproduction. J Reprod Fert 1995; 49(suppl.):423–435.

Kennaway DJ, Royles P. Circadian rhythms of 6-sulphatoxy melatonin, cortisol and electrolyte excretion at the summer and winter solstices in normal men and women. Acta Endocrinol 1986; 113:450–456.

Kilduff TS, Krilowicz B, Milsom WK, et al. Sleep and mammalian hibernation: homologous adaptations and homologous processes? Sleep 1993; 16:372–386.

Klemfuss H. Rhythms and the pharmacology of lithium. Pharm Ther 1992; 56:53–78.

Kramlinger KG, Post RM. Ultra-rapid and ultradian cycling in bipolar affective illness. Br J Psychiatry 1996; 168:314–323.

Kripke DF. Phase-advance theories for affective illnesses. In: Wehr TA, Goodwin FK, eds. Circadian Rhythms in Psychiatry. Pacific Grove, CA: Boxwood Press, 1983:41–69.

Kripke DF, Mullaney DJ, Gabriel S. The chronopharmacology of antidepressant drugs. In: Reinberg A, Smolensky M, Labrecque G, eds. Annual Review of Chronopharmacology. Vol 2. Oxford: Pergamon Press, 1986:275–289.

Kukopulos A, Reginaldi D, Laddomada P, et al. Course of the manic-depressive cycle and changes caused by treatment. Pharmakopsychiatrie Neuro-Psychopharmakologie 1980; 13:156–167.

Labrecque G, Vanier M-C. Biological rhythms in pain and in the effects of opioid analgesics. Pharm Ther 1995; 68:129–147.

Labrecque G, Bureau J-P, Reinberg AE. Biological rhythms in the inflammatory response and in the effects of non-steroidal anti-inflammatory drugs. Pharm Ther 1995; 66:285–300.

Lakowski B, Hekimi S. Determination of life-span in *Caenorhabditis elegans* by four clock genes. Science 1996; 272:1010–1013.

Lam RW, Gorman CP, Michalon M, et al. Multicenter, placebo-controlled study of fluoxetine in seasonal affective disorder. Am J Psychiatry 1995; 152:1765–1770.

Lam RW, Zis AP, Grewal A, et al. Effects of rapid tryptophan depletion in patients with seasonal affective disorder in remission after light therapy. Arch Gen Psychiatry 1996; 53:41–44.

Leibenluft E. Do gonadal steroids regulate circadian rhythms in humans? J Affective Disord 1993; 29:175–181.

Leibenluft E. Women with bipolar illness: clinical and research issues. Am J Psychiatry 1996; 153:163–173.

Leibenluft E, Moul DE, Schwartz PJ, et al. A clinical trial of sleep deprivation in combination with antidepressant medication. Psychiatry Res 1993; 46:213–227.

Leibenluft E, Fiero PL, Rubinow DR. Effects of the menstrual cycle on dependent variables in mood disorder research. Arch Gen Psychiatry 1994; 51:761–781.

Lester D. Suicide and the menstrual cycle. Medical Hypotheses 1990; 31;197–199.

Levitt AJ, Joffe RT, Moul DE, et al. Side effects of light therapy in seasonal affective disorder. Am J Psychiatry 1993; 150:650–652.

Lewy AJ. Effects of light on human melatonin production and the human circadian system. Prog Neuropsychopharmacol Biol Psychiatry 1983; 7:551–556.

Lewy AJ, Sack RL. Intensity, wavelength and timing: three critical parameters for chronobiologically active light. In: Kupfer DJ, Monk TH, Barchas JD, eds. Biological Rhythms and Mental Disorders. New York: Guilford Press, 1988:197–217.

Lewy AJ, Nurnberger JI, Wehr TA, et al. Supersensitivity to light: possible trait marker for manic-depressive illness. Am J Psychiatry 1985; 142:725–727.

Lewy AJ, Ahmed S, Sack RL. Phase shifting the human circadian clock using melatonin. Behav Brain Res 1996; 73:131–134.

Lewy AJ, Wehr TA, Goodwin FK, et al. Manic depressive patients may be supersensitive to light. Lancet 1981; i:383–384.

Liu C, Gillette MU. Cholinergic regulation of the suprachiasmatic nucleus circadian rhythm via a muscarinic mechanism at night. J Neurosci 1996; 16:744–751.

Lyman CP. Pharmacological aspects of mammalian hibernation. Pharmacol Ther 1984; 25:371–393.

MacKinnon IL, MacKinnon PCB, Thomson AD. Lethal hazards of the luteal phase of the menstrual cycle. Br Med J 1959; 1:1015–1017.

Madden PAF, Heath AC, Rosenthal NE, et al. Seasonal changes in mood and behaviour. Arch Gen Psychiatry 1996; 53:47–55.

Mayeda A, Nurnberger J Jr. Melatonin and circadian rhythms in bipolar mood disorders. In: Shafii M, Shaffii SL, eds. Biological Rhythms, Mood Disorders, Light Therapy, and the Pineal Gland. Washington, DC: APA, 1990:119–137.

Mazurek MF, Rosebush PI. Circadian pattern of acute, neuroleptic-induced dystonic reactions. Am J Psychiatry 1996; 153:708–710.

McKinlay JB, McKinlay SM, Brambilla D. The relative contributions of endocrine changes and social circumstances of depression in mid-aged women. J Health Soc Behav 1987; 28:345–363.

McMillan MJ, Pihl RO. Premenstrual depression: a distinct entity. J Abnorm Psychol 1987; 96:149–154.

Merikangas KR, Foeldenyi M, Angst J. The Zurich Study. XIX. Patterns of menstrual disturbances in the community: results of the Zurich Cohort Study. Eur Arch Psychiatry Clin Neurosci 1993; 243:23–32.

Minors DS. Chronobiology: its importance in clinical medicine. Clin Science 1985; 69:369–376.

Mizukawa R, Ishiguro S, Takada H, et al. Long-term observation of a manic-depressive patient with rapid cycles. Biol Psychiatry 1991; 29:671–678.

Moline ML, Pollak CP, Monk TH, et al. Age-related differences in recovery from simulated jet lag. Sleep 1992; 15:28–40.

Moltke von LL, Greenblatt DJ, Harmatz JS, et al. Cytochromes in psychopharmacology. J Clin Psychopharmacol 1994; 14:1–4.

Moore RY. Vision without sight. N Engl J Med 1995; 332:54–55.

Mrosovsky N. Seasonal affective disorder, hibernation, and annual cycles in animals: chipmunks in the sky. J Biol Rhythms 1988; 3:189–207.

Mrosovsky N, Reebs SG, Honrado GI, et al. Behavioral entrainment of circadian rhythms. Experientia 1989; 45:696–702.

Mrosovsky N, Salmon PA, Menaker M, et al. Nonphotic phase shifting in hamster clock mutants. J Biol Rhythms 1992; 7:41–49.

Myers MP, Wager-Smith K, Rothenfluh-Hilfiker A, et al. Light-induced degradation of *timeless* and entrainment of the drosophila circadian clock. Science 1996; 271:1736–1740.

Myers BL, Badia P. Changes in circadian rhythms and sleep quality with aging: mechanisms and interventions. Neurosci Biobehav Rev 1995; 19:553–571.

Nagayama H. Chronopharmacology of psychotropic drugs: circadian rhythms in drug effects and its implications to rhythms in the brain. Pharm Ther 1993; 59:31–54.

Offord DR, Boyle MH, Szatmari P, et al. Ontario child health study. II. Six month prevalence of disorder and rates of service utilization. Arch Gen Psychiatry 1987; 44:832–836.

Paffenbarger RS. Epidemiological aspects of mental illness associated with child-bearing. In: Brockington IF, Kumar R, eds. Motherhood and Mental Illness. New York: Grune and Stratton, 1982:19–36.

Pearlstein TB, Frank E, Rivera-Tovar A, et al. Prevalence of axis I and axis II disorders in women with late luteal phase dysphoric disorder. J Affective Disord 1990; 20:129–134.

Pévet P, Masson-Pévet M, Hermès MLHJ, et al. Photoperiod, pineal gland, vaso-pressinergic innervation and timing of hibernation. In: Malan A, Canguilhem B, eds. Living in the Cold. II. John Libbey Eurotext, London, 1989:43–51.

Piercy J, Lack L. Daily exercise can shift the endogenous circadian phase. Sleep Res 1988; 17:393.

Pittendrigh CS. The photoperiodic phenomena: seasonal modulation of the "day within." J Biol Rhythms 1988; 3:173–188.

Platz C, Kendell RE. A matched control follow-up and family study of "puerperal psychoses." Br J Psychiatry 1988; 153:90–94.

Pohl H, Giedke H. Natural hibernation—an animal model for seasonal affective disorder? J Therm Biol 1987; 12:125–130.

Post RM, Weiss SR, Smith M, et al. Stress, conditioning, and the temporal aspects of affective disorders. Ann NY Acad Sci 1995; 771:677–696.

Preskorn SH, Alderman J, Chung M, et al. Pharmacokinetics of desipramine coadministered with sertraline or fluoxetine. J Clin Psychopharmacol 1994; 14:90–98.

Price WA, DiMarzio L. Premenstrual tension syndrome in rapid-cycling bipolar affective disorder. J Clin Psychiatry 1986; 47:415–417.

Prosser RA, Dean RR, Edgar DM, et al. Serotonin and the mammalian circadian system. I. *In vitro* phase shifts by serotonergic agonists and antagonists. J Biol Rhythms 1993; 8:1–16.

Radloff LS. The use of the center for epidemiological studies depression scale in adolescents and young adults. Special issue: the emergence of depressive symptoms during adolescence. J Youth Adol 1991; 20:149–166.

Ramcharan S, Love EJ, Fick GH, Goldfien A. The epidemiology of premenstrual symptoms in a population-based sample of 2650 urban women. J Clin Epidemiol 1992; 45:377–392.

Reiter RJ. Melatonin: the chemical expression of darkness. Mol Cellular Endocrinol 1991; 79:C153–C158.

Reme C, Terman M, Wirz-Justice A. Are deficient retinal photoreception renewal mechanisms involved in the pathogenesis of winter depression? Arch Gen Psychiatry 1990; 47:878–879.

Reyner LA, Horne JA. Gender- and age-related differences in sleep determined by home-recorded sleep logs and altimetry from 400 adults. Sleep 1995; 18:127–134.

Riemann D, Hohagen F, König A, et al. Advanced vs. normal sleep timing: effects on depressed mood after response to sleep deprivation in patients with a major depressive disorder. J Affective Disord 1996; 37:121–128.

Rivera-Tovar AD, Frank E. Late luteal phase dysphoric disorder in young women. Am J Psychiatry 1990; 147:1634–1636.

Rosenthal NE, Sack DA, Gillin JC, et al. Seasonal affective disorder: a description of the syndrome and preliminary findings with light therapy. Arch Gen Psychiatry 1984; 41:72–80.

Rusak B, Bina KG. Neurotransmitters in the mammalian circadian system. Annu Rev Neurosci 1990; 13:387–401.

Rusak B, Robertson HA, Wisden W, et al. Light pulses that shift rhythms induce gene expression in the suprachiasmatic nucleus. Science 1990; 248:1237–1240.

Sack DA, Nurnberger J, Rosenthal NE, et al. Potentiation of antidepressant medications by phase advance of the sleep-wake cycle. Am J Psychiatry 1985; 142:606–608.

Sack DA, Rosenthal NE, Parry BL, et al. Biological rhythms in psychiatry. In: Meltzer HY, ed. Psychopharmacology: The Third Generation of Progress. New York: Raven Press, 1987:669–685.

Sack DA, Duncan W, Rosenthal NE, et al. The timing and duration of sleep in partial sleep deprivation therapy of depression. Acta Psychiatr Scand 1988; 77:219–224.

Sack RL, Blood ML, Ormerod GM, et al. Oral melatonin reverses the alerting effects of nocturnal bright light exposure in humans. Sleep Res 1992; 21:49.

Schmidt PJ, Rubinow DR. Menopause-related affective disorders: a justification for further study. Am J Psychiatry 1991; 148:844–852.

Schwartz WJ. A clinician's primer on the circadian clock: its localization, function, and resetting. Adv Int Med 1993; 38:81–106.

Schwitzer J, Neudorfer C, Blecha HG, et al. Mania as a side effect of phototherapy. Biol Psychiatry 1990; 28:532–534.

Seeman MV, Lang M, The role of estrogens in schizophrenia gender differences. Schizophrenia Bull 1990; 16:185–194.

Shanahan TL, Czeisler CA. Light exposure induces equivalent phase shifts of the endogenous circadian rhythms of circulating plasma melatonin and core body temperature in men. J Clin Endocrinol Metab 1991; 73:227–235.

Sherwin BB. Affective changes with estrogen and androgen replacement therapy in surgically menopausal women. J Affective Disord 1988; 14:177–187.

Sherwin BB. The impact of different doses of estrogen and progestin on mood and sexual behavior in postmenopausal women. J Clin Endocrinol Metab 1991; 72:336–343.

Sherwin BB, Gelfand MM. Sex steroids and affect in the surgical menopause: a double-blind, cross-over study. Psychoneuroendocrinology 1985; 10:325–335.

Silverstone T, Romans S, Hunt N, et al. Is there a seasonal pattern of relapse in bipolar affective disorders? Br J Psychiatry 1995; 167:58–60.

Smolensky MH, McGovern JP, Scott PH, et al. Chronobiology and asthma. II. Body-time-dependent differences in the kinetics and effects of bronchodilator medications. J Asthma 1987; 24:91–134.

Sothern RB, Slover GP, Morris RW. Case report: circannual and menstrual rhythm characteristics in manic episodes and body temperature. Biol Psychiatry 1993; 33:194–203.

Souêtre E, Salvati E, Belugou J-L, et al. Circadian rhythms in depression and recovery: evidence for blunted amplitude as the main chronobiological abnormality. Psychiatry Res 1989; 28:263–278.

Speroff L, Glass RH, Kase NG. Clinical Gynecologic Endocrinology and Infertility. 5th ed. Baltimore: Williams and Wilkins, 1994:141–181.

Steiner M. Premenstrual dysphoric disorder: an update. Gen Hosp Psychiatry, 1996; 18:244–250.

Steiner M, Dunn EJ. The psychobiology of female-specific mood disorders. Infertil Reprod Med Clin NA 1996; 7:297–313.

Steiner M, Werstiuk ES, Seggie J. Dysregulation of neuroendocrine crossroads: depression, circadian rhythms, and the retina—a hypothesis. Prog Neuro-Psychopharmacol Biol Psychiatry 1987; 11:267–278.

Steiner M, Brown GM, Goldman S. Nocturnal melatonin and cortisol secretion in newly admitted psychiatric inpatients. Eur Arch Psychiatry Neurol Sciences 1990; 240:21–27.

Stout AL, Steege JF. Psychological assessment in women seeking treatment for premenstrual syndrome. J Psychosom Research 1985; 29:621–629.

Takahashi JS. Molecular neurobiology and genetics of circadian rhythms in mammals. Annu Rev Neurosci 1995; 18:531–553.

Tam EM, Lam RW, Levitt AJ. Treatment of seasonal affective disorder: a review. Can J Psychiatry 1995; 40:457–466.

Tanner JM. Growth at Adolescence. 2nd ed. Oxford: Blackwell Scientific Publications, 1962.

Targum SD, Caputo KP, Ball SK. Menstrual cycle phase and psychiatric admissions. J Affective Disord 1991; 22:49–53.

Terman M. On the question of mechanism in phototherapy for seasonal affective disorder: considerations of clinical efficacy and epidemiology. J Biol Rhythms 1988; 3:155–172.

Terman M, Terman JS, Quitkin FM, et al. Light therapy for seasonal affective disorder: a review of efficacy. Neuropsychopharmacology 1989; 2:1–22.

Terman M, Lewy AJ, Dijk D-J, et al. Light treatment for sleep disorders: consensus report. IV. Sleep phase and duration disturbances. J Biol Rhythms 1995; 10:135–147.

Thompson C, Stinson D, Smith A. Seasonal affective disorder and season-dependent abnormalities of melatonin suppression by light. Lancet 1990; i:703–706.

Tosini G, Menaker M. Circadian rhythms in cultured mammalian retina. Science 1996; 272:419–421.

Touitou Y, Haus E. Aging of the human endocrine and neuroendocrine time structure. Annals NY Acad Sci 1994; 378–397.

Turek FW, Penev P, Zhang Y, et al. Effects of age on the circadian system. Neurosci Biobehav Rev 1995; 19:53–58.

Van den Hoofdakker RH. Chronobiological theories of nonseasonal affective disorders and their implications for treatment. J Biol Rhythms 1994; 9:157–183.

Vanezis P. Deaths in women of reproductive age and relationship with menstrual cycle phase: an autopsy study of cases reported to the coroner. Forens Sci Int 1990; 47:39–57.

Vollmann J, Berger M. Sleep deprivation with consecutive sleep-phase advance therapy in patients with major depression: a pilot study. Biol Psychiatry 1993; 33:54–57.

Walker JM, Berger RJ. Sleep as an adaptation for energy conservation functionally related to hibernation and shallow torpor. Prog Brain Res 1980; 53:255–278.

Wehr TA. Effects of wakefulness and sleep on depression and mania. In: Montplaisir J, Godbout R, eds, Sleep and Biological Rhythms: Basic Mechanisms and Applications to Psychiatry. New York: Oxford University Press, 1990:42–86.

Wehr TA. Sleep-loss as a possible mediator of diverse causes of mania. Br J Psychiatry 1991; 159:576–578.

Wehr TA. Seasonal vulnerability to depression: implications for etiology and treatment. Encephale 1992; 18:479–483.

Wehr TA, Rosenthal NE. Seasonality and affective illness. Am J Psychiatry 1989; 146:829–839.

Wehr TA, Jacobsen FM, Sack DA, et al. Phototherapy of seasonal affective disorder. Arch Gen Psychiatry 1986; 43:870–875.

Wehr TA, Sack DA, Rosenthal NE, et al. Rapid cycling affective disorder: contributing factors and treatment responses in 51 patients. Am J Psychiatry 1988; 145:179–184.

Wehr TA, Giesen HA, Schulz, PM, et al. Contrasts between symptoms of summer depression and winter depression. J Affective Disord 1991; 23:173–183.

Weibel L, Follenius M, Spiegel K, et al. Comparative effect of night and daytime sleep on the 24-hour cortisol secretory profile. Sleep 1995; 18:549–556.

Weissman MM. The myth of involutional melancholia. JAMA 1979; 242:742–744.

Weissman MM, Olfson M. Depression in women: implications for health care research. Science 1995; 269:799–801.

Weissman MM, Bland R, Joyce PR, et al. Sex differences in rates of depression: cross-national perspectives. J Affective Disord 1993; 29:77–84.

Wever RA. Use of light to treat jet lag: differential effects of normal and bright artificial light on human circadian rhythms. Ann NY Acad Sci 1985; 453:282–304.

Wever RA. Characteristics of circadian rhythms in human functions. J Neural Transm 1986; 21(suppl):323–373.

Wirz-Justice A. Biological rhythms in mood disorders. In: Bloom FE, Kupfer DJ, eds. Psychopharmacology: The Fourth Generation of Progress. New York: Raven Press, 1995:999–1017.

Wirz-Justice A, Campbell IC. Antidepressant drugs can slow or dissociate circadian rhythms. Experientia 1982; 38:1301–1309.

Wirz-Justice A, Bucheli C, Graw P, et al. How much light is antidepressant? [letter]. Psychiatry Res 1986; 17:75–77.

Wirz-Justice A, Graw P, Kräuchi K, et al. Light therapy in seasonal affective disorder is independent of time of day or circadian phase. Arch Gen Psychiatry 1993; 50:929–937.

Wirz-Justice A, Graw P, Kräuchi K, et al. "Natural" light treatment of seasonal affective disorder. J Affective Disord 1996; 37:109–120.

Wisner KL, Peindl KS, Hanusa BH. Psychiatric episodes in women with young children. J Affective Disord 1995; 34:1–11.

Wolk SI, Weissman MM. Women and depression: an update. In: Oldham JM, Riba MB. APA Review of Psychiatry. Vol 14. Washington, DC: APA, 1995:227–259.

Wu JC, Bunney WE. The biological basis of an antidepressant response to sleep deprivation and relapse: review and hypothesis. Am J Psychiatry 1990; 147:14–21.

Yonkers KA, White K. Premenstrual exacerbation of depression: one process or two? J Clin Psychiatry 1992; 53:289–292.

Youngs DD. Some misconceptions concerning the menopause. Obstet Gynecol 1990; 75:881–883.

Zacharias L, Wurtman RJ. Blindness: its relation to age of menarche. Science 1964; 144:1154–1155.

Zhang Y, Kornhauser JM, Zee PC, et al. Effects of aging on light-induced phase-shifting of circadian behavioral rhythms, fos expression and CREB phosphorylation in the hamster suprachiasmatic nucleus. Neurosci 1996; 70:951–961.

6
Neuropeptides in Bipolar Disorder

Emile D. Risby, Kelly Hartline, Michael J. Owens, and Charles B. Nemeroff
Emory University School of Medicine, Atlanta, Georgia

I. INTRODUCTION

It has been estimated that there are 50–75 biologically active neuropeptides in the central nervous system (CNS). Many of these neuropeptides have a close neuroanatomical and functional relationship with monoamine neurotransmitters; they exert direct CNS effects (Stout et al., 1995). Primary or secondary dysfunction in one or more of these CNS neuropeptide systems has now been reported in a number of psychiatric syndromes. In this chapter, we review the data and theoretical implications concerning neuropeptide abnormalities in patients with bipolar disorder. Neuropeptides that have been measured in biological tissues and fluids in patients with mood disorders include corticotropin-releasing factor, vasopressin, opioid peptides, neurotensin, somatostatin, growth hormone, cholecystokinin, neuropeptide Y, and thyrotropin-releasing hormone.

II. CORTICOTROPIN-RELEASING FACTOR

Neurons containing corticotropin-releasing factor (CRF) are heterogeneously distributed throughout the brain and are neuroanatomically positioned to mediate limbic and cortical responses to stress (Swanson et al., 1983; Merchenthaler et al., 1984; Stout et al., 1995). An overview of the preclinical research data reveals that CRF coordinates the behavioral, endocrine, autonomic, and immune responses to stress (Owens et al., 1991; Souza, 1995).

161

What is the theoretical basis for positing CRF abnormalities in bipolar disorder? Abnormalities in noradrenergic (Siever, 1987), serotonergic (Asberg, 1976; Roy, 1989; Gibbons, 1986; Meltzer, 1987; Mann, 1986; Arora, 1989; Yates, 1990), and/or cholinergic (Carroll, 1980; Risch, 1981; Gillin, 1980; McCarley, 1982) neurotransmission have been reported in patients with mood disorders. Most studies demonstrate stimulatory effects of cholinergic and serotonergic neurons on CRF release (Plotsky et al., 1989; Owens and Nemeroff, 1991). Central administration of CRF to rats increases the firing rate of noradrenergic neurons and elicits fearful or anxiety-like behaviors (reviewed by Stout et al., 1995). CRF appears to produce a variety of behavioral effects in laboratory animals reminiscent of the signs and symptoms of major depression. For example, central administration of CRF to rats diminishes sexual behavior (Sirinathsinghji, 1987), decreases food consumption (Britton, 1982, 1986; Gosnell, 1983), and decreases social interactions without decreasing locomotion (Dunn, 1987). Central administration of CRF to infant rhesus monkeys mimics the behavioral despair syndrome observed after maternal separation (Kalin, 1989, 1990). There is considerable evidence that the mood disorders are stress-sensitive, and stress is a potent stimulus for CRF release. Furthermore, CRF is the major physiological regulator of the synthesis and release of adrenocorticotropic hormone (ACTH), which has repeatedly been demonstrated to be abnormally regulated in unipolar depression (reviewed by Stout et al., 1995) as well as bipolar depression. Therefore, both preclinical and clinical data suggest that alterations in CRF neurons may be present in patients with bipolar disorder.

The vast majority of studies on CRF in mood disorders have focused on patients with unipolar depression. Dysregulation of the hypothalamic-pituitary-adrenal (HPA) axis in major depression remains one of the most consistent findings in biological psychiatry (Rothschild, 1993). In patients with major depression, a correlation appears to exist between nonsuppression of cortisol on the dexamethasone suppression test (DST) (a measure of HPA axis hyperactivity) and a blunted ACTH response to CRF (Krishnan et al., 1993). Moreover, there is a 23% decrease in the density of CRF receptors in the frontal cortex of suicide victims relative to control brains. The above data are consistent with down-regulation of CRF receptors in frontal cortex in depression in response to increased CRF synaptic availability (Nemeroff et al., 1988). Most (but not all) studies have found elevated CRF concentrations in cerebrospinal fluid (CSF) of depressed patients (Nemeroff et al., 1984b; Arato et al., 1989; Banki et al., 1987; Davis, 1988; Roy, 1992). The elevated CSF CRF concentrations appear to be state-dependent, because with clinical improvement they decrease toward normal (reviewed in Plotsky et al., 1995).

Collectively, the data suggest that there is hypersecretion of one or more CRF-containing circuits in major depression.

The data on CRF abnormalities in bipolar disorders are not as strong as those for unipolar depression. Several (but not all) studies have reported that HPA axis activity, as measured by the dexamethasone suppression test, (DST) is increased in mixed or dysphoric mania (reviewed by Swann et al., 1992; Carroll, 1979; Evans and Nemeroff, 1983; Stokes, 1984). In euphoric mania, however, the DST is usually normal. There are no reports of increased CSF CRF in acutely manic patients. Banki et al. (1992) reported elevated CSF CRF concentrations in unipolar depressed patients, but normal CSF CRF levels in manics. Berrettini et al. (1987b) measured CSF CRF levels in normal controls and euthymic bipolar patients on and off lithium, and found no difference in CRF concentrations among the three groups. Furthermore, Gold et al. (1984) reported that, in contrast to depressed patients who exhibited a blunted ACTH response to CRF, manic patients exhibited an ACTH and cortisol response indistinguishable from that of normal controls.

Collectively, these observations suggest that state-dependent HPA dysfunction does exist in patents with bipolar disorder. HPA hyperactivity has been observed in both the depressed and the dysphoric manic phases of bipolar disorder, yet documentation of CRF abnormalities in bipolar disorder is lacking. If there is an abnormality of CRF in bipolar disorders, it is most likely to be increased CRF secretory activity in bipolar depression and mixed mania. It is possible that the HPA abnormalities may have different etiologies in the two phases of the illness (e.g.,) hypersecretion of CRF in depression and decreased feedback inhibition of ACTH in dysphoric mania). Whatever the etiology, the increased HPA activity appears to resolve with remission of the mixed-mania or depressive episode (Greden, 1983; Sachar, 1973).

III. VASOPRESSIN

Arginine vasopressin (AVP) is a nonapeptide neurohypophysial hormone, synthesized mainly in the supraoptic and paraventricular hypothalamic nuclei, that regulates fluid and electrolyte balance, particularly in response to dehydration (reviewed by Stout, 1995). However, the existence of extrahypothalamic AVP projections, and the effects of AVP on the firing rate of hippocampal neurons, suggest that this peptide also functions as a primary neurotransmitter (Muhlethaler et al., 1982). Moreover, AVP can influence memory, pain sensitivity, circadian rhythms, and REM sleep (Reus, 1978). It has been demonstrated that AVP synthesis and release and its coexpression in CRF-containing neurons are dramatically increased following stress (reviewed by Stout et al., 1995). Furthermore, AVP contributes to HPA axis regulation by potentiating the effects of CRF on ACTH release (Whitnall, 1993; Antoni, 1993) and independently possessing ACTH-releasing activity (Gibbs, 1986). In view of the role of stress in the pathophysiology of depression, and the reported abnormalities in the HPA axis in patients with mood disorders, it seems plausible that there may be alterations in AVP neural circuits as well. However, low, not elevated, levels of CSF AVP have been reported in depressed patients (Gold et al., 1984; Gjerris et al., 1985), just the opposite of what would be expected if AVP contributed to HPA axis hyperactivity in depression. However, CSF AVP concentrations may not reflect the activity of hypothalamic AVP-containing neurons. Berrettini et al. (1987b) found no differences in CSF AVP levels between euthymic bipolar patients and controls. However, as in the case of the HPA dysregulation, abnormalities in AVP neurons may be state-dependent. Indeed, Radsheer et al. (1995) have reported that in postmortem brain tissue from depressed patients, including bipolar depressed patients, the number of hypothalamic neurons expressing AVP is markedly increased when compared to controls.

IV. OPIOID PEPTIDES

The opioid peptides comprise three sets of homologous peptide classes (Olson et al., 1992). β-endorphin is a 31-amino-acid peptide derived from the ACTH precursor proopiomelanocortin (POMC); the enkephalins and dynorphins are shorter peptides, each having its own large precursor prohormones coded for by specific genes. These endogenous opioids may play a major role in the brain's response to stress; various stressors induce changes in opioid concentrations in the hypothalamus and other brain regions.

Given that CRF is a major physiological regulator of the synthesis and release of β-endorphin (Owens, 1991), that CRF–opioid interactions appear to be common to many stress responses (Kawata et al., 1982), and that CSF CRF levels are elevated in depression, it seems reasonable to suspect that there are detectable abnormalities of central opioids in patients with mood disorders. Indeed, like the ACTH response, the β-endorphin response to exogenously administered CRF is blunted in depressed patients (Young et al., 1995). Acute administration of morphine has been used as an animal model of mania (Gessa, 1995). Administration of β-endorphin to depressed patients has been reported to produce transient improvements in some subjects (Kline et al., 1977; Kline and Lehman, 1979), although these findings have not been confirmed by others. In a small study by Angst et al. (1979), four of six depressed patients who were administered β-endorphin developed mania or hypomania. The above data would suggest that mania is associated with elevated endogenous opiate activity. However, carbamazepine, used in the treatment of mania, potentiates opiate-induced locomotor activity in mice (Katz, 1979). Furthermore, carbamazepine does not appear to alter CSF opioid activity (Post, 1981). Despite the suggestion that increased endogenous opioid activity may be associated with mania and low opioid activity associated with depression, the current literature does not provide strong evidence supporting a major role of endogenous opioids in the pathophysiology of bipolar disorder.

V. NEUROTENSIN

Neuroendocrine and biochemical data suggest that neurotensin (NT) may play a role in the CNS's response to various stressful stimuli. For example, NT activates the HPA axis (reviewed by Stout, 1995). The intimate functional and anatomical association between NT and dopamine-containing neurons in the brain (including the mesocortical dopamine system) suggests that NT may be involved in the pathophysiology of certain psychiatric disorders, particularly schizophrenia. To date, only one study has assessed NT in patients with bipolar disorders. In that study, CSF levels of NT in euthymic bipolar patients (both unmedicated and lithium-treated) were not different from those in normal controls (Berrettini et al., 1987b).

VI. SOMATOSTATIN

Somatostatin (SRIF), a tridecapeptide, is widely distributed throughout the CNS. SRIF-containing nerve terminals and/or cell bodies have been found in such diverse brain regions as the limbic system, cortex, hypothalamus, striatum, locus ceruleus, and septal nuclei (Rubinow, 1995, 1992). SRIF is the major physiological inhibitor of growth-hormone secretion; it also inhibits the secretion of TSH and of CRF-stimulated ACTH (Plotsky, 1995). Central administration of SRIF has been observed to alter cholinergic, dopaminergic, noradrenergic, and serotonergic neurotransmission. Electrophysiological studies have demonstrated both inhibitory and excitatory effects of SRIF. There is evidence linking SRIF to kindled seizures within the limbic system, a mechanism posited to underlie the pathogenesis of bipolar disorder (Rubinow et al., 1987). Behavioral effects of centrally administered SRIF include changes in sleep patterns, food consumption, locomotor activity, and memory processes (reviewed by Stout, 1995; Rubinow, 1995, 1992). Furthermore, there are data to suggest that increased SRIF activity may enhance learning and SRIF depletion may diminish cognitive performance (Vecsei and Widerlov, 1990; Walsh et al., 1985). It is notable that abnormalities in each of the above behaviors also occur in patients with depression.

Multiple investigators have reported decreases in CSF SRIF levels in both unipolar and bipolar depressed subjects (Kling, 1993; Bissette et al., 1986; Sunderland, 1987; Davis, 1988; Molchan, 1991; Gerner and Yamada, 1982; Rubinow, 1995, 1992, 1983). Repeated measures of CSF SRIF concentrations in patients in different affective states have demonstrated that the lowest SRIF values were obtained during depression and are lower than those obtained during mania or euthymia (Rubinow, 1995, 1986). However, low CSF SRIF levels do not appear to be a useful diagnostic measure because CSF SRIF concentrations do not appear to correlate with the severity of the depression, and similar decreases in CSF SRIF have been reported in a number of neurological disorders, including Alzheimer's disease and Huntington's disease, in the absence of psychiatric comorbidity (Rubinow, 1983).

Both increased and normal CSF SRIF concentrations have been reported in manic patients. Sharma et al. (1995) reported that patients with mania had higher CSF SRIF concentrations than did patients with schizophrenia or schizoaffective disorder. Consistent with this finding is the observation that selective serotonin uptake inhibitors—which, like all antidepressants, may induce mania—increase CSF SRIF levels, while the anticonvulsant (and antimanic) carbamazepine decreases CSF SRIF levels (Plotsky, 1995; Rubinow et al., 1985). Recently, Zachrisson et al. (1995) reported that chronic lithium treatment in rats produces an increase in SRIF mRNA expression in layers IV–VI of the entorhinal cortex and in the lateral caudate-putamen. Berrettini et al. (1987b) found no differences in CSF SRIF concentrations between controls, unmedicated euthymic bipolar patients, and lithium-treated euthymic bipolar patients. Thus, elevated CSF SRIF levels may be a state-dependent feature of mania or a nonspecific response to stress that returns to normal when the mood disorder resolves.

Although a recent study by Banki et al. (1992) did not find any differences in SRIF levels among patients with depression and mania and normal controls, an overview of the extant literature reveals that most studies report decreases in CSF SRIF levels in depression and elevated CSF SRIF levels in mania. The abnormal CSF concentrations of SRIF return to normal with resolution of the affective episode (reviewed by Sharma et al., 1995; Rubinow, 1983).

VII. GROWTH HORMONE

Stimulation of central α_2-adrenergic receptors is a potent stimulator of growth-hormone (GH) release (Martin et al., 1978). In vitro studies indicate that acetylcholine inhibits the release of SRIF, the major physiological inhibitor of GH release from the hypothalamus (Richardson, 1990); thus, the release of GH is also partly under cholinergic control (Ross et al., 1987). Because noradrenergic and cholinergic neurotransmission have been postulated to be dysregulated in mood disorders, abnormalities in GH secretion might also be expected in these patients.

There are no reports of abnormalities in basal levels of GH in depression or mania (Dinan et al., 1994). GH release following the administration of the acetylcholinesterase inhibitor pyridostigmine is enhanced in patients with major depression (O'Keane et al., 1992) and mania (Dinan et al., 1994). Thus, cholinergically mediated GH release appears to be enhanced in both depression and mania. In contrast, at least five independent studies have demonstrated a blunted GH response to the α_2-agonist clonidine in endogenously depressed patients compared to controls (reviewed by Willner, 1985). GH release in response to the noradrenergic tricyclic antidepressant desipramine is reported to be blunted in unipolar and bipolar depressed patients (Laakmann, 1980; Sawa et al., 1980) as well as in mania (Dinan et al., 1994; Ansseau et al., 1988; Dinan et al., 1991). Therefore, noradrenergic-mediated release of GH via clonidine and desipramine appears to be blunted in both depression and mania.

The GH response to insulin using a standard insulin tolerance test (ITT) has also been reported to be abnormal in patients with mood disorders. The insulin-induced release of GH appears to be mediated via noradrenergic mechanisms (Siever et al., 1982; Laakmann et al., 1986). Most studies using the ITT in unipolar depression have reported either a diminished GH response or no difference compared to controls (reviewed by Amsterdam et al., 1991). Studies comparing unipolar and bipolar depressives have reported no differences in the peak GH response to insulin between the two groups (Koslow et al., 1982; Amsterdam et al., 1983). However, a study by Amsterdam et al. (1991), comparing unipolar depressives, bipolar depressives, and hypomanic patients, revealed that the centered cumulative GH response (similar to the area under the curve) to the ITT was diminished in the hypomanic patients compared to the bipolar and unipolar depressed patients and healthy controls. The bipolar depressed patients had the highest centered cumulative GH response of the four groups while the hypomanics had the smallest increase. These data, while not consistent with other studies, suggest that the ITT-mediated GH response in bipolar patients is dependent on the phase of the bipolar illness.

In summary, the majority of the research indicates that the cholinergic-mediated release of GH is enhanced and the noradrenergic-mediated release of GH is blunted in acutely ill bipolar patients.

VIII. CHOLECYSTOKININ

Cholecystokinin (CCK) is a 33-amino-acid peptide hormone that is synthesized by the small intestine and exerts complex effects on gastrointestinal physiology. Peptides of the gastrin–cholecystokinin family are also known to be present in the central nervous system. High concentrations of CCK are found in the cortex, amygdala, hippocampus, and septum. Cholecystokinin is extensively colocalized with opioid peptides as well as dopamine. Preclinical data support an anxiogenic role for CCK acting at central CCK receptors (Harro et al., 1993). In rats, the central administration of CCK produces fear and behavior arousal, and decreases exploratory behavior. Similarly, CCK produces fearful behavior in primates and appears to be anxiogenic in humans as well (Bradwejn et al., 1990, 1991). However, the close anatomical relationship of CCK with several dopamine pathways and the limbic system also suggest a putative role for these peptides in the pathophysiology of mood disorders (Verbanck, 1984).

To date, there has been only one study that measured CSF CCK levels in patients with mood disorders. Verbanck et al. (1984) studied 51 controls and 18 unipolar and 12 bipolar depressed patients and found a decrease in CSF CCK immunoreactivity in the bipolar depressed patients compared to the controls. There were no differences between controls and unipolar depressed patients. Although the authors do not report on the statistical comparison of unipolar versus bipolar patients, the CCK mean for the unipolar depressives was 3.4 ± 0.5 pmol/L, while the CCK mean for the bipolar patients was lower, at 2.8 ± 0.6 pmol/L. The clinical significance of low CSF CCK concentrations is unclear at this time.

IX. NEUROPEPTIDE Y

Neurons displaying neuropeptide Y (NPY)-like immunoreactivity are abundant in the CNS, most notably in limbic areas and the cerebral cortex (De

Quidt, 1986; Hendry, 1993; Aoki, 1990). NPY exerts a strong influence on hypothalamic functions that are reported to be dysregulated in depression, such as circadian rhythms, HPA axis, and food intake. For example, central administration of NPY stimulates appetite as well as the production and release of CRF (Haas, 1987; Tsagarakis, 1989; Liposits, 1988). Consistent with the preclinical data, decreases in central NPY levels have been reported in the CSF of depressed patients (Widerlov et al., 1988) and in postmortem brain tissue of suicide victims (Widdowson et al., 1992). However, decreased CSF NPY levels have not been consistently reported in depressed patients (Wilderlov, 1988; Widdowson, 1992; Berrettini, 1987b). Zachrisson et al. (1995) reported that chronic lithium treatment in rats produces an increase in NPY mRNA expression in the hippocampus, layers II–III of the entorhinal cortex, nucleus accumbens shell, and the medial caudate-putamen. Currently, the role, if any, of NPY in bipolar disorder is unclear.

X. THYROTROPIN-RELEASING HORMONE

Specific, high-affinity thyrotropin-releasing hormone (TRH) receptors have been characterized and found to be widely distributed in the CNS (Nemeroff, 1990; Manaker et al., 1986; Sharif, 1989). There is a large body of data to support a role of the tripeptide TRH as a neurotransmitter or neuromodulator (Nemeroff, 1990). TRH modulates several other neurotransmitter systems, including those that utilize dopamine, serotonin, and acetylcholine (Griffiths, 1985; Nemeroff, 1984a). Studies have demonstrated the colocalization of TRH in neurons containing other neurotransmitters such as serotonin, substance P, the enkephalins, dopamine, NPY, histamine, and GH (Mason et al., 1995). TRH has been shown to arouse hibernating animals and to antagonize the sedation, motor impairment, and hypothermia produced by ethanol and other CNS depressants (Nemeroff, 1984a). TRH is believed to stimulate locomotor activity by activation of the mesolimbic dopamine system (Collu et al., 1992).

Approximately 25–30% of depressed patients have a blunted TSH response to TRH (Loosen, 1987; Nemeroff, 1990; Howland, 1993). It is unclear if this 25–30% represents a distinct subgroup of depressed patients. Although it has not been consistently validated, psychopathological features reported to be associated with the blunted TSH response include suicidality, agitation, and panic (Corrigan et al., 1992). One hypothesis to explain the blunted TSH response to TRH found in depressed patients is hypersecretion of hypothalamic TRH, which leads to desensitization of pituitary TRH receptors (Mason, 1995). In support of the hypersecretion hypothesis, CSF TRH has been reported to be increased in patients with major depression (Banki et al., 1988). The elevations in CSF TRH may be specific to depression—it has not been reported in Alzheimer's disease, anxiety disorders, or alcoholism (Fossey et al., 1993; Roy et al., 1990).

While a blunted TSH response to TRH occurs in some depressed patients, an exaggerated response occurs in others. These patients may have subclinical hypothyroidism. Current data suggest that depressed patients with subclinical hypothyroidism have more cognitive impairment, resistance to antidepressants, and, if bipolar, a greater tendency for rapid cycling (Haggerty, 1990).

The conflicting data on the TSH response to TRH make a unifying theory of the role of TRH in mood disorders difficult to posit. There are no comprehensive studies of TRH in mania. Further studies on the role of TRH in mood disorders are certainly warranted.

XI. DISCUSSION

There are several reports of abnormal concentrations of central neuro-transmitters in mood disorders. However, the role of neuropeptides in the pathophysiology of mood disorders remains unclear, particularly in bipolar disorder. Detera-Wadleigh (1987) used restriction-fragment-length polymor-phisms (RFLPs) to perform a linkage analysis in an attempt to associate, at a molecular level, reported abnormalities in the concentrations of numerous neuropeptides in patients with mood disorders, including bipolar disorder. They did not find an association between the polymorphic alleles of SRIF or NPY with mood disorders. Their finding suggests that previously observed alterations in the levels of these neuropeptides may have resulted from secondary events, and are not a reflection of an obvious genetic mutation. Nonetheless, these biologically active neuropeptides obviously have effects on brain functioning, and further exploration of their roles in neuropsychi-atric disorders is clearly warranted.

ACKNOWLEDGMENTS

This work was supported by grants NIMH MH-42088, MH-39415, MH-51761, MH-00870, and NIDA DA-09492.

REFERENCES

Amsterdam JD, Maislin G. Hormonal responses during insulin-induced hypoglycemia in manic-depressed, unipolar depressed, and healthy control subjects. J Clin Endocrinol Metab 1991; 73(3):541–547.

Amsterdam JD, Winokur A, Lucki I, Caroff SN, Snyder P, Rickels K. A neuroendocrine test battery in bipolar patients and healthy subjects. Arch Gen Psychiatry 1983; 40:515–521.

Angst J, Autenrieth V, Brem F, Kovkkov M, Meyer H, Stassen HH, Storck U. In: Usdin E, Bunney WE Jr, Kline NS, Endorphins eds. in Mental Health Research. New York: Macmillan, 1979:518–528.

Annseau M, vonFrenckell R, Cergontaine JL, Papart P, Franck G, Timsit-Berthier M, Geenen V, Legros JJ. Neuroendocrine evaluation of catecholaminergic neurotransmission in mania. Psychiatry Res 1998; 22:193–206.

Antoni FA. Vasopressinergic control of pituitary adrenocorticotropin secretion comes of age. Frontiers Neuroendocrinol 1993; 14:76–122.

Aoki C, Pickel VM. Neuropeptide Y in cortex and striatum: ultrastructural distribution and coexistence with classical neurotransmitters and neuropeptides. Ann NY Acad Sci 1990; 611:186–205.

Arato M, Banki CM, Bissette G, Nemeroff CB. Elevated CSF CRF in suicide victims. Biol Psychiatry 1989; 25:355–359.

Arora RC, Meltzer HY. Serotonergic measures in the brains of suicide victims: 5-HT_2 binding sites in the frontal cortex of suicide victims and control subjects. Am J Psychiatry 1989; 146:730–736.

Asberg M, Thoren L, Traskman P. Serotonin depression: a biochemical subgroup within the affective disorders. Science 1976; 191:478–480.

Axelrod J, Reisine TD. Stress hormones: their interaction and regulation. Science 1984; 224:452–459.

Banki CM, Bissette G, Arato M, O'Connor L, Nemeroff CB. CSF corticotropin-releasing factor-like immunoreactivity in depression and schizophrenia. Am J Psychiatry 1987; 144:873–877.

Banki CM, Bissette G, Arato M, Nemeroff CB. Elevation of immunoreactive CSF TRH in depressed patients. Am J Psychiatry 1988; 145:1526–1531.

Banki CM, Karmacsi L, Bissette G, Nemeroff CB. Cerebrospinal fluid neuropeptides in mood disorder and dementia. J Affective Disord 1992; 25:39–46.

Bartalena L, Placidi GF, Martino E, et al. Nocturnal serum thyrotropin (TSH) surge and the TSH response to TSH-releasing hormone: dissociated behavior in untreated depressives. J Clin Endocrinol Metab 1990; 71:650–655.

Berrettini WH, Doran AR, Kelsoe J, Roy A, Pickar D. Cerebrospinal fluid neuropeptide Y in depression and schizophrenia. Neuropsychopharmacology 1987a; 1:81–83.

Berrettini WH, Nurnberger JI Jr, Zerbe RL, Gold PW, Chrousos GP, Tomai T. CSF neuropeptides in euthymic bipolar patients and controls. Br J Psychiatry 1987b; 150:208–212.

Bissette G, Widerlov E, Walleus H, Karlsson I, Eklund K, Forsman A, Nemeroff CB. Alterations in cerebrospinal fluid concentrations of somatostatin-like immunoreactivity in neuropsychiatric disorders. Arch Gen Psychiatry 1986; 43:1148–1154.

Bradwejn J, Koszycki D, Meterissian G. Cholecystokinin tetrapeptide-induced panic attacks in patients with panic disorder. Can J Psychiatry 1990; 35:83–85.

Bradwjn J, Koszycki D, Bourin M. Dose ranging study of the effect of CCK in healthy volunteers. J Psychiatry Neurosci 1991; 16:260–264.

Britton DR, Koob GF, Rivier J, Vale W. Intraventricular corticotropin-releasing factor enhances behavioral effects of novelty. Life Sci 1982; 31:363–367.

Britton KT, Lee G, Dana R, Risch SC, Koob GF. Activating and "anxiogenic" effects of corticotropin-releasing factor are not inhibited by blockade of the pituitary-adrenal system with dexamethasone. Life Sci 1986; 39:1281–1286.

Carroll BJ. Neuroendocrine function in mania. In: Shopsin B, Manic Illness. New York: Raven Press, 1979:163–176.

Carroll BJ, Greden JF, Haskett R. Neurotransmitter studies of neuroendocrine pathology in depression. Acta Psychiatrica Scand 1980; 61(suppl 280):183–199.

Collu M, D'Aquila PS, Gessa GL, Serra G. TRH activates mesolimbic dopamine system: behavioral evidence. Behav Pharmacol 1992; 3:639–641.

Corrigan MHC, Gillette GM, Quade D, Garbutt JC. Panic, suicide, and agitation: independent correlates of the TSH response to TRH in depression. Biol Psychiatry 1992; 31:984–982.

Davis KL, Davidson M, Yang R-K, et al. CSF somatostatin in Alzheimer's disease, depressed patients, and control subjects. Biol Psychiatry 1988; 24:710–712.

De Quidt ME, Emson PC. Distribution of neuropeptide Y-like immunoreactivity in the rat central nervous system. II. Immunohistochemical analysis. Neuroscience 1986; 18:545–618.

Delfs JR, Dichter MA. Effects of somatostatin on mammalian cortical neurons in culture. J Neurosci 1983; 1176–1188.

Detera-Wadleigh Sevilla D. Neuropeptide gene polymorphisms in affective disorders and schizophrenia. J Psychiat Res 1987; 21(4):581–587.

Dinan TG, Yatham L, Barry S, Keane OV. Blunting of noradrenergic stimulated growth hormone release in mania. Am J Psychiatry 1991; 148:936–938.

Dinan TG, Keane VO, Thakore J. Pyridostigmine induced growth hormone release in mania: focus on the cholinergic/somatostatin system. Clin Endocrinol 1994; 40:93–96.

Dunn AJ, File SE. Corticotropin-releasing factor has an anxiogenic action in the social interaction test. Horm Behav 1987; 21:193–202.

Evans DL, Nemeroff CB. The dexamethasone suppression test in mixed bipolar disorder. Am J Psychiatry 1983; 140:615–617.

Fadda P, Tortorella A, Fratta W. Sleep deprivation decreases μ and δ opioid receptor binding in the rat limbic system. Neurosci Lett 1991; 129:315–317.

Fadda P, Martellotta MC, DeMontis MG, Gessa GI, Fratta W. Dopamine D_1 and opioid receptor binding changes in the limbic system of sleep deprived rats. Neurochem Int 1992; 20(suppl):153S–156S.

Fossey MD, Lydiard RB, Ballenger JC, Laraia MT, Bissette G, Nemeroff CB. Cerebrospinal fluid thyrotropin-releasing hormone concentrations in patients with anxiety disorders. J Neuropsychiat Clin Neurosci 1993; 5:335–337.

Garcia-Sevilla JA, Magnusson T, Carlsson A. Effect of intracerebroventricularly administered somatostatin on brain monoamine turnover. Brain Res 1978; 155:159–164.

Gerner RH, Yamada T. Altered neuropeptide concentrations in cerebrospinal fluid of psychiatric patients. Brain Res 1982; 238:298–302.

Gessa GL, Pani L, Serra G, Fratta W. Animal models of mania. Adv Biochem Psychopharmacol 1995; 49:43–66.

Gibbons RD, Davis JM. Consistent evidence for a biological subtype of depression characterized by low CSF monoamine levels. Acta Psychiatr Scand 1986; 74:8–12.

Gibbs DM. Vasopressin and oxytocin: hypothalamic modulators of the stress response: a review. Psychoneuroendocrinology 1986; 11:131–140.

Gillin JC, Sitaram N, Duncan WC, Gershon Es, Nurnberger J, Post RM, Murphy DL, Wehr T, Goodwin FK, Birney WL. Sleep disturbance in depression: diagnostic potential and pathophysiology. Psychopharmacol Bull 1980; 16:40–42.

Gjerris A, Rafaelson OJ, Vendsborg P, Fahrenkrug J, Rehfeld JF. Vasoactive intestinal polypeptide decreased in cerebrospinal fluid (CSF) in atypical depression: vasoactive intestinal polypeptide, cholecystokinin and gastrin in CSF in psychiatric disorders. J Affective Disord 1984; 7:325–337.

Gjerris A, Hammer M, Vendsborg P, Christensen NJ, Rafaelsen OJ. Cerebrospinal fluid vasopressin—changes in depression. Br J Psychiatry 1985; 147: 696–701.

Gold PW, Goodwin FK. Vasopressin in affective illness. Lancet 1978; i:1233–1235.

Gold PW, Chrolsos G, Kellner C, Post R, Roy A, Avcernos P, Schulte H, Oldfield E, Loriaux DL. Psychiatric implications of basic and clinical studies with corticotropin releasing factor. Am J Psychiatry 1984; 141:619–627.

Gosnell BA, Morley JE, Levine AS. A comparison of the effects of corticotropin-releasing factor and sauvagine on food intake. Pharmacol Biochem Behav 1983; 19:771–775.

Greden JF, Gardner R, King D, Grunhaus L, Carroll BJ, Kraunfol Z. Dexamethasone suppression tests in antidepressant treatment of melancholia. Arch Gen Psychiatry 1983; 40:493–500.

Griffiths EC. Thyrotropin releasing hormone: endocrine and central effect Psychoneuroendocrinology 1985; 225–235.

Haas DA, George SR. Neuropeptide Y administration acutely increases hypothalamic corticotropin-releasing factor immunoreactivity: lack of effect in other rat brain regions. Life Sci 1987; 41:2728–2731.

Haggerty JJ Jr, Garbutt JC, Evans DL, Simon JS, Nemeroff CB. Subclinical hypothyroidism: a review of neuropsychiatric aspects. Int J Psychiatry Med 1990; 20:193–208.

Harro J, Vasar E, Bradwejn J. CCK in animal and human research on anxiety. Trends Pharmacol Sci 1993; 14:244–249.

Heilig M, Koob GF, Ekman R, Britton KT. Corticotropin-releasing factor and neuropeptide Y: role in emotional integration. Trends Neurosci 1994; 17:80–85.

Hendry JHC. Organization of neuropeptide Y neurons in the mammalian central nervous system. In: Colmers WF, Wahlestedt C, eds. The Biology of Neuropeptide Y and Related Peptides. Totowa, NJ: Humana Press, 1993; 65–156.

Howland RH. Thyroid dysfunction in refractory depression: implications for pathophysiology and treatment. J Clin Psychiatry 1993; 54:47–54.

Kaji H, Chihara K, Minamitani N, Kodarna H, Yarahara N, Fauita T. Release of VIP into CSF of the fourth ventricle of the rat: involvement of a cholinergic mechanism. Brain Res 1983; 269:303–310.

Kalin NH. Behavioral and endocrine studies of corticotropin-releasing hormone in primates. In: Corticotropin-Releasing Factor: Basic and Clinical Studies of a Neuropeptide. DeSouza EB, Nemeroff CB, eds. Boca Raton: CRC Press, 1990:275–289.

Kalin NH, Shelton SE, Barksdale CM. Behavioral and physiologic effects of CRH administered to infant primates undergoing maternal separation. Neuropsychopharmacology 1989; 2:97–104.

Katz RJ, Schmaltz K. Facilitation of opiate- and enkephalin-induced motor activity in the mouse by phenytoin sodium and carbamazepine. Psychopharmacology 1979; 65:65.

Kawata M, Hashimoto K, Takahara J, Sano Y. Immunohistochemical demonstration of the localization of corticotropin releasing factor–containing neurons in the hypothalamus of mammals including primates. Anat Embryol 1982; 165:303–313.

Kline NS, Lehmann HE. In: Usdin E, Bunney WE Jr, Kline NS, eds. Endorphins in Mental Health Research. New York: Macmillan, 1979:500–517.

Kline NS, Li CH, Lehmann HE, Lajtha A, Laski E, Cooper T. Beta-endorphin-induced changes in schizophrenic and depressed patients. Arch Gen Psychiatry 1977; 34:1111–1113.

Kling MA, Rubinow DR, Doran AR, et al. Cerebrospinal fluid immunoreactive somatostatin concentrations in patients with Cushing's disease and major depression: relationship to indices of corticotropin-releasing hormone and cortisol secretion. Neuroendocrinology 1993; 57:79–88.

Koslow SH, Stokes PE, Mendels J, Ramsey A, Casper R. Insulin tolerance test: human growth hormone response and insulin resistance in primary unipolar depressed, bipolar depressed and control subjects. Psychol Med 1982; 12:45–55.

Krishnan KRR, Rayasam K, Reed DR, et al. The corticotropin releasing factor stimulation test in patients with major depression: relationship to dexamethasone suppression test results. Depression 1993; 1:133–136.

Laakmann, G. Effects of antidepressants on the secretion of pituitary hormones in healthy subjects, neurotic depressive patients and endogenous depressive patients. Nervenarzi 1980; 51:725–732.

Laakmann G, Zygan K, Schoen HW, Weiss A, Wittmann M, Meissner R, Blaschke D. Effect of receptor blockers (methysergide, propranolol, phentolamine, yohimbine and prazosin) on desipramine-induced pituitary hormone stimulation in humans. I. Growth hormone. Psychoneuroendocrinology 1986; 11:447–461.

Liposits Z, Sievers L, Paul WK. Neuropeptide-Y and ACTH-immunoreactive innervation of corticotropin releasing factor (CRF)-synthesizing neurons in the hypothalamus of the rat: an immunocytochemical analysis at the light and electron microscopic levels. Histochemistry 1988; 88:227–234.

Loh HH, Smith AP. Molecular characterization of opioid receptors. Ann Rev Pharmacol Toxicol 1990; 30:123–147.

Loosen PT. Pituitary-thyroid axis in affective disorders. In: Meltzer HY, ed. Psychopharmacology: The Third Generation of Progress. New York: Raven Press, 1987:629–636.

Lundberg JM, Anggard A, FahrenKrug J, Hokfelt T, Mutt V. VIP in cholinergic neurons of exocine glands: functional significance of coexisting neurotransmitters for vasodilation and secretion. Proc Natl Acad Sci 1980; 77:1651–1655.

Maeda K, Yoshimoto Y, Yamadori A. Blunted TSH and unaltered PRL responses to TRH following repeated administration of TRH in neurologic patients: a replication of neuroendocrine features of major depression. Biol Psychiatry 1993; 33:277–283.

Manaker S, Eichen A, Winokur A, Rhodes CH, Rainbow TC. Autoradiographic localization of thyrotropin releasing hormone receptor in human brain. Neurology 1986; 36:641–646.

Mann JJ, Stanley M, McBride PA, McEwen BS. Increased serotonin$_2$ and beta-adrenergic receptor binding in the frontal cortices of suicide victims. Arch Gen Psychiatry 1986; 43:945–959.

Martin JB, Brazeau P, Tannenbaum GS, Willoughby JO, Epelbaum J, Terry LC, Durand D. Neuroendocrine organization of growth hormone regulation. In: Reichlin S, Baldessarini R, Martin JB, eds. The Hypothalamus. New York: Raven Press, 1978:329-355.

McCarley RW. REM sleep and depression: common neurological control mechanisms. Am J Psychiatry 1982; 139:565–570.

Meltzer HY, Lowy MT. The serotonin hypothesis of depression. In: Meltzer HY, ed. Psychopharmacology: The Third Generation of Progress. New York: Raven Press, 1987:513–526.

Merchenthaler I. Corticotropin-releasing factor (CRF)-like immunoreactivity in the rat central nervous system: extrahypothalamic distribution. Peptides 1984; 5:53–69.

Molchan SE, Lawlor BA, Hill JL, et al. CSF monoamine metabolites and somatostatin in Alzheimer's disease and major depression. Biol Psychiatry 1991; 29:1110–1118.

Muhlethaler M, Dreifuss JJ, Gahwiler BH. Vasopressin excites hippocampal neurons. Nature 1982; 296:749–751.

Nadi NS, Nurnberger JI Jr, Gershon ES. Muscarinic cholinergic receptors on skin fibroblasts in familial affective disorders. N Engl J Med 1984; 311:252–230.

Nemeroff CB. The relevance of thyrotropin-releasing hormone to psychiatric disorders. In: Nemeroff CB, ed. Neuropeptides and Psychiatric Disorders. Washington, DC: American Psychiatric Association Press, 1990:15–28.

Nemeroff CB, Kalivas PW, Golden RN. Behavioral effects of hypothalamic hypophysiotropic hormones: neurotensin, substance P and other neuropeptides. Pharmacol Ther 1984a; 24:1–56.

Nemeroff CB, Widerlov E, Bissette G, Walleus H, Karlsson I, Eklund K, Kilts CD, Loosen PT, Vale W. Elevated concentrations of CSF corticotropin-releasing factor-like immunoreactivity in depressed patients. Science 1984b; 226:1342–1344.

Nemeroff CB, Owens MJ, Bissette G, Andorn AC, Stanley M. Reduced corticotropin-releasing factor binding sites in the frontal cortex of suicide victims. Arch Gen Psychiatry 1988; 45:577–579.

O'Keane V, O'Flynn K, Lucey J, Dinan TG. Pyridostigmine induced growth hormone responses in healthy and depressed subjects: evidence for cholinergic supersensitivity in depression. Psycho Med 1992; 22:55–60.

Olson GA, Olson RD, Kastin AJ. Endogenous opioids: 1992. Peptides 1993; 14:1339–1378.

Owens MJ, Nemeroff CB. The physiology and pharmacology of corticotropin-releasing factor. Pharmaco Rev 1991; 43:425–473.

Patel YC. General aspects of the biology and function of somatostatin. In: Weil CM, Mulle EE, Thorner MO, eds. Basic and Clinical Aspects of Neuroscience. Vol 4. Berlin: Springer-Verlag, 1992:1–16.

Plotnikoff NP, Prange AJ Jr, Breese GR, Anderson MS, Wilson IC. Thyrotropin releasing hormone: enhancement of DOPA activity by a hypothalamic hormone. Science 1972; 178:417–418.

Plotsky PM, Cunningham ET Jr, Widmaier EP. Catecholaminergic modulation of corticotropin-releasing factor and adrenocorticotropin secretion. Endocr Rev 1989; 10:437–458.

Post RM, Pickar D, Naber D, Ballenger JC, Uhde, TW, Bunney WE Jr. Effect of carbamazepine on CSF opioid activity: relationship to antidepressant response. Psychiatry Res 1981; 5:59–66.

Raadsheer FC, Van Heerikhuize JJ, Lucassen PJ, Hoogendijk WJ, Tilders FJ, Swaab DF. Corticotropin-releasing hormone mRNA levels in the paraventricular nucleus of patients with Alzheimer's disease and depression. Am J Psychiatry 1995; 152:1372–1376.

Richardson SB, Hollander CS, D'Eletto R, Greenleaf PW, Thaw C. Acetylcholine inhibits the release of somatostatin from the hypothalamus in vitro. Endocrinology. 1990; 107:122–129.

Risch SC, Cohen PM, Janowsky DS, Gillin JC. Physostigmine induction of depressive symptomatology in normal human subjects. J Psychiat Res 1981; 4:89–94.

Ross RJM, Tsagarakis S, Grossman A, Besser GM. GH feedback occurs through modulation of hypothalamic somatostatin under cholinergic control: studies with pyridostigmine and GHRH. Clin Endocrinol 1987; 27:727–733.

Rothschild AJ. The dexamethasone suppression test in psychiatric disorders. Psychiatry Ann 1993; 23:662–670.

Roy A. Hypothalamic-pituitary-adrenal axis function and suicidal behavior in depression. Biol Psychiatry 1992; 32:812–816.

Roy A, DeJong J, Linnoila M. Cerebrospinal fluid monoamine metabolites and suicidal behavior in depressed patients. Arch Gen Psychiatry 1989; 46:609–612.

Roy A, Bissette G, Nemeroff CB. Cerebrospinal fluid thyrotropin-releasing hormone concentrations in alcoholics and normal controls. Biol Psychiatry 1990; 28:767–772.

Rubinow DR. Cerebrospinal fluid somatostatin and psychiatric illness. Biol Psychiatry 1986; 21:341–365.

Rubinow DR, Gold PW, Post RM, Ballenger JC, Cowdry R, Bollinger J, Reichlin S. CSF somatostatin in affective illness. Arch Gen Psychiatry 1983; 40:409–412.

Rubinow DR, Post RM, Gold PW, Ballenger JC, Reichlin S. Effects of carbamazepine on CSF somatostatin. Psychopharmacology 1985; 85:210–213.

Rubinow DR, Post RM, Davis C, Doran A. Somatostatin and depression. In: Reichlin S, ed. Somatostatin: Basic and Clinical Status. New York: Plenum, 1987.

Rubinow DR, Davis CL, Muller EE, Thorner MO, eds. Somatostatin: Basic and Clinical Aspects of Neuroscience. Vol 4. Berlin: Springer-Verlag, 1992:29–42.

Sachar EJ, Hellman L, Roffwarg HP, Halpern FS, Fukushima KK, Gallagher TF. Disrupted 24 hour patterns of cortisol secretion in psychotic depression. Arch Gen Psychiatry 1973; 28:19–24.

Sawa Y, Odo S, Nakazawa T. Growth hormone secretion by tricyclic and non-tricyclic antidepressants in healthy volunteers and depressives. In: Langer SZ, Takahashi R, Segawa T, Briley M, eds. New Vistas in Depression. New York: Pergamon Press, 1980:309–315.

Sharif NA. Quantitative autoradiography of TRH receptors in discrete brain regions of different mammalian species. Ann NY Acad Sci 1989; 553:147–175.

Siever JL. Role of noradrenergic mechanisms in the etiology of the affective disorders. In: Meltzer HY, ed. Psychopharmacology: Third Generation of Progress. New York: Raven Press, 1987:493–504.

Sharma RP, Bissette G, Janicak PG, Davis JM, Nemeroff CB. Elevation of CSF somatostatin concentrations in mania. Am J Psychiatry 1995; 152:1807–1809.

Siever LJ, Uhde TW, Silberman EK, Jimerson DC, Aloi JA, Post RM, Murphy DL. Growth hormone response to clonidine as a probe of noradrenergic receptor responsiveness in affective disorder patients and controls. Psychiatry Res 1982; 6:171–183.

Sirinathsinghji DJS. Inhibitory influence of corticotropin-releasing factor on components of sexual behavior in the male rat. Brain Res 1987; 407:185–190.

Sitaram N, Nurnberger JI Jr, Gersjpm ES, Gillin JC. Faster cholinergic REM sleep induction in euthymic patients with primary affective illness. Science 1980; 208:200–202.

Stokes PE, Stoll PM, Koslow SH, et al. Pretreatment DST and hypothalamic-pituitary-adrenocortical function in depressed patients and comparison groups. Arch Gen Psychiatry 1984; 41:257–267.

Stout SC, Kilts CD, Nemeroff CB. Neuropeptides and stress: preclinical findings and implications for pathophysiology. In: Friedman M, Deutsch AY, Charney DL, eds. Neurobiological Consequences of Stress: From Normal Adaptation to Post-traumatic Stress Disorders. New York: Raven Press, 1995:103–123.

Sunderland T, Rubinow DR, Tariot PN, et al. CSF somatostatin in patients with Alzheimer's disease, older depressed patients, and age-matched control subjects. Am J Psychiatry 1987; 144:1313–1316.

Swann AC, Stokes PE, Casper R, Secunda SK, Bowden CL, Berman N. Hypothalamic-pituitary-adrenocortical function in mixed and pure mania. Acta Psychiatr Scand 1992; 85:270–274.

Swanson LW, Sawchenko PE, Rivier J, Vale W. Organization of ovine corticotropin-releasing factor immunohistochemical study. Neuroendocrinology 1983; 36:165–186.

Tsagarakis S, Rees LH, Besser GM, Grossman A. Neuropeptide-Y stimulates CRF-41 release from rat hypothalami in vitro. Brain Res 1989; 502:167–170.

Vecsei L, Widerlov E. Effects of somatostatin-28 and some of its fragments and analogs on open-field behavior, barrel rotation, and shuttle box learning in rats. Psychoneuroendocrinology 1990; 15:139–145.

Verbanck PMP, Lotstra F, Giles P, Linkowski P, Mendlewicz J, Vanderhaeghen JJ. Reduced cholecystokinin immunoreactivity in the cerebrospinal fluid of patients with psychiatric disorders. Life Sci 1984; 34:67–72.

Walsh TJ, Emerich DF, Winokur A, Banki C, Bissette G, Nemeroff CB. Intrahippocampal injection of cysteamine depletes somatostatin and produces cognitive impairments in the rat. Neurosci Abstr 1985; 11:621.

Whitnall MH. Regulation of the hypothalamic corticotropin-releasing hormone neurosecretory system. Progress Neurobiol 1993; 40:573–629.

Widdowson PS, Ordway GA, Halaris AE. Reduced neuropeptide Y concentrations in suicide brain. J Neurochem 1992; 59:73–80.

Widerlov E, Lindstrom LH, Wahlestedt C, Ekman R. Neuropeptide Y and peptide YY as possible cerebrospinal markers for major depression and schizophrenia, respectively. J Psychiat Res 1988; 22(1):69–79.

Willner P. Depression: A Psychobiological Synthesis. New York: Wiley 1985:228–229.

Yates M, Leake A, Candy JM, Fairburn AF, McKeith IG, Ferrier IN. 5-HT$_2$ receptor changes in major depression. Biol Psychiatry 1990; 27:489–496.

Young EA, Akil H, Roger F, Haskett R, Watson SJ. Evidence against changes in corticotrophic CRF receptors in depressed patients. Biol Psychiatry 1995; 37:355–363.

Zachrisson O, Mathe AA, Stenfors C, Lindefors N. Region-specific effects of chronic lithium administration on neuropeptide Y and somatostatin mRNA expression in the rat brain. Neurosci Lett 1995; 194:89–92.

7

Neuroanatomical Models and Brain Imaging Studies

Terence A. Ketter
Stanford University School of Medicine, Stanford, California

Mark S. George
Medical University of South Carolina, Charleston, South Carolina, and National Institute of Mental Health, National Institutes of Health, Bethesda, Maryland

Tim A. Kimbrell, Mark W. Willis, Brenda E. Benson, and Robert M. Post
National Institute of Mental Health, National Institutes of Health, Bethesda, Maryland

I. INTRODUCTION

The last decade has seen dramatic advances in understanding the neural substrates of emotional experiences and mood disorders. While older animal, postmortem, and lesion studies were useful in developing neuroanatomical models of these substrates, recent brain imaging methods have allowed direct testing of hypotheses generated by these models in healthy volunteers and patients with mood disorders. Such studies have the potential to bridge the fields of human neuroanatomy, basic neurochemistry, and clinical phenomenology, and in so doing provide an integrated perspective of the regional neurobiological substrates of emotional experiences both in health and in mental illnesses.

This chapter focuses on the emerging consensus and recent findings of brain imaging studies in mood disorders, with particular emphasis on

179

bipolar illness, and their implications for the hypothesis that prefrontal and anterior paralimbic dysfunction contributes importantly to the mediation of these conditions.

II. NEUROANATOMICAL MODELS OF NEURAL SUBSTRATES OF EMOTIONS

A. The Limbic Lobe and Limbic System

For over a century, there has been interest in midline cerebral structures as possible mediators of emotional experiences. Broca (1) focused on the *great limbic lobe* as a midline cortical limbus (border) around the brainstem in mammals (Figure 1). Papez (2) proposed a corticothalamic mechanism of emotion in which hypothalamus, cingulate, and hippocampus were central.

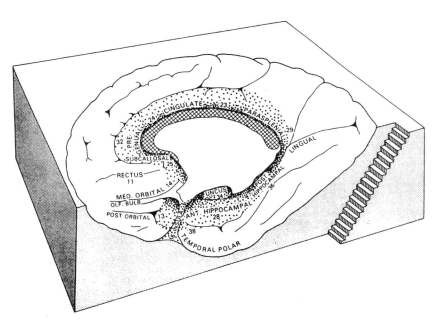

Figure 1 The limbic lobe (limbic cortex). Three-dimensional cartoon of human brain showing subdivisions of the limbic *lobe* (stipple). Numbers refer to cytoarchitectonic areas of Brodmann. The limbic *system* includes these cortical areas as well as closely related brainstem structures. Anterior paralimbic and cortical structures are emerging as being particularly important to emotional processes and disorders (see text). (From Ref. 4.)

He suggested that hypothalamus was the site of origin of emotional impulses, which were output to mamillary body and thence to anterior thalamus and on to cingulate. In addition, Papez saw the cingulate as the putative receptive region for experiencing emotion, which through cortical projections could add affective valence to other cerebral processes. In his classic paper, he discussed differential parallel corticothalamic circuits for emotional, cognitive, and motor processing, a model that, with refinements, is still hypothesized more than half a century later.

MacLean (3,4) introduced the term *limbic system* to describe cortex of the limbic lobe and closely related brainstem structures.

B. Basal Ganglia-Thalamocortical Circuits

Because anterior thalamic (anterodorsal, anteroventral, and anteromedial) nuclei have extensive connections with limbic structures, they have been referred to as the *limbic thalamus* (5–7). The fornix and mammillothalamic tract provide limbic input to these nuclei, which in turn project to cingulate cortex. Yakovlev and colleagues (8) noted thalamolimbic connections (Figure 2) in which clusters of adjacent nuclei in the anterior portion of the thalamus projected to components of the limbic system in a topographic fashion. They focused on segmenting the limbic system into medial (parahippocampal) and lateral (orbitoinsular) sectors, each receiving efferents from clusters of adjacent thalamic nuclei. However, in a similar fashion, the limbic system may be segmented into anterior and posterior components (as described below), each receiving efferents from different thalamic nuclei. Thus, for the anterior limbic system, the ventral anterior nucleus pars magnocellularis projects to insula, medial dorsal nucleus pars magnocellularis to orbitofrontal cortex, and anterior medial nucleus to anterior cingulate, while for the posterior limbic system, the lateral dorsal nucleus projects to the posterior cingulate. In addition, anterior paralimbic structures such as the amygdala and anterior cingulate project to the medial dorsal nucleus, while posterior limbic structures such as the posterior cingulate and hippocampus project to the lateral dorsal, anteroventral, and anteromedial nuclei.

Alexander and colleagues (9,10) described a series of basal ganglia-thalamocortical circuits, three of which involve anterior cerebral structures with particular relevance to psychiatric disorders. The *limbic circuit* involves anterior paralimbic structures, going from anterior cingulate and medial orbitofrontal cortices to ventral striatum (*limbic striatum*—nucleus accumbens and olfactory tubercle), to ventral pallidum, to medial dorsal nucleus of thalamus, and back to anterior cingulate and medial orbitofrontal cortices (Figure 3, left). This circuit may serve as a positive feedback loop, while a

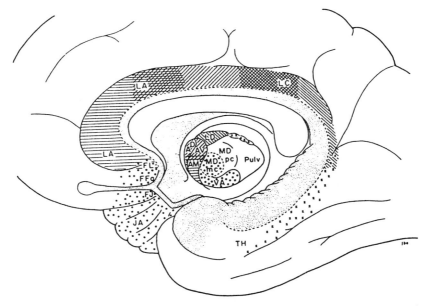

Figure 2   The limbic thalamus and its projections. Cartoon of medial structures in the human brain showing the thalamic nuclei with projections to limbic cortex. Thalamic nuclei include: AM = anteromedial; AD = anterodorsal; AV = anteroventral; LD = lateral dorsal; VA = ventral anterior; MDmc/MDpc = medial dorsal pars magnocellularis/parvicellularis. Cortical areas are indicated according to von Economo and Koskinas. (From Ref. 8.)

side loop involving the subthalamic nucleus may allow it to also serve as a negative feedback loop.

This model extends the limbic concept by including basal ganglia structures (ventral striatum and pallidum) whose limbic associations have been appreciated relatively recently (11). In keeping with its limbic nature, this circuit receives substantial inputs from the amygdala at several points. However, this circuit fails to include the important anterior thalamic nuclei mentioned above, which, by virtue of their limbic associations, have been referred to as limbic thalamus (7). Functional imaging studies already suggest that structures in this limbic circuit contribute to the mediation of physiological emotional experience. Furthermore, as described below, elements of this circuit appear to function abnormally in affective disorders.

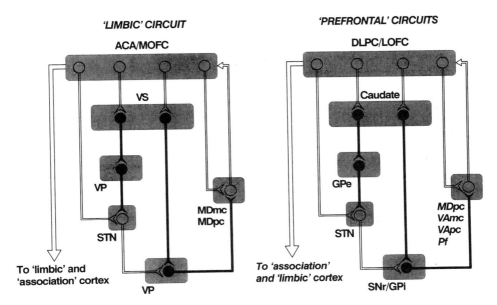

Figure 3 Anterior basal ganglia-thalamocortical circuits. (Left) Limbic circuit. (Right) Prefrontal (dorsolateral and lateral orbitofrontal) circuits. Solid lines indicate inhibitory (GABAergic) connections. Open (double) lines indicate excitatory (glutamatergic) connections. ACA = anterior cingulate area; MOFC = medial orbitofrontal cortex; DLPC = dorsolateral prefrontal cortex; LOFC = lateral orbitofrontal cortex; VS = ventral striatum; VP = ventral pallidum; STN = subthalamic nucleus; MDmc/MDpc = Medial dorsal nucleus of thalamus pars magnocellularis/parvicellularis; GPe/GPi = globus pallidus external/internal segment; SNr = substantia nigra pars reticulata; VAmc/VApc = ventral anterior nucleus of thalamus pars magnocellularis/parvicellularis; Pf = parafascicular nucleus. (From Ref. 10.)

The *lateral orbitofrontal circuit* is from lateral orbitofrontal cortex to caudate, to globus pallidus, to substantia nigra, to medial dorsal nucleus of thalamus, and back to lateral orbitofrontal cortex (Figure 3, right). Imaging studies suggest that dysfunction of structures in this circuit may be important in obsessive-compulsive disorder (12,13). Similarly, the *dorsolateral prefrontal circuit* is from dorsolateral prefrontal cortex to caudate, to globus pallidus, to substantia nigra, to medial dorsal nucleus of thalamus, and back to dorsolateral prefrontal cortex (Figure 3, right). Dysfunction of structures in this circuit may contribute to the clinical profiles of schizophrenia and mood disorders.

C. Prefrontal and Anterior Paralimbic Model

Although the connections between hippocampus and posterior cingulate noted in Papez's review have continued to receive attention, there has been increasing acknowledgment of the importance of the amygdala in affective processes (14). Recent evidence suggests that the limbic system may be segmented into anterior and posterior components based on differences in cytoarchitecture, connections, and functions (15,16). The anterior (amygdalocentric) limbic system—which includes the amygdala; septum; orbitofrontal, insular, and anterior cingulate cortices; and ventral striatum—may be considered more related to affective, motivational, and endocrine functions. In contrast, the posterior (hippocampocentric) limbic system—which includes the hippocampus; posterior parietal, posterior parahippocampal, and posterior cingulate cortices; and the dorsal striatum—may be more related to learning and memory (16–18). In accordance with this model, the anterior (executive) cingulate has been proposed to mediate higher functions such as affect, attention, semantic processing, and vocalization, while the posterior (evaluative) cingulate may mediate motor and sensory functions (15).

Thus, the last century has seen a progressively more fine-grained analysis of putative substrates of emotional experience. Currently, a circuit involving prefrontal, anterior paralimbic, and related subcortical structures appears to be a useful refinement. Below we discuss structural and functional brain imaging studies in healthy volunteers and mood (especially bipolar) disorders, with emphasis on how these studies relate to a prefrontal and anterior paralimbic model.

III. STRUCTURAL BRAIN IMAGING STUDIES

A. Computerized Tomography and Magnetic Resonance Imaging

Computerized tomography (CT) was the first modern brain-imaging method. Ionizing radiation is transmitted through tissues and detected by sensors. With the aid of computers, the resulting data is processed to generate sets of transaxial (horizontal) slices (tomograms), which reflect cerebral structures. This is a relatively inexpensive technology, but it involves the risk of ionizing radiation and yields images with limited spatial resolution.

Magnetic resonance imaging (MRI) involves placing paramagnetic (having an odd atomic number) elements such as hydrogen (^{1}H) in strong magnetic fields, exciting them (forcing into a higher energy state) with pulses of electromagnetic radiation, and then detecting energy released when these elements relax (return to a lower energy state). MRI has several advantages over CT: 1) no ionizing radiation, 2) greater spatial resolution, 3) less artifact from bone, 4) ability to acquire not only transaxial but also coronal and sagittal images, and 5) ability to be modified to yield a variety of images. The latter include T1-weighted images, which reflect neuroanatomy, and T2-weighted images, which reflect neuropathology. As described below, MRI methods can be further extended to generate functional brain images.

The ability to perform serial assessments of cerebral gross anatomy in living patients represents a dramatic methodological advance over post-mortem pathological studies. Structural brain imaging can detect brain abnormalities in some secondary mood disorders and differences between groups of patients with primary psychiatric disorders and healthy controls, but cannot diagnose primary mood disorders in individual patients.

There is now a substantial structural imaging literature in mood disorders. Recent observations, consensus findings, and results of meta-analyses in this area, with emphasis on findings in bipolar disorder, are reviewed below. Readers interested in details of individual structural imaging studies are referred to prior review articles (19–23).

B. Lateral Ventricular Enlargement and Sulcal Prominence in Primary Mood Disorders

Increased lateral ventricular enlargement is often reported in groups of mood disorder patients compared to healthy controls (Figure 4) (24,25). The ventricular brain ratio (VBR), the most commonly reported measure of lateral ventricular size, is typically assessed by determining the percentage of the whole brain area occupied by the lateral ventricles, in the slice in which the lateral ventricles have their greatest size. Increased prominence of sulci and fissures is also often reported in mood disorders (24,25). This is usually assessed by rating the prominence of the interhemispheric or Sylvian fissures or frontal or temporal lobe sulci. There are conflicting data regarding third ventricular enlargement in mood disorders (26–29), and its possible relationships with dexamethasone suppression status and post-dexamethasone cortisol (27,30,31). In patients with schizophrenia, lateral ventricular enlargement appears to be linked to third ventricular dilatation but not to sulcal atrophy (24). This suggests that in schizophrenia, lateral ventricular enlargement may represent a neuropathological process related to third ventricular dilatation yet independent of sulcal atrophy. The relationships between these abnormalities in mood disorders remain to be determined.

The major findings of increased lateral ventricular enlargement and sulcal prominence in mood disorder patients compared to controls have been

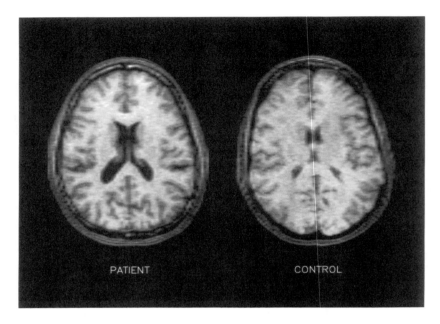

Figure 4 Lateral ventricular dilatation in a patient with bipolar disorder. (Left) T1-weighted cerebral MRI of a 27-year-old man with bipolar disorder. (Right) Similar image from a 27-year-old healthy male control. Note the enlarged lateral ventricles in the bipolar patient. Although lateral ventricular dilatation in this particular case is striking, and occurs more often in mood disorder patients than in healthy controls, this is not a uniform finding, and hence cannot be used to diagnose mood disorders in individual patients.

observed in many, but not all studies (24,25). Potentially confounding influences that could contribute to the variability of findings include age, nutritional status, comorbid alcohol abuse, somatic therapies, and heterogeneity of mood disorders. Narrative and "vote-counting" (keeping a tally of studies with significant and nonsignificant findings) reviews appear to offer overly conservative conclusions because these methods penalize studies with low statistical power (32). Recently, meta-analysis methods have provided important insights into structural imaging findings in mood disorders (24,25,33).

Raz and Raz (24) reported meta-analyses that indicated that mood disorder patients compared to controls had increased lateral ventricular enlargement (from 18 studies) and sulcal prominence (from seven studies). The composite effects for these findings were moderate to small in magnitude (+0.55 and +0.42, respectively). The corresponding effect sizes for schizophrenia (+0.70 and +0.35, respectively) did not differ significantly from those for mood disorders.

More recently, Elkis and associates (25) reported meta-analyses that similarly indicated that mood disorder patients compared to healthy controls had increased ventricular enlargement (from 29 studies) and sulcal prominence (from 10 studies) (Table 1). The composite effects for these findings were highly significant ($p < 0.001$), but again moderate to small in magnitude (+0.44 and +0.42, respectively), and were not systematically related to gender or illness polarity. In addition, they noted that schizophrenia patients had greater ventricular enlargement than mood disorder patients. The composite effect size for this finding was highly significant ($p < 0.002$) but small in magnitude (−0.2) and was not systematically related to gender or illness polarity. There were too few studies to draw conclusions regarding differences in sulcal enlargement between mood disorder and schizophrenia patients. Thus, generalized structural brain abnormalities in mood disorder patients may be less different from those in schizophrenia patients than from

Table 1   Summary of Elkis and Associates' Meta-Analyses of Studies of Ventricular Enlargement and Sulcal Prominence in Mood Disorders

Hypothesis	No. of studies	% Uni- polar	No. sig. studies	No. nonsig. studies	No. sig. not reported	Composite effect size	p for effect size
More ventricular enlargement in mood disorders than in healthy controls	29	58.4	11	15	3	+0.437	0.001
More sulcal prominence in mood disorders than in healthy controls	10	58.5	3	5	2	+0.421	0.001
Less ventricular enlargement in mood disorders than in schizophrenia	11	31.3	0	11	0	-0.201	0.002
Less sulcal prominence in mood disorders than in schizophrenia	3	—	0	3	0	a	a

aInsufficient data. (From Ref. 25)

those in controls, supporting a continuum model of mood and schizophrenic disorders (19,24,25).

Follow-up studies suggest that ventricular enlargement may increase with disease duration, perhaps in excess of the increase noted with normal aging (34,35). Increased ventricular enlargement in bipolar (particular male) compared to unipolar patients (36,37) has been reported, but other groups have failed to find this difference (27,38). Furthermore, as noted above, in Elkis and colleagues' meta-analysis, ventricular enlargement was not systematically related to polarity or gender. Investigators have also found that ventricular enlargement generally failed to have significant relationships with severity of mood symptoms as assessed by mood rating scales (39–41), and was only inconsistently related to psychotic symptoms (27,28,40,42–45) or cognitive dysfunction (28,44–49). Furthermore, ventricular enlargement also appeared to be unrelated to dexamethasone suppression status and post-dexamethasone cortisol in most studies (27,31,41,43,50,51), although one study (52) reported a trend and another (53) a significant relationship. However, ventricular enlargement has been reported to be related to pre-dexamethasone plasma cortisol (54) and urinary free cortisol (55), although the latter finding was not replicated in another study (56). Thus, although ventricular enlargement appears to occur in mood disorders, it probably has at most modest relationships with clinical parameters.

C. Subcortical Hyperintensities in Primary Mood Disorders

Subcortical hyperintensities (SCHs), which are also fancifully referred to as unidentified bright objects (UBOs), appear as bright areas in periventricular white, deep white, or subcortical gray matter on T2-weighted MRI images. Both bipolar (37,57–60) and elderly unipolar (61–68) mood disorder patients have been reported to have increased SCHs compared to controls. SCHs may (69,70) or may not (37) also be increased in psychoses. These lesions vary with age, and may be related to a number of factors including hypertension, carotid arteriosclerosis, arteriolar hyalinization, and dilated perivascular spaces, but their exact significance in mood disorder patients remains to be determined. For example, SCHs do not appear to be related to dexamethasone-suppression status or post-dexamethasone cortisol levels (31,53,71).

Dupont and associates (60) recently reported that younger bipolar patients but not similarly aged unipolar patients or controls had increased volumes of abnormal white matter. The distribution of SCHs in bipolar patients appeared relatively frontal compared to similarly aged unipolar patients and controls, but not significantly different from older controls matched for abnormal white-matter volume. Total volume of abnormal white matter appeared to be associated with increased cognitive impairment, increased rate of psychiatric illness in family, and onset after adolescence. This study did not find ventricular enlargement, but suggested that thalamic volume could be increased in bipolar patients and decreased in unipolar ones.

Altshuler and colleagues (33) recently reported increased periventricular SCHs in bipolar I but not bipolar II patients compared to healthy controls; in the same article they reviewed eight studies comparing SCHs in a total of 198 bipolar I disorder patients and 307 healthy controls. Four studies found significantly increased SCHs in bipolar patients compared to controls, three found more limited evidence of a relationship, and one suggested no relationship. A meta-analysis of these eight studies yielded a common odds ratio of 3.3 for the presence of any SCH in bipolar I patients versus healthy controls ($p < 0.00001$).

D. Other Structural Changes in Primary Mood Disorders

In contrast to the above, the literature concerning other structural changes in mood disorders is less extensive. Decreased frontal (72), caudate (73), putamen (74), and brainstem and cerebellar vermis (75) areas or volumes in mood disorder patients compared to controls have been reported in some studies, while others have failed to replicate these findings (29,59,76–78). Coffman and associates (79) found a trend toward decreased mean frontal area in midsagittal MRI slices in bipolar patients, which correlated with the degree of impairment on neuropsychological testing. Bipolar patients have been reported to have decreased temporal lobe areas (80) (relative to cerebellum) and volumes (81). However, other groups failed to find altered temporal lobe areas (82) or volumes (83) in bipolar disorder. Corpus callosum size has been reported decreased in bipolar (79,84) and unchanged (85) or increased in the anterior and posterior quadrants (86) in unipolar patients. Pituitary enlargement has been reported in mood disorder patients (87), and may be related to degree of adrenal escape from suppression by dexamethasone (88).

Healthy volunteers have cerebral asymmetry with right wider than left frontal lobes, and left wider than right occipital lobes. In schizophrenia, increased incidence of reversal of this cerebral asymmetry pattern has been reported in some but not other studies. In mood disorder patients, three studies found no evidence (89–91) and one study (26) a trend toward an increased incidence of reversed cerebral asymmetry.

E. Structural Changes in Secondary Mood Disorders

The high prevalence of mood disorder symptoms in patients with stroke, Huntington's disease, Parkinson's disease, traumatic brain injury, epilepsy, multiple sclerosis, and brain tumors has fueled interest in a provocative but at times controversial literature concerning the neuroanatomy of secondary mood disorders.

Thus, the risk of depression may be greater after anterior compared to posterior and left compared to right strokes, while the risk of mania may be greater after right compared to left strokes (92,93). Basal ganglia strokes may also be associated with secondary depression (94). The profound basal ganglia damage noted in Huntington's disease and Parkinson's disease and the high prevalence of mood symptoms in these disorders also provides support of a role for basal ganglia dysfunction in secondary depressions (95–98). After traumatic brain injury, left dorsolateral prefrontal and/or left basal ganglia lesions may increase the risk of depression (99), while right temporal basal polar lesions may increase the risk of mania (100). The risk of secondary depression in patients with epilepsy may be greater with left than with right temporal lobe lesions (101). Temporal (102) and left frontal lobe (103) lesions may also increase the risk of depression secondary to multiple sclerosis, although a recent study failed to replicate these findings (104). Finally, frontal lobe brain tumors may be associated with secondary depression (105,106).

F. Summary of Structural Imaging Findings

Taken together, the structural imaging literature reviewed above suggests that primary mood disorders may be associated with increased ventricular enlargement, sulcal widening, and subcortical hyperintensities. However, in general, these findings appear to lack consistent relationships with clinical parameters. Further study is required to assess whether structural abnormalities in primary mood disorders are confined to these rather regionally nonspecific findings or extend to more specific prefrontal, limbic, and basal ganglia-thalamocortical circuit abnormalities suggested by neuroanatomical models. The structural imaging literature provides some support of such specific prefrontal, temporal, and basal ganglia abnormalities (perhaps left more than right) in a variety of secondary mood syndromes, in a fashion consistent not only with the neuroanatomical models discussed above but also with the functional imaging observations in primary and secondary mood disorders discussed below.

IV. FUNCTIONAL BRAIN IMAGING STUDIES

A. Positron Emission Tomography and Single Photon Emission Computed Tomography

Positron emission tomography (PET) uses radiotracers that emit antimatter (positrons), which annihilate electrons to emit photon pairs moving in opposite directions. PET radiolabels such as oxygen-15, carbon-11, and fluorine-18 have short half-lives and thus generally require expensive on-site production facilities (i.e., a cyclotron). Commonly used PET radiotracers include fluorine-18-deoxyglucose ([18]FDG) for determination of the cerebral metabolic rate for glucose (CMRglu) and oxygen-15 water ($H_2{}^{15}O$) for determination of cerebral blood flow (CBF). Other tracers allow more specific cerebral biochemical measures such as neurotransmitters and receptors but are even more technically challenging and expensive to produce.

Single photon emission computed tomography (SPECT) uses radiotracers that directly emit photons. This method lacks the spatial resolution of PET and does not generally yield quantitative (absolute) data, but is substantially less expensive. SPECT radiotracers include technetium-99m-hexamethylpropyleneamineoxime (^{99m}Tc-HMPAO), technetium-99m-exametazime (^{99m}Tc-EMZ), and iodine-123-N-isopropyl-4-iodo-amphetamine (^{123}I-IMP) for determination of relative CBF, and a variety of iodine-123-labeled compounds for determination of receptors.

B. PET Studies in Healthy Volunteers

Functional imaging studies in healthy subjects yield important contributions to our understanding of the neural substrates of emotion. Assessments of regional cerebral function in healthy volunteers provide bases for comparison with mood disorder patients. For example, anterior cerebral structures are commonly very active (hyperfrontality) in health, and much less active (hypofrontality) in affective illness (Figures 5 and 6). Since cerebral function may vary with age and gender, it is important to match patients with healthy controls on these parameters.

Also, the induction of affective arousal in healthy volunteers may indicate neuroanatomical structures contributing to affective shifts. For example, induction of transient emotions (sadness, happiness, anger, and anxiety) by recall of affectively congruous events has been associated with changes in anterior paralimbic function (107,108). Animal studies have demonstrated that the local anesthetic procaine is a selective limbic activator, and in humans acute intravenous procaine yields diverse affective and

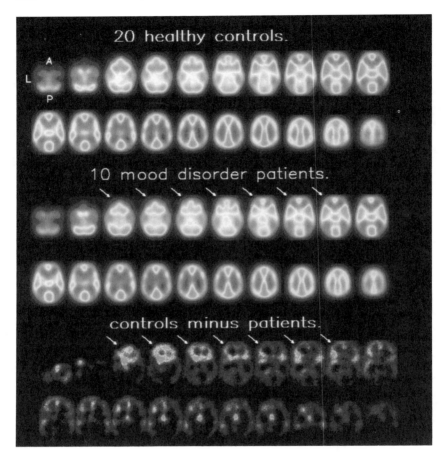

Figure 5 Hypofrontality in primary mood disorders: mean images. (Top) Mean of smoothed stereotactically normalized $H_2{}^{15}O$ PET scans of 20 healthy controls at rest with eyes closed. Note normal hyperfrontality in these scans (prominent red in anterior regions of first row). (Center) Similar images for 10 age- and gender-matched medication-free mood disorder patients. Note relative hypofrontality (yellow rather than red in anterior regions, indicated by arrows) in these scans. (Bottom) Enhanced subtraction (controls minus patients) images showing regions with lower mean activity in patients. Arrows indicate regions with hypofrontality in patients. Absolute cerebral blood flow rates are indicated by colors (lowest = blue < green < yellow < red = highest). L = left; A = anterior; P = posterior.

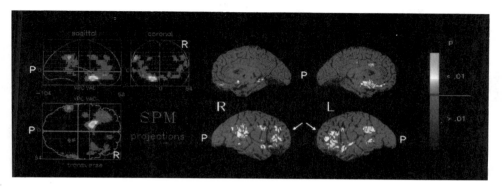

Figure 6 Hypofrontality in primary mood disorders: statistical parametric map. The same data as in Figure 5 (bottom) but subjected to a test of statistical inference. Images show voxels with significantly (voxel by voxel unpaired t-tests, $p < 0.01$, not corrected for multiple comparisons) lower CBF at rest in 10 mood disorder compared to 20 healthy controls. (Left) See-through projections—colors indicate voxels with significantly lower CBF in patients. Note the similarity of the transverse projection to the mean subtraction images in Figure 5 (bottom). (Right) Cortical renderings—yellow and red indicate voxels with significantly lower CBF in patients. Arrows indicate regions with hypofrontality in patients. L = Left; R = Right; P = Posterior. The images in Figures 5 and 6 reflect the most commonly observed findings in PET studies of primary depression (see text) and are remarkably similar to the findings of Bench and colleagues (175), who used nearly identical scan acquisition and image-processing methodology. Data analyzed using SPM software produced by MRC Cyclotron Unit, Hammersmith Hospital, London.

psychosensory symptoms in concert with increased temporal lobe fast EEG activity and increases in ACTH, cortisol, and prolactin but not growth hormone. We recently found that procaine's clinical effects are also accompanies by robust changes in global and anterior paralimbic CBF (109). Moreover, different CBF responses to procaine were related to various clinical responses. Figure 7 shows the concordant anterior paralimbic activation patterns observed with induction of acute affective changes by neuropsychological [self-induced sadness (107)] and pharmacological [procaine (109)] methods. This concordance extended even to regional correlational relationships, as left amygdala activation correlated with the degree of negative affect (self-induced sadness and procaine-induced dysphoria) and deactivation with the intensity of positive affect (self-induced happiness and procaine-induced euphoria). Other neuropsychological studies have explored discrete components of affective processing. For example, matching of facial

SADNESS INDUCTION   PROCAINE ACTIVATION

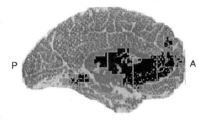
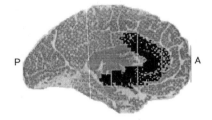

11 Healthy Women   32 Healthy Volunteers

Figure 7 Anterior paralimbic activation accompanies both neuropsychologically and pharmacologically induced acute affective changes in healthy volunteers. Statistical parametric maps (SPMs) of CBF activation rendered on the mesial aspect of the left hemisphere. (Left) Regions activated during transient self-induced sadness in 11 healthy women. (Right) Regions activated during acute intravenous procaine-induced affective symptoms in 32 healthy volunteers. Note the concordance of anterior paralimbic activation patterns with these two methods of inducing affective changes.

emotional expression has been associated with anterior paralimbic (right anterior cingulate and inferior frontal) activation, which does not occur with facial-identity matching or spatial-object-relationship matching (110).

In the following sections, we review functional imaging studies in primary and secondary affective disorders, which in many cases demonstrate functional disruptions in anterior paralimbic structures and anterior basal gangliathalamocortical circuits. Since this chapter emphasizes recent functional imaging studies, readers interested in earlier studies may wish to refer to prior review articles (23,111,112).

C. Decreased Anterior Cerebral Blood Flow and Metabolism In Primary Depression

Over the last decade, a substantial and largely consistent literature has described CBF and metabolic abnormalities in primary depression patients compared to controls. The majority of studies have noted decreased anterior paralimbic and cortical activity in depression (Figures 5,6, and 8). In the literature between 1984 and 1995, we found a total of 38 papers and abstracts

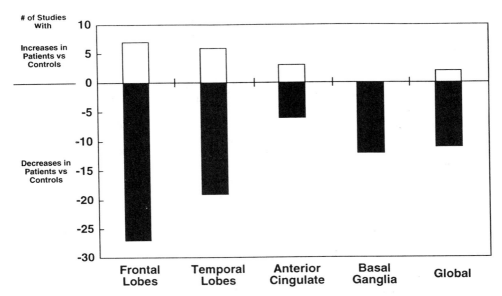

Figure 8 Summary findings of 36 controlled studies of CBF and metabolism in primary depression. Bars indicate the number of studies reporting increased (light bars above the horizontal axis) and decreased (dark bars below the horizontal axis) CBF or metabolism in patients with primary depression compared to controls. Prefrontal and anterior paralimbic abnormalities were consistently noted in mood disorders with some variability in the direction of the abnormality.

comparing CBF and metabolism in a total of 576 mood disorder patients with 590 healthy controls (references available upon request). Half (19) of these reports studied cerebral glucose metabolism as assessed by [18]FDG, while the other half studied cerebral blood flow by H_2[15]O, ^{99m}Tc-HMPAO, ^{99m}Tc-EMZ, ^{123}I-IMP, or other tracers. Only two studies (113,114) failed to find significant differences between mood disorder patients and controls. However, this may be biased by the lower likelihood of publication of negative studies. As noted in Figure 8, the remaining studies found abnormal (decreased much more often than increased) cerebral activity in anterior paralimbic, cortical, and subcortical structures (prefrontal > temporal > basal ganglia > anterior cingulate) in primary depression (Figures 5 and 6). As mentioned above, this sort of "vote-counting" analysis probably offers overly conservative conclusions because it penalizes studies with low statistical power (32).

Table 2 Negative Correlations Between Hamilton Depression Ratings and Cerebral Blood Flow and Metabolism in Primary Depression

Study	Region	r	p
Baxter et al., 1989 (126)	L DLPF/hemisphere	−0.49[a]	0.0002
	R DLPF/hemisphere	−0.41	0.005
O'Connell et al., 1989 (137)	FL/cerebellum	−0.32[a]	0.001
	TL/cerebellum	−0.45	0.001
Schlegel et al., 1989 (173)	L TL	−0.44	0.05
Kanaya and Yonekawa, 1990 (61)	Cerebrum/cerebellum	−0.58	0.01
Kumar et al., 1991 (174)	Cerebrum/cerebellum	−0.75	0.01
Austin et al., 1992 (158)	R FL/occipital	−0.37[a]	0.05
Cohen et al., 1992 (127)	M PF	−0.95[a]	0.02
Drevets et al., 1992 (119)	L PF/global	−0.62[a]	0.05
Yazici et al., 1992 (157)	L PF/slice	−0.68[a]	0.006
	M PF/slice	−0.58	0.02
O'Connell et al., 1995 (138)	FL/cerebellum	−0.34[a]	0.01

[a]Seven studies with significant negative correlations between frontal activity and severity of depression.
L = left; R = right; M = mesial; FL = frontal lobe; TL = temporal lobe; PF = prefrontal; DLPF = dorsolateral prefrontal.

Thus, there is now overwhelming evidence of prefrontal cortical deficits in primary depression. The 27 studies reporting frontal decreases included 419 patients, while the seven studies with frontal increases included only 56 patients. Moreover, severity of depression ratings often correlated with the degree of decrease in cerebral activity (Table 2), in contrast to the generally negative findings of studies attempting to relate depression severity to structural imaging findings noted above. Most studies did not report lateralized cerebral functional changes in primary depression, and only very weak pluralities of studies reported left lateralized frontal and temporal hypoactivity in primary depression.

In addition, recent studies suggest blunted anterior paralimbic CBF increases in mood disorder patients compared to healthy controls during neuropsychological activation with facial emotion recognition (115), Stroop interference (stating colors of ink of words that spell out discordant colors, e.g., saying "blue" when observing the word "red" printed in blue ink) (116), transient sadness-self-induction (117) tasks, and pharmacological activation with acute intravenous procaine (118).

The few studies reporting increased anterior cerebral activity in primary depression tended to include patients with affective illness subtypes with unique phenomenological, pathophysiological, and treatment-response characteristics. Mood disorders are heterogeneous, and clinical distinctions and subtypes include unipolar versus bipolar, nonpsychotic versus psychotic, seasonal versus nonseasonal, familial versus nonfamilial, pure versus complicated (comorbid anxiety, substance abuse, or other disorders), episodic versus chronic, mild versus severe, and melancholic (anorexic, insomnic, agitated, loss of mood reactivity) versus atypical (hyperphagic, hypersomnic, retarded, preserved mood reactivity). In addition, covert and inadequately defined state-versus-trait differences and treatment carryover effects may contribute to heterogeneity (Figure 9).

Increased cerebral activity compared to controls has been reported in familial pure depressive disorder (119), bipolar II patients with summer seasonal affective disorder (120), bipolar I depression (121), and responders to sleep deprivation (122,123) and antidepressant responders to carbamazepine (124). The brain regions with increased activity in these subtypes tended to be the same (prefrontal and anterior paralimbic) areas where decreases were noted in the majority of studies, suggesting that in these subtypes, different or opposing biochemical disruptions may occur in these structures, which are involved in the mediation of emotional experience. This is further supported by differential clinical responses in some of these subtypes. For example, patients with anterior limbic hyperactivity (compared to those without this marker) may be more likely to have antidepressant responses to sleep deprivation or carbamazepine, interventions that appear to decrease cerebral activity. Of interest, many responders to either of these interventions have bipolar illness. Our group has found that bipolar I depression may be associated with hypermetabolism, bipolar II depression with heterogeneous metabolic patterns, and unipolar depression with hypometabolism (Figure 9) (121).

D. Mood States, Treatments, and Cerebral Blood Flow and Metabolism in Primary Mood Disorders

Reports of euthymic compared to depressed patients, controlling for medication status, have generally found that with euthymia there is attenuation (or resolution) of many of the abnormalities observed in depression (119,125). Residual abnormalities in medication-free euthymic patients may represent possible trait markers of depressive illnesses (119). Treatment responders compared with their depressed pretreatment baseline also generally showed attenuation (or resolution) of pretreatment cerebral functional abnormalities with various therapies, including medication (61,124,126), light (127), and sleep deprivation (122,123). However, successful electroconvulsive therapy appeared to further exacerbate decreased anterior cerebral activity (128).

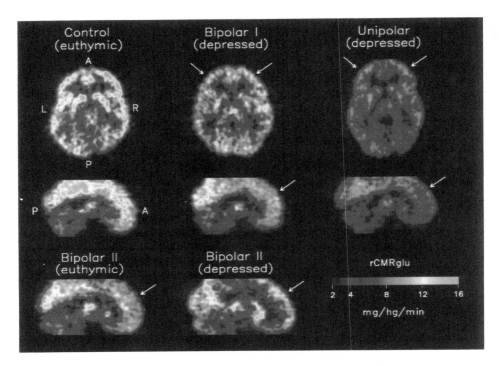

Figure 9 Heterogeneity in primary mood disorders. (Top row) Transaxial slices of 18FDG PET scans of (left) a euthymic healthy control, (center) a depressed bipolar I patient, and (right) a similarly depressed unipolar patient while performing a simple, continuous auditory-discrimination task. Subjects are matched for age and gender. (Center row) Midsagittal slices of the same subjects as in the top row. (Bottom row) Midsagittal slices of 18FDG PET scans of a patient with rapid-cycling bipolar II disorder in (left) euthymic and (right) depressed mood states. Arrows indicate hypofrontality, a common finding in PET studies of primary mood disorders. Color scale indicates absolute cerebral metabolic rates. L = left; R = right; A = anterior; P = posterior.

Comparisons of baseline (pretreatment) cerebral function in patients who later respond or fail to respond to therapy suggest possible baseline markers of treatment responses that may offer important insights into the heterogeneity of mood disorders, and perhaps may even someday be used to more effectively target treatment in refractory illness. Thus, anterior limbic hyperactivity may be a baseline marker for patients who obtain antidepressant responses to sleep deprivation (122,123). In addition, preliminary data from our group suggest that baseline temporal hypermetabolism and frontal hypometabolism may be markers for patients who respond to carbamazepine and nimodipine, respectively (124).

E. Ligand-Mediated and Neurotransmitter-Targeted PET and SPECT Studies in Primary Mood Disorders

PET and SPECT studies using more biochemically specific radiotracers have also noted differences between mood disorder patients and controls. However, this literature is much less extensive than the CBF and metabolism literature, and most of these findings require replication. Unipolar patients may have diffusely decreased cerebral uptake of monoamine precursors (L-5-hydroxytryptophan and L-3,4-dihydroxyphenylalanine), and increased mesial prefrontal L-5-hydroxytryptophan utilization (129). Also, in patients with unipolar mood disorders, serotonin 5-HT$_2$ receptors may have greater right than left inferior prefrontal asymmetry and be increased in parietal lobe (130). Psychotic (but not nonpsychotic) bipolar patients may have increased caudate dopamine D$_2$ receptors (Figure 10), with the degree of D$_2$ increases correlating with psychosis ratings (131). In another report (132), while baseline D$_2$ receptors in depressed bipolar II patients did not differ from those in

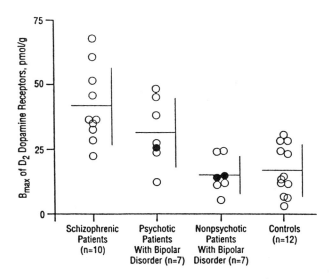

Figure 10 Increased caudate dopamine D$_2$ receptors in psychotic (but not nonpsychotic) bipolar patients. (From Ref. 131.)

controls, responders (but not nonresponders) after sleep deprivation had decreased basal ganglia D_2 binding, suggesting enhanced dopamine release with response. Bipolar patients may have decreased frontal (but not striatal) D_1 receptors (133), while in refractory depression prefrontal, temporal, cingulate, and caudate mu opiate receptors may be increased (134).

F. PET and SPECT Studies in Primary Mania

The few CBF and metabolism studies in primary mania have had variable and at times conflicting findings. Global cerebral metabolism in medication-free hypomanic or euthymic bipolars may not differ from healthy controls but be increased compared to bipolars in depressed or mixed states (135). Kishimoto and colleagues (136) noted widespread increases in ^{11}C-glucose uptake in three medication-free manic patients compared to controls, and in contrast to widespread decreases in nine unipolar depressed patients. O'Connell and colleagues reported that 11 manic patients had increased (globally normalized) temporal lobe CBF compared to controls, in a fashion similar to patients with schizophrenia (137,138) and atypical psychosis (137). Also, decreased normalized frontal and basal ganglia rCBF was noted in both mania and schizophrenia patients compared to controls (138). Moreover, across mixed subjects (schizophrenia, mania, and controls), mania ratings had positive correlations with caudate ($r = 0.25$; $n = 100$; $p < 0.01$)(137) and right temporal ($r = 0.41$; $n = 48$; $p < 0.01$) CBF (138). In contrast, Migliorelli and colleagues (139) found that five medication-free manic patients had decreased right temporal basal cortical rCBF (normalized to cerebellum) compared to controls as well as (right less than left) temporal basal and (basal less than dorsal) right temporal CBF asymmetries. Their group found a trend toward a negative correlation ($r = -0.86$; $n = 5$; $p = 0.06$) between mania ratings and right basotemporal rCBF.

There have also been very few studies of primary mania using more biochemically specific imaging methods. The report of increased caudate dopamine D_2 receptors in psychotic but not nonpsychotic bipolar patients mentioned above was in a sample of predominantly manic (11/14) neuro-leptic-free or naive patients (131). Also, as noted below, MRS studies have reported increased PMEs in mania, and a positive correlation between cerebral lithium levels and antimanic responses.

G. PET and SPECT Studies in Secondary Mood Disorders

There is also a substantial literature documenting anterior cerebral hypoac-tivity in secondary depressions. Patients with depression secondary to diverse

Table 3 Cerebral Blood Flow and Metabolism in Secondary Depression

Study	Frontal	Temporal/other	Primary disorder
Mayberg et al., 1991 (140)		↓ Temporal, anterior cingulate	Stroke
Bromfield et al., 1992 (141)	↓		Complex partial seizures
Mayberg et al., 1990 (142)	↓[a]	↓ Caudate	Parkinson's disease
Mayberg et al., 1992 (143)	↓		Huntington's disease
Renshaw et al., 1992 (144)	↓		Acquired immuno-deficiency syndrome
Baxter et al., 1989 (126)	↓[a]		Obsessive-compulsive disorder
Andreason et al., 1992 (145)	↓[a]		Bulimia
Volkow et al., 1991 (146)	↓[a]		Cocaine abuse

[a]Four studies with significant negative correlations between frontal activity and severity of depression.

↓ = Decreased cerebral activity in depressed patients compared to controls.

neurological and medical disorders—stroke (140), epilepsy (141), Parkinson's (142) and Huntington's (143) diseases, acquired immunodeficiency syndrome (144)—or other psychiatric disorders—obsessive compulsive disorder (126), bulimia (145), cocaine abuse (146)—have consistently had anterior cerebral hypoactivity compared to either healthy controls or controls matched for the primary illness (Table 3). In addition, the degree of anterior cerebral hypoactivity has often correlated with the severity of rated depression. Hence, anterior cerebral hypoactivity may represent a common substrate of depressive symptoms independent of illness etiology.

Also, Mayberg et al. (147) found that patients after right- (but not left-) sided strokes had a greater ipsilateral than contralateral asymmetry in serotonin 5-HT$_2$ receptors in undamaged temporal and parietal regions. In addition, in left-sided strokes the ipsilateral/contralateral temporal lobe 5-HT$_2$ receptor ratio correlated inversely with depression scores, suggesting that a failure to up-regulate ipsilateral 5-HT$_2$ receptors after left-sided strokes could be related to the development of secondary depression.

There is a paucity of functional imaging studies in secondary mania. Starkstein and colleagues (148) reported right temporal lobe hypometabolism in three patients with mania secondary to stroke. Thus, preliminary functional imaging findings in mania and depression secondary to stroke are in convergence with other clinical and structural imaging evidence that left-sided lesions may be associated with secondary depression and right-sided lesions with secondary mania. However, this evidence of lateralization in secondary mood disorders should be considered with caution in view of the limited data, as well as the apparent lack of robust lateralization in primary depression.

H. Magnetic Resonance Spectroscopy Studies in Primary Mood Disorders

Magnetic resonance spectroscopy (MRS) uses modified structural MRI scanners to study resonance spectra of compounds containing paramagnetic (having an odd atomic number) elements. Proton or ^{1}H MRS allows determination of lactate, glutamate, aspartate, gamma-aminobutyric acid, creatinine, choline, and N-acetylaspartate. Lithium ([7]Li) and fluorine (^{19}F) MRS can assess cerebral concentrations of lithium and fluorinated drugs, respectively. Phosphorous (^{31}P) MRS allows determination of high-energy phosphates, intracellular pH and free magnesium, and some phospholipids, including phosphomonoesters (PMEs—putative cell-membrane "building blocks") and phosphodiesters (PDEs—putative cell-membrane "breakdown products").

An emerging MRS literature is beginning to suggest biochemically specific abnormalities in mood disorder patients, and allow assessment of brain concentrations of lithium and fluorinated medications. Proton (^{1}H) MRS studies suggest increased basal ganglia (but not occipital) choline, N-acetylaspartate (NAA), and inositol (relative to phosphocreatine-creatine) in bipolar patients on lithium (149), and increased basal ganglia choline but not NAA (relative to creatine) in depressed unipolars (150). Nefazodone therapy decreased basal ganglia choline in these unipolars (150).

Lithium ([7]Li) MRS studies in primarily bipolar patients have fairly consistently reported brain lithium concentrations to be about one-half of serum lithium levels. Across nine studies, the mean brain/serum lithium ratio was 0.54 (standard deviation 0.11; range 0.40 to 0.77). Moreover, improvement in manic symptoms may correlate with brain lithium ($r = 0.64$; Figure 11) and brain/serum lithium ratio ($r = 0.60$), but not serum lithium or lithium dose/weight (151). Also, brain lithium concentrations may correlate better with serum ($r = 0.66$) than with red blood cell ($r = 0.33$) lithium levels (152). Preliminary evidence suggests that brain lithium concentrations may need to be at least 0.2 mM (151,153) for adequate therapeutic effects.

Phosphorous (^{31}P) MRS studies of medicated and unmedicated euthymic bipolar patients have found decreased frontal phosphomonoesters (PMEs—putative cell membrane "building blocks") and increased phosphodiesters (PDEs—putative cell membrane "breakdown products"), while manic or depressed bipolars had increased PMEs (154,155). Despite lithium's inhibitory effect on the inositol phosphatase pathway, lithium therapy failed

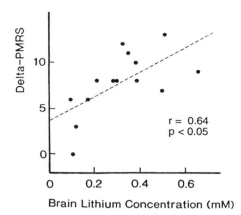

Figure 11 Cerebral lithium concentrations correlate with antimanic responses. Brain lithium levels assessed by ^{7}Li (lithium-7) MRS. (From Ref. 151.)

to alter PMEs (which include an inositol phosphate component) in schizophrenic and schizoaffective patients (156).

I. Summary of Functional Imaging Findings

In both primary and secondary depression, a substantial PET and SPECT literature supports decreased prefrontal and anterior paralimbic CBF and metabolism, which may often correlate with severity of depression and normalize with successful therapy. Some variable findings have been reported, often in specific primary mood disorder subtypes. Further study is needed to follow up on preliminary findings suggesting that functional changes in bipolar depression may differ from those in unipolar depression.

The limited literature describing CBF and metabolism in manic patients has inconsistencies that indicate a need for further studies. Interestingly, for both depression and mania, abnormalities in prefrontal and anterior paralimbic function are consistently reported, with the direction of the abnormality appearing to be the main source of variability across studies. Thus, differential abnormalities in prefrontal and anterior paralimbic CBF and metabolism may occur across different subtypes of affective illness, and perhaps even across different illness phases.

Studies using more specific biochemical techniques have reported intriguing findings in mood disorders, but generally require replication. Radiotracer methods offer good spatial resolution but involve substantial cost, while MRS methods may be less expensive but thus far have limited spatial resolution. Methodological advances will hopefully yield techniques with the combination of acceptable cost and adequate spatial resolution. This could in the next decade allow extension of the insights derived from CBF and metabolism studies in the last decade.

V. SIMILARITIES AND DIFFERENCES BETWEEN MOOD DISORDERS AND SCHIZOPHRENIA

A. Clinical Similarities

There are important areas of overlap between mood disorders and schizophrenia. Clinically, affective psychoses most resemble positive symptoms of schizophrenia, and retarded (bipolar) depressions most resemble negative symptoms. Patients with schizophrenia may develop secondary depressions, and, in some cases, presentations are sufficiently mixed to warrant a schizoaffective diagnosis. Medication responses also overlap, with traditional antipsychotics being helpful in mania and psychotic depression, and mood-stabilizer augmentation occasionally being helpful in schizophrenia. The serotonin-dopamine antagonists (atypical antipsychotics) bridge neurotransmitter systems classically associated with mood disorders and schizophrenia, and may also have dual efficacy in these illnesses.

B. Similarities and Differences in Brain Imaging Studies

There are also overlapping abnormalities of cerebral structure and function. Increased ventricular enlargement and sulcal prominence is noted in both disorders. However, ventricular enlargement may be slightly greater in schizophrenia than in mood disorders (25). Frontal hypoactivity occurs in both illnesses, which in mood disorders is related to the degree of depression (126,127,138,157,158) and in schizophrenia is related to negative symptoms (159–162). Furthermore, in a large sample of 40 depression and 30 schizophrenia patients, Dolan and colleagues (163) found that decreased normalized dorsolateral prefrontal rCBF was related to poverty of speech, independent of diagnosis. Thus, overlap in phenomenology may help explain some of the overlap in imaging findings in these disorders. Although rest and continuous performance task (CPT) studies indicate similar frontal deficits in the two disorders, during the Wisconsin Card Sort frontal activation was blunted in schizophrenia but preserved in depression (164).

Basal ganglia disturbances at rest may also differentiate the two disorders, as activity may be increased in schizophrenia and decreased in depression (61,126,135,165–169)—but possibly increased in mania (138). Treatment-naive schizophrenia patients may lack hypofrontality but do have basal ganglia hyperactivity (170). O'Connell et al. (138) recently noted frontal decreases and basal ganglia and temporal increases in normalized rCBF in both mania and schizophrenia, with the temporal lobe increases being more prevalent in manic patients. Patients with schizophrenia have been reported to have increased caudate D_2 receptors (171), and the same finding occurred in psychotic but not nonpsychotic bipolars. Despite the methodological controversy concerning caudate D_2 increases in schizophrenia (172), these preliminary results suggest that imaging methods can detect cerebral functional concomitants of important clinical overlaps between mood disorders and schizophrenia.

VI. CONCLUSION

Neuroanatomical research, structural brain imaging, and functional brain imaging studies provide converging evidence suggesting that prefrontal and anterior paralimbic structures may contribute importantly to the mediation of normal emotion, and that dysfunction of these structures may be important in mood disorders. Thus far, structural abnormalities in primary mood disorders appear to lack regional specificity, while those in secondary mood disorders appear consistent with such a neuroanatomical model. Furthermore, in both primary and secondary depression, the PET and SPECT literature supports altered (predominantly decreased) prefrontal and anterior paralimbic CBF and metabolism. In contrast with structural changes, cerebral functional abnormalities appear to be more consistently related to important clinical measures, such as the degree of depression at the time of the scan.

Technological refinements to enhance spatial and temporal resolution, decrease or eliminate exposure to ionizing radiation (such as functional or flow MRI and more sensitive scanners), and increase biochemical specificity (such as MRS and new PET and SPECT radiotracers) should allow further advances in our knowledge of the neuroanatomical substrates of mood disorders. Although the present methodology has already yielded a preliminary map of the functional neuroanatomy of mood disorders consistent with predictions of Broca, Papez, MacLean, and Alexander, much more clinical work is now needed to provide advances in the critical areas of illness heterogeneity and clinical response prediction.

REFERENCES

1. Broca P. Anatomie comparée des circonvolutions cérébrales: le grand lobe limbique et la scissure limbique dans la série des mammifères. Rev Anthropol 1878; 1:385–498.

2. Papez JW. A proposed mechanism of emotion. Arch Neurol Psychiatry 1937; 38:725–743.

3. MacLean P. Some psychiatric implications of physiological studies on frontotemporal portion of limbic system (visceral brain). Electroencephalog Clin Neurophysiol 1952; 4:407–418.

4. MacLean PD. The Triune Brain in Evolution: Role in Paleocerebral Functions. New York: Plenum Press, 1990.

5. Clarke WEI, Boggon RH. On the connections of the anterior nucleus of the thalamus. J Anat 1933; 67:215–226.

6. Rose JE, Woolsey CN. Structure and relations of limbic cortex and anterior thalamic nuclei in rabbit and cat. J Comp Neurol 1948; 89:279–347.

7. Bentivoglio M, Kultas-Ilinsky K, Ilinsky I. Limbic thalamus: structure, intrinsic organization, and connections. In: Vogt BA, Gabriel M, eds. Neurobiology of Cingulate Cortex and Limbic Thalamus: A Comprehensive Handbook. Boston: Birkhauser, 1993:71–122.

8. Yakovlev PI, Locke S, Angevine JB Jr. The limbus of the cerebral hemisphere, limbic nuclei of the thalamus, and the cingulum bundle. In: Purpura DP, Yahr MD, eds. The Thalamus. New York: Columbia University Press, 1966:77–97.

9. Alexander GE, DeLong MR, Strick PL. Parallel organization of functionally segregated circuits linking basal ganglia and cortex. Annu Rev Neurosci 1986; 9:357–81.

10. Alexander GE, Crutcher MD, DeLong MR. Basal ganglia-thalamocortical circuits: parallel substrates for motor, oculomotor, prefrontal and limbic functions. Prog Brain Res 1990; 85:119–146.

11. Nauta WJH. Circuitous connections linking cerebral cortex, limbic system, and corpus striatum. In: Doane BK, Livingston KE, eds. The Limbic System: Functional Organization and Clinical Disorders. New York: Raven Press, 1986:43–54.

12. Insel TR. Toward a neuroanatomy of obsessive-compulsive disorder. Arch Gen Psychiatry 1992; 49:739–744.

13. Baxter LR Jr. Neuroimaging studies of human anxiety disorders: cutting paths of knowledge through the field of neurotic phenomena. In: Bloom FE, Kupfer DJ, eds. Psychopharmacology: The Fourth Generation of Progress. New York: Raven Press, 1995:1287–1299.

14. LeDoux JE. Emotion and the limbic system concept. Concepts Neurosci 1991; 2:169–199.

15. Vogt BA, Finch DM, Olson CR. Functional heterogeneity in cingulate cortex: the anterior executive and posterior evaluative regions. Cereb Cortex 1992; 2:435–443.

16. Devinsky O, Morrell MJ, Vogt BA. Contributions of anterior cingulate cortex to behaviour. Brain 1995; 118:279–306.

17. MacLean P, Delgado JMR. Electrical and chemical stimulation of frontopolar portion of limbic system in the waking animal. Electroencephalog Clin Neurophysiol 1953; 5:91–100.

18. Mesulam MM. Neural substrates of behavior: the effects of brain lesions upon mental state. In: Nicholi AM, ed. The New Harvard Guide to Psychiatry. Cambridge, MA: Harvard University Press, 1988:91–128.

19. Jeste DV, Lohr JB, Goodwin FK. Neuroanatomical studies of major affective disorders. A review and suggestions for further research. Br J Psychiatry 1988; 153:444–459.

20. Nasrallah HA, Coffman JA, Olson SC. Structural brain-imaging findings in affective disorders: an overview. J Neuropsychiatry Clin Neurosci 1989; 1:21–6.

21. Schlegel S. Computed tomography in affective disorders. In: Hauser P, ed. Brain Imaging in Affective Disorders. Washington, DC: American Psychiatric Press, 1991:1–24.

22. Hauser P. Magnetic resonance imaging in primary affective disorder. In: Hauser P, ed. Brain Imaging in Affective Disorders. Washington; DC: American Psychiatric Press, 1991:25–53.

23. Sackeim HA, Prohovnik I. Brain imaging studies of depressive disorders. In: Mann JJ, Kupfer DJ, eds. The Biology of Depressive Disorders. New York: Plenum, 1993:205–258.

24. Raz S, Raz N. Structural brain abnormalities in the major psychoses: a quantitative review of the evidence from computerized imaging. Psychol Bull 1990; 108:93–108.

25. Elkis H, Friedman L, Wise A, Meltzer HY. Meta-analyses of studies of ventricular enlargement and cortical sulcal prominence in mood disorders: comparisons with controls or patients with schizophrenia. Arch Gen Psychiatry 1995; 52:735–746.

26. Tanaka Y, Hazama H, Fukuhara T, Tsutsui T. Computerized tomography of the brain in manic-depressive patients—a controlled study. Folia Psychiat Neurol Jpn 1982; 36:137–143.

27. Schlegel S, Kretzschmar K. Computed tomography in affective disorders. I. Ventricular and sulcal measurements. Biol Psychiatry 1987; 22:4–14.

28. Dewan MJ, Haldipur CV, Lane EE, Ispahani A, Boucher MF, Major LF. Bipolar affective disorder. I. Comprehensive quantitative computed tomography. Acta Psychiat Scand 1988; 77:670–676.

29. Strakowski SM, Wilson DR, Tohen M, Woods BT, Douglass AW, Stoll AL. Structural brain abnormalities in first-episode mania. Biol Psychiatry 1993; 33:602–609.

30. Mukherjee S, Schnur DB, Lo ES, Sackeim HA, Cooper TB. Post-dexamethasone cortisol levels and computerized tomographic findings in manic patients. Acta Psychiatr Scand 1993; 88:145–148.

31. Coffey CE, Wilkinson WE, Weiner RD, Ritchie JC, Aque M. The dexamethasone suppression test and quantitative cerebral anatomy in depression. Biol Psychiatry 1993; 33:442–449.

32. Hedges LV, Olkin I. Statistical Methods for Meta-analysis. Orlando, FL: Academic Press, 1985.

33. Altshuler LL, Curran JG, Hauser P, Mintz J, Denikoff K, Post R. T_2 hyperintensities in bipolar disorder: magnetic resonance imaging comparison and literature meta-analysis. Am J Psychiatry 1995; 152:1139–1144.

34. Vita A, Sacchetti E, Cazzullo CL. A CT follow-up study of cerebral ventricular size in schizophrenia and major affective disorder. Schizophrenia Res 1988; 1:165–166.

35. Woods BT, Yurgelun-Todd D, Benes FM, Frankenburg FR, Pope HG Jr, McSparren J. Progressive ventricular enlargement in schizophrenia: comparison to bipolar affective disorder and correlation with clinical course. Biol Psychiatry 1990; 27:341–352.

36. Andreasen NC, Swayze VW II, Flaum M, Alliger RJ, Cohen G. Ventricular abnormalities affective disorder: clinical and demographic correlates. Am J Psychiatry 1990; 147:893–900.

37. Swayze VW II, Andreasen NC, Alliger RJ, Ehrhardt JC, Yuh WT. Structural brain abnormalities in bipolar affective disorder: ventricular enlargement and focal signal hyperintensities. Arch Gen Psychiatry 1990; 47:1054–1059.

38. Dolan RJ, Calloway SP, Mann AH. Cerebral ventricular size in depressed subjects. Psychol Med 1985; 15:873–878.

39. Luchins DJ, Lewine RR, Meltzer HY. Lateral ventricular size, psychopathology, and medication response in the psychoses. Biol Psychiatry 1984; 19:29–44.

40. Schlegel S, Frommberger U, Buller R. Computerized tomography (CT) in affective disorders: relationship with psychopathology. Psychiatry Res 1989; 29:271–272.

41. Van den Bossche B, Maes M, Brussaard C, et al. Computed tomography of the brain in unipolar depression. J Affective Disord 1991; 21:67–74.

42. Luchins DJ, Meltzer HY. Ventricular size and psychosis in affective disorder. Biol Psychiatry 1983; 18:1197–1198.

43. Targum SD, Rosen LN, DeLisi LE, Weinberger DR, Citrin CM. Cerebral ventricular size in major depressive disorder: association with delusional symptoms. Biol Psychiatry 1983; 18:329–336.

44. Nasrallah HA, McCalley-Whitters M, Pfohl B. Clinical significance of large cerebral ventricles in manic males. Psychiatry Res 1984; 13:151–156.

45. Pearlson GD, Garbacz DJ, Tompkins RH, et al. Clinical correlates of lateral ventricular enlargement in bipolar affective disorder. Am J Psychiatry 1984; 141:253–256.

46. Kellner CH, Rubinow DR, Post RM. Cerebral ventricular size and cognitive impairment in depression. J Affective Disord 1986; 10:215–219.

47. Rabins PV, Pearlson GD, Aylward E, Kumar AJ, Dowell K. Cortical magnetic resonance imaging changes in elderly inpatients with major depression. Am J Psychiatry 1991; 148:617–620.

48. Schlegel S, Maier W, Philipp M, Heuser I, Aldenhoff J. The association between psychopathological aspects and CT measurements in affective disorders. Pharmacopsychiatry 1988; 21:416–417.

49. Abas MA, Sahakian BJ, Levy R. Neuropsychological deficits and CT scan changes in elderly depressives. Psychol Med 1990; 20:507–520.

50. Standish-Barry HM, Hale AS, Honig A, Bouras N, Bridges PK, Bartlett JR. Ventricular size, the dexamethasone suppression test and outcome of severe endogenous depression following psychosurgery. Acta Psychiatr Scand 1985; 72:166–171.

51. Dewan MJ, Haldipur CV, Boucher M, Major LF. Is CT ventriculomegaly related to hypercortisolemia? Acta Psychiatr Scand 1988; 77:230–231.

52. Rothschild AJ, Benes F, Hebben N, et al. Relationships between brain CT scan findings and cortisol in psychotic and nonpsychotic depressed patients. Biol Psychiatry 1989; 26:565–575.

53. Rao VP, Krishnan KR, Goli V, et al. Neuroanatomical changes and hypothalamo-pituitary-adrenal axis abnormalities. Biol Psychiatry 1989; 26:729–732.

54. Schlegel S, von Bardeleben U, Wiedemann K, Frommberger U, Holsboer F. Computerized brain tomography measures compared with spontaneous and suppressed plasma cortisol levels in major depression. Psychoneuroendocrinology 1989; 14:209–216.

55. Kellner CH, Rubinow DR, Gold PW, Post RM. Relationship of cortisol hypersecretion to brain CT scan alterations in depressed patients. Psychiatry Res 1983; 8:191–197.

56. Risch SC, Lewine RJ, Kalin NH, et al. Limbic-hypothalamic-pituitary-adrenal axis activity and ventricular-to-brain ratio studies in affective illness and schizophrenia. Neuropsychopharmacology 1992; 6:95–100.

57. Dupont RM, Jernigan TL, Butters N, et al. Subcortical abnormalities detected in bipolar affective disorder using magnetic resonance imaging: clinical and neuropsychological significance. Arch Gen Psychiatry 1990; 47:55–59.

58. Figiel GS, Krishnan KR, Rao VP, et al. Subcortical hyperintensities on brain magnetic resonance imaging: a comparison of normal and bipolar subjects. J Neuropsychiatry Clin Neurosci 1991 3:18–22.

59. Aylward EH, Roberts-Twille JV, Barta PE, et al. Basal ganglia volumes and white matter hyperintensities in patients with bipolar disorder. Am J Psychiatry 1994; 151:687–693.

60. Dupont RM, Jernigan TL, Heindel W, et al. Magnetic resonance imaging and mood disorders: localization of white matter and other subcortical abnormalities. Arch Gen Psychiatry 1995; 52:747–755.

61. Kanaya T, Yonekawa M. Regional cerebral blood flow in depression. Jpn J Psychiatry Neurol 1990; 44:571–576.

62. Krishnan KR, Goli V, Ellinwood EH, France RD, Blazer DG, Nemeroff CB. Leukoencephalopathy in patients diagnosed as major depressive. Biol Psychiatry 1988; 23:519–522.

63. Krishnan KR, McDonald WM, Doraiswamy PM, et al. Neuroanatomical substrates of depression in the elderly. Eur Arch Psychiatry Clin Neurosci 1993; 243:41–46.

64. Brown FW, Lewine RJ, Hudgins PA, Risch SC. White matter hyperintensity signals in psychiatric and nonpsychiatric subjects. Am J Psychiatry 1992; 149:620–625.
65. Coffey CE, Figiel GS, Djang WT, Cress M, Saunders WB, Weiner RD. Leukoencephalopathy in elderly depressed patients referred for ECT. Biol Psychiatry 1988; 24:143–161.
66. Coffey CE, Figiel GS, Djang WT, Saunders WB, Weiner RD. White matter hyperintensity on magnetic resonance imaging: clinical and neuroanatomic correlates in the depressed elderly. J Neuropsychiatry Clin Neurosci 1989; 1:135–144.
67. Coffey CE, Figiel GS, Djang WT, Weiner RD. Subcortical hyperintensity on magnetic resonance imaging: a comparison of normal and depressed elderly subjects. Am J Psychiatry 1990; 147:187–189.
68. Lesser IM, Miller BL, Boone KB, et al. Brain injury and cognitive function in late-onset psychotic depression. J Neuropsychiatry Clin Neurosci 1991; 3:33–40.
69. Botteron KN, Figiel GS, Zorumski CF. Electroconvulsive therapy in patients with late-onset psychosis and structural brain changes. J Geriatr Psychiatry Neurol 1991; 4:44–47.
70. Miller BL, Lesser IM, Boone K, et al. Brain white-matter lesions and psychosis. Br J Psychiatry 1989; 155:73–78.
71. Deicken RF, Reus VI, Manfredi L, Wolkowitz OM. MRI deep white matter hyperintensity in a psychiatric population. Biol Psychiatry 1991; 29:918–922.
72. Coffey CE, Wilkinson WE, Weiner RD, et al. Quantitative cerebral anatomy in depression: a controlled magnetic resonance imaging study. Arch Gen Psychiatry 1993; 50:7–16.
73. Krishnan KR, McDonald WM, Escalona PR, et al. Magnetic resonance imaging of the caudate nuclei in depression: preliminary observations. Arch Gen Psychiatry 1992; 49:553–557.
74. Husain MM, McDonald WM, Doraiswamy PM, et al. A magnetic resonance imaging study of putamen nuclei in major depression. Psychiatry Res 1991; 40:95–99.
75. Shah SA, Doraiswamy PM, Husain MM, et al. Posterior fossa abnormalities in major depression: a controlled magnetic resonance imaging study. Acta Psychiatr Scand 1992; 85:474–479.
76. Swayze VW 2nd, Andreasen NC, Alliger RJ, Yuh WT, Ehrhardt JC. Subcortical and temporal structures in affective disorder and schizophrenia: a magnetic resonance imaging study. Biol Psychiatry 1992; 31:221–240.
77. Yates WR, Jacoby CG, Andreasen NC. Cerebellar atrophy in schizophrenia and affective disorder. Am J Psychiatry 1987; 144:465–467.
78. Raine A, Lencz T, Reynolds G, et al. An evaluation of structural and functional prefrontal deficits in schizophrenia: MRI and neuropsychological measures. Psychiatry Res 1992; 45:123–137.
79. Coffman JA, Bornstein RA, Olson SC, Schwarzkopf SB, Nasrallah HA. Cognitive impairment and cerebral structure by MRI in bipolar disorder. Biol Psychiatry 1990; 27:1188–1196.

80. Hauser P, Altshuler LL, Berrettini W, Dauphinais ID, Gelernter J, Post RM. Temporal lobe measurement in primary affective disorder by magnetic resonance imaging. J Neuropsychiatry Clin Neurosci 1989; 1:128–134.

81. Altshuler LL, Conrad A, Hauser P, et al. Reduction of temporal lobe volume in bipolar disorder: a preliminary report of magnetic resonance imaging [letter]. Arch Gen Psychiatry 1991; 48:482–483.

82. Johnstone EC, Owens DG, Crow TJ, et al. Temporal lobe structure as determined by nuclear magnetic resonance in schizophrenia and bipolar affective disorder. J Neurol Neurosurg Psychiatry 1989; 52:736–741.

83. Harvey I, Persaud R, Ron MA, Baker G, Murray RM. Volumetric MRI measurements in bipolars compared with schizophrenics and healthy controls. Psychol Med 1994; 24:689–699.

84. Hauser P, Dauphinais ID, Berrettini W, DeLisi LE, Gelernter J, Post RM. Corpus callosum dimensions measured by magnetic resonance imaging in bipolar affective disorder and schizophrenia. Biol Psychiatry 1989; 26:659–668.

85. Husain MM, Figiel GS, Lurie SN, et al. MRI of corpus callosum and septum pellucidum in depression [letter]. Biol Psychiatry 1991; 29:300–301.

86. Wu JC, Buchsbaum MS, Johnson JC, et al. Magnetic resonance and positron emission tomography imaging of the corpus callosum: size, shape and metabolic rate in unipolar depression. J Affective Disord 1993; 28:15–25.

87. Krishnan KR, Doraiswamy PM, Lurie SN, et al. Pituitary size in depression. J Clin Endocrinol Metab 1991; 72:256–259.

88. Axelson DA, Doraiswamy PM, Boyko OB, et al. In vivo assessment of pituitary volume with magnetic resonance imaging and systematic stereology: relationship to dexamethasone suppression test results in patients. Psychiatry Res 1992; 44:63–70.

89. Weinberger DR, DeLisi LE, Perman GP, Targum S, Wyatt RJ. Computed tomography in schizophreniform disorder and other acute psychiatric disorders. Arch Gen Psychiatry 1982; 39:778–783.

90. Tsai L, Nasrallah HA, Jacoby CG. Hemispheric asymmetries on computed tomographic scans in schizophrenia and mania. Arch Gen Psychiatry 1983; 39:1286–1289.

91. Dewan MJ, Haldipur CV, Lane EE, Donnelly MP, Boucher MF, Major LF. Normal cerebral asymmetry in bipolar patients. Biol Psychiatry 1987; 22:1058–1066.

92. Starkstein SE, Robinson RG. Affective disorders and cerebrovascular disease. Br J Psychiatry 1989; 154:170–182.

93. Stern RA, Bachmann DL. Depressive symptoms following stroke. Am J Psychiatry 1991; 148:351–356.

94. Mendez MF, Adams NL, Lewandowski KS. Neurobehavioral changes associated with caudate lesions. Neurology 1989; 39:349–354.

95. Folstein SE, Folstein MF. Psychiatric features of Huntington's disease: recent approaches and findings. Psychiatr Dev 1983; 1:193–205.

96. Caine ED, Shoulson I. Psychiatric syndromes in Huntington's disease. Am J Psychiatry 1983; 140:728–733.

97. Horn S. Some psychological factors in Parkinsonism. J Neurol Neurosurg Psychiatry 1974; 37:27–31.

98. Mindham RH. Psychiatric symptoms in Parkinsonism. J Neurol Neurosurg Psychiatry 1970; 33:188–191.

99. Federoff JP, Starkstein SE, Forrester AW, et al. Depression in patients with acute traumatic brain injury. Am J Psychiatry 1992; 149:918–923.

100. Jorge RE, Robinson RG, Starkstein SE, Arndt SV, Forrester AW, Geisler FH. Secondary mania following traumatic brain injury. Am J Psychiatry 1993; 150:916–921.

101. Altshuler LL, Devinsky O, Post RM, et al. Depression, anxiety, and temporal lobe epilepsy: laterality of focus and symptoms. Arch Neurol 1990; 47:284–288.

102. Honer WG, Hurwitz T, Li DKB, et al. Temporal lobe involvement in multiple sclerosis patients with psychiatric disorders. Arch Neurol 1987; 44:187–190.

103. George MS, Kellner CH, Bernstein H, Goust JM. A magnetic resonance imaging investigation into mood disorders in multiple sclerosis. J Nerv Mental Dis 1994; 182:410–412.

104. Moller A, Wiedemann G, Rohde U, Backmund H, Sonntag A. Correlates of cognitive impairment and depressive mood disorder in multiple sclerosis. Acta Psychiatr Scand 1994; 89:117–121.

105. Direkze M, Bayliss SG, Cutting JC. Primary tumours of the frontal lobe. Br J Clin Pract 1971; 25:207–213.

106. Kanakaratnam G, Direkze M. Aspects of primary tumours of the frontal lobe. Br J Clin Pract 1976; 30:220–221.

107. George MS, Ketter TA, Parekh PI, Horwitz B, Herscovitch P, Post RM. Brain activity during transient sadness and happiness in healthy women. Am J Psychiatry 1995; 152:341–351.

108. Kimbrell TA, George MS, Parekh PI, Ketter TA, Herscovitch P, Post RM. Regional brain activity during self-induced anger and anxiety. 50th Annual Meeting of the Society of Biological Psychiatry, Miami, May 17–20, 1995. Abstr 93. Biol Psychiatry 1995; 37(9):617.

109. Ketter TA, Andreason PJ, George MS, et al. Anterior paralimbic mediation of procaine-induced emotional and psychosensory experiences. Arch Gen Psychiatry 1996; 53:59–69.

110. George MS, Ketter TA, Gill DS, et al. Brain regions involved in recognizing facial emotion or identity: an oxygen-15 PET study. J Neuropsychiatry Clin Neurosci 1993; 5:384–394.

111. Dolan RJ, Friston KJ. Positron emission tomography in psychiatric and neuropsychiatric disorders. Sem Neurol 1989; 9:330–337.

112. Baxter LR Jr. PET studies of cerebral function in major depression and obsessive-compulsive disorder: the emerging prefrontal consensus. Ann Clin Psychiatry 1991; 3:103–109.

113. Kling AS, Metter EJ, Riege WH, Kuhl DE. Comparison of PET measurement of local brain glucose metabolism and CAT measurement of brain atrophy in chronic schizophrenia and depression. Am J Psychiatry 1986; 143:175–180.

114. Maes M, Dierckx R, Meltzer HY, et al. Regional cerebral blood flow in unipolar depression measured with Tc-99m-HMPAO single photon emission computed tomography: negative findings. Psychiatry Res 1993; 50:77–88.

115. George MS, Ketter TA, Gill D, Marangell LB, Pazzaglia PJ, Post RM. Blunted CBF with emotion recognition in depression. 146th Annual Meeting of the American Psychiatric Association, San Francisco, May 22–27, 1993. Abstr NR114.

116. George MS, Ketter TA, Parekh PI, et al. Mood disorder subjects have blunted cingulate activation during a response interference task (the Stroop). J Neuropsychiatry. In press.

117. George MS, Kimbrell T, Parekh PI, et al. Actively depressed subjects have difficulty inducing, and blunted limbic rCBF during, transient sadness. 148th Annual Meeting of the American Psychiatric Association, Miami, May 20–25, 1995. Abstr NR167.

118. Ketter TA, Andreason PJ, George MS, Pazzaglia PJ, Marangell LB, Post RM. Blunted CBF response to procaine in mood disorders. 146th Annual Meeting of the American Psychiatric Association, San Francisco, May 22–27, 1993. Abstr NR297.

119. Drevets WC, Videen TO, Price JL, Preskorn SH, Carmichael ST, Raichle ME. A functional anatomical study of unipolar depression. J Neurosci 1992; 12:3628–3641.

120. Goyer PF, Schulz PM, Semple WE, et al. Cerebral glucose metabolism in patients with summer seasonal affective disorder. Neuropsychopharmacology 1992; 7:233–240.

121. Ketter TA, George MS, Andreason PJ, et al. rCMRglu in unipolar versus bipolar depression. 147th Annual Meeting of the American Psychiatric Association, Philadelphia, May 21–26, 1994. Abstr NR444.

122. Ebert D, Feistel H, Barocka A. Effects of sleep deprivation on the limbic system and the frontal lobes in affective disorders: a study with Tc-99m-HMPAO SPECT. Psychiatry Res 1991; 40:247–251.

123. Wu JC, Gillin JC, Buchsbaum MS, Hershey T, Johnson JC, Bunney WE. Effect of sleep deprivation on brain metabolism of depressed patients. Am J Psychiatry 1992; 149:538–543.

124. Ketter TA, George MS, Parekh PI, et al. PET imaging and psychotropic response prediction in mood disorders. 148th Annual Meeting of the American Psychiatric Association, Miami, May 20–25, 1995. Paper Session 19, Paper 58.

125. Post RM, DeLisi LE, Holcomb HH, Uhde TW, Cohen R, Buchsbaum MS. Glucose utilization in the temporal cortex of affectively ill patients: positron emission tomography. Biol Psychiatry 1987; 22:545–553.

126. Baxter LR Jr, Schwartz JM, Phelps ME, et al. Reduction of prefrontal cortex glucose metabolism common to three types of depression. Arch Gen Psychiatry 1989; 46:243–250.

127. Cohen RM, Gross M, Nordahl TE, Semple WE, Oren DA, Rosenthal N. Preliminary data on the metabolic brain pattern of patients with winter seasonal affective disorder. Arch Gen Psychiatry 1992; 49:545–552.

128. Nobler MS, Sackeim HA, Prohovnik I, et al. Regional cerebral blood flow in mood disorders. III. Treatment and clinical response. Arch Gen Psychiatry 1994; 51:884–897.

129. Agren H, Reibring L, Hartvig P, et al. Monoamine metabolism in human prefrontal cortex and basal ganglia: PET studies using [β-11C]L-5-hydroxytryptophan and [β-11C]L-DOPA in healthy volunteers and patients with unipolar major depression. Depression 1993; 1:71–81.

130. D'haenen H, Bossuyt A, Mertens J, Bossuyt-Piron C, Gijsemans M, Kaufman L. SPECT imaging of serotonin$_2$ receptors in depression. Psychiatry Res 1992; 45:227–237.

131. Pearlson GD, Wong DF, Tune LE, et al. In vivo D2 dopamine receptor density in psychotic and not nonpsychotic patients with bipolar disorder. Arch Gen Psychiatry 1995; 52:471–477.

132. Ebert D, Feistel H, Kaschka W, Barocka A, Pirner A. Single photon emission computerized tomography assessment of cerebral dopamine D2 receptor blockade in depression before and after sleep deprivation—preliminary results. Biol Psychiatry 1994; 35:880–885.

133. Suhara T, Nakayama K, Inoue O, et al. D1 dopamine receptor binding in mood disorders measured by positron emission tomography. Psychopharmacology 1992; 106:14–18.

134. Mayberg HS, Dannals RF, Ross CA, Wilson AA, Ravert HT, Frost JJ. Mu opiate receptor binding is increased in depressed patients measured by PET and C-11-carfentanil. 30th Annual Meeting of the American College of Neuropsychopharmacology, Dec 9–13, 1991. Abstr, p 61.

135. Schwartz JM, Baxter LR Jr, Mazziotta JC, Gerner RH, Phelps ME. The differential diagnosis of depression: relevance of positron emission tomography studies of cerebral glucose metabolism to the bipolar–unipolar dichotomy. JAMA 1987; 258:1368–1374.

136. Kishimoto H, Takazu O, Ohno S, et al. 11C-glucose metabolism in manic and depressed patients. Psychiatry Res 1987; 22:81–88.

137. O'Connell RA, Van Heertum RL, Billick SB, et al. Single photon emission computed tomography (SPECT) with [123I]IMP in the differential diagnosis of psychiatric disorders. J Neuropsychiatry Clin Neurosci 1989; 1:145–153.

138. O'Connell RA, Van Heertum RL, Luck D, et al. Single-photon emission computed tomography of the brain in acute mania and schizophrenia. J Neuroimaging 1995; 5:101–104.

139. Migliorelli R, Starkstein SE, Teson A, et al. SPECT findings in patients with primary mania. J Neuropsychiatry Clin Neurosci 1993; 5:379–383.

140. Mayberg HS, Starkstein SE, Morris PL, et al. Remote cortical hypometabolism following focal basal ganglia injury: relationship to secondary changes in mood. Abstr 540S. Neurology 1991; 41:266.

141. Bromfield EB, Altshuler L, Leiderman DB, et al. Cerebral metabolism and depression in patients with complex partial seizures. Arch Neurol 1992; 49:617–623.

142. Mayberg HS, Starkstein SE, Sadzot B, et al. Selective hypometabolism in the inferior frontal lobe in depressed patients with Parkinson's disease. Ann Neurol 1990; 28:57–64.

143. Mayberg HS, Starkstein SE, Peyser CE, Brandt J, Dannals RF, Folstein SE. Paralimbic frontal lobe hypometabolism in depression associated with Huntington's disease. Neurology 1992; 42:1791–1797.

144. Renshaw PF, Johnson KA, Worth JL, et al. New onset depression in patients with AIDS dementia complex (ADC) is associated with frontal lobe perfusion defects on HMPAO-SPECT scan. 31st Annual Meeting of the American College of Neuropsychopharmacology, San Juan, Puerto Rico, Dec 14–18, 1992. Abstract, p 94.

145. Andreason PJ, Altemus M, Zametkin AJ, King AC, Lucinio J, Cohen RM. Regional cerebral glucose metabolism in bulimia nervosa. Am J Psychiatry 1992; 149:1506–1513.

146. Volkow ND, Fowler JS, Hitzemann R, Wolf AP. Abnormal dopamine brain activity in cocaine abusers. 30th Annual Meeting of the American College of Neuropsychopharmacology, Dec 9–13, 1991. Abstract, p 30.

147. Mayberg HS, Robinson RG, Wong DF, et al. PET imaging of cortical S2 serotonin receptors after stroke: lateralized changes and relationship to depression. Am J Psychiatry 1988; 145:937–943.

148. Starkstein SE, Mayberg HS, Berthier ML, et al. Mania after brain injury: neuroradiological and metabolic findings. Ann Neurol 1990; 27:652–659.

149. Sharma R, Venkatasubramanian PN, Barany M, Davis JM. Proton magnetic resonance spectroscopy of the brain in schizophrenic and affective patients. Schizophr Res 1992; 8:43–49.

150. Charles HC, Lazeyras F, Krishnan KR, Boyko OB, Payne M, Moore D. Brain choline in depression: in vivo detection of potential pharmacodynamic effects of antidepressant therapy using hydrogen localized spectroscopy. Prog Neuropsychopharmacol Biol Psychiatry 1994; 18:1121–1127.

151. Kato T, Inubushi T, Takahashi S. Relationship of lithium concentrations in the brain measured by lithium-7 magnetic resonance spectroscopy to treatment response in mania. J Clin Psychopharmacol 1994; 14:330–335.

152. Kato T, Shioiri T, Inubushi T, Takahashi S. Brain lithium concentrations measured with lithium-7 magnetic resonance spectroscopy in patients with affective disorders: relationship to erythrocyte and serum concentrations. Biol Psychiatry 1993; 33:147–152.

153. Gyulai L, Wicklund SW, Greenstein R, et al. Measurement of tissue lithium concentration by lithium magnetic resonance spectroscopy in patients with bipolar disorder. Biol Psychiatry 1991; 29:1161–1170.

154. Kato T, Takahashi S, Shioiri T, Inubushi T. Alterations in brain phosphorous metabolism in bipolar disorder detected by in vivo 31P and 7Li magnetic resonance spectroscopy. J Affective Disord 1993; 27:53–59.

155. Deicken RF, Fein G, Weiner MW. Abnormal frontal lobe phosphorus metabolism in bipolar disorder. Am J Psychiatry 1995; 152:915–918.

156. Keshavan MS, Pettegrew JW, Panchalingam KS. Membrane phospholipids and lithium response in schizophrenia: a 31P-MRS study. Abstract VIII.B.1. Schizophrenia Res 1992; 6:134.
157. Yazici KM, Kapucu O, Erbas B, Varoglu E, Gulec C, Bekdik CF. Assessment of changes in regional cerebral blood flow in patients with major depression using the 99mTc-HMPAO single photon emission tomography method. Eur J Nucl Med 1992; 19:1038–1043.
158. Austin MP, Dougall N, Ross M, et al. Single photon emission tomography with 99mTc-exametazime in major depression and the pattern of brain activity underlying the psychotic/neurotic continuum. J Affective Disord 1992; 26:31–43.
159. DeLisi LE, Buchsbaum MS, Holcomb HH, et al. Clinical correlates of decreased anteroposterior metabolic gradients in positron emission tomography (PET) of schizophrenic patients. Am J Psychiatry 1985; 142:78–81.
160. Kishimoto H, Kuwahara H, Ohno S, et al. Three subtypes of chronic schizophrenia identified using 11C-glucose positron emission tomography. Psychiatry Res 1987; 21:285–292.
161. Volkow ND, Wolf AP, Van Gelder P, et al. Phenomenological correlates of metabolic activity in 18 patients with chronic schizophrenia. Am J Psychiatry 1987; 144:151–158.
162. Liddle PF, Friston KJ, Frith CD, Hirsch SR, Jones T, Frackowiak RS. Patterns of cerebral blood flow in schizophrenia. Br J Psychiatry 1992; 160:179–186.
163. Dolan RJ, Bench CJ, Liddle PF, et al. Dorsolateral prefrontal cortex dysfunction in the major psychoses: symptom or disease specificity? J Neurol Neurosurg Psychiatry 1993; 56:1290–1294.
164. Berman KF, Doran AR, Pickar D, Weinberger DR. Is the mechanism of prefrontal hypofunction in depression the same as in schizophrenia? Regional cerebral blood flow during cognitive activation. Br J Psychiatry 1993; 162:183–192.
165. Baxter LR Jr, Phelps ME, Mazziotta JC, et al. Cerebral metabolic rates for glucose in mood disorders: studies with positron emission tomography and fluorodeoxyglucose F 18. Arch Gen Psychiatry 1985; 42:441–447.
166. Hurwitz TA, Clark C, Murphy E, Klonoff H, Martin WR, Pate BD. Regional cerebral glucose metabolism in major depressive disorder. Can J Psychiatry 1990; 35:684–688.
167. Kumar A, Newberg A, Alavi A, Berlin J, Smith R, Reivich M. Regional cerebral glucose metabolism in late-life depression and Alzheimer disease: a preliminary positron emission tomography study. Proc Natl Acad Sci USA 1993; 90:7019–7023.
168. Mayberg HS, Lewis PJ, Regenold W, Wagner HN Jr. Paralimbic hypoperfusion in unipolar depression. J Nucl Med 1994; 35:929–934.
169. Goodwin GM, Austin MP, Dougall N, et al. State changes in brain activity shown by the uptake of 99mTc-exametazime with single photon emission tomography in major depression before and after treatment. J Affective Disord 1993; 29:243–253.

170. DeLisi LE, Holcomb HH, Cohen RM, et al. Positron emission tomography in schizophrenic patients with and without neuroleptic medication. J Cereb Blood Flow Metab 1985; 5:201–206.

171. Wong DF, Wagner HN, Tune LE, et al. Positron emission tomography reveals elevated D2 dopamine receptors in drug-naive schizophrenics. Science 1986; 234:1558–1563.

172. Farde L, Wiesel FA, Stone-Elander S, et al. D2 dopamine receptors in neuroleptic-naive schizophrenic patients: a positron emission tomography study with [11C]raclopride. Arch Gen Psychiatry 1990; 47:213–219.

173. Schlegel S, Aldenhoff JB, Eissner D, Lindner P, Nickel O. Regional cerebral blood flow in depression: associations with psychopathology. J Affective Disord 1989; 17:211–218.

174. Kumar A, Mozley D, Dunham C, et al. Semiquantitative I-123 IMP SPECT studies in late onset depression before and after treatment. Int J Geriatr Psychiatry 1991; 6:775–777.

175. Bench CJ, Friston KJ, Brown RG, Scott LC, Frackowiak RS, Dolan RJ. The anatomy of melancholia—focal abnormalities of cerebral blood flow in major depression. Psychol Med 1992; 22:607–615.

8
Linkage Studies of Bipolar Syndromes

Wade H. Berrettini
University of Pennsylvania, Philadelphia, Pennsylvania

I. INTRODUCTION

In this chapter, the genetic epidemiological evidence (twin, family, and adoption studies) that bipolar (BP) disorders are heritable are discussed. Attempts to localize genes that increase risk for BP disorders through molecular genetic linkage techniques are reviewed.

Geneticists have used the term *complex* to describe partially inherited syndromes that are common in the general population (risk of 1% or more), genetically heterogeneous, and characterized by reduced penetrance and/or prominent environmental influence (as determined from the monozygotic twin concordance rate). The term *complex* is used to distinguish these syndromes from Mendelian disorders, which are rare in the general population, and in which a single gene explains most (if not all) of the total variance in disease development within the population. BP disorder is a complex syndrome.

Family, twin and adoption studies have indicated the existence of genetic predisposition (for review, see Ref. 1). Heritability estimates (from twin studies) of BP illness vary from ~60 to 80% (1). This evidence for heritability of BP disorder has immediate clinical application, in genetic counseling, for example. Additionally, the heritability of BP disorder can (and should) shape the choice of pharmacotherapy for a BP or unipolar (UP) patient, if a similarly affected first-degree relative has had a good response to a certain medication regimen.

II. FAMILY STUDIES

Multiple-family studies of BP illness and UP disorder have been conducted over the past 30 years. More recent studies, using rigorously controlled methods, with modern diagnostic criteria and validated semistructured interviews (2–13), show familial aggregation for the disorder of the proband. The risk for BP and other disorders varies widely among family studies, for both relatives of BP probands and relatives of control probands, primarily because different diagnostic criteria are used.

Further, these studies report increased risk for UP illness among the first-degree relatives of BP patients compared to the risk for first-degree relatives of unaffected individuals. Similarly, these studies show an increased risk for BP disorder among the first-degree relatives of UP patients compared to the risk for BP disorder among first-degree relatives of unaffected individuals. These results support the hypothesis that UP and BP disorders may share some common genetic susceptibility factors. This hypothesis is also supported by twin studies.

III. TWIN STUDIES

Twin studies reveal evidence for heritability (Table 1). Monozygotic (MZ) twin-pair concordance is approximately 65% compared to the 14% figure for dizygotic (DZ) twin pairs, a significant difference. Just as general population risk will vary with diagnostic criteria, so will twin-concordance figures vary widely. As can be seen from Table 1, within a given study, the MZ twin concordance is consistently greater than DZ twin concordance. Because these figures are not age-corrected, they represent a conservative estimate of heritability. The probands include BP and UP patients.

Concordance in MZ twins increases with severity of the probands' diagnosis as follows: BPI probands, 80% concordance; BPII probands, 78% concordance; UP probands with three or more episodes, 59% concordance; and UP probands with fewer than three episodes, 33% concordance (20,21). A representative statistic for heritability from twin studies is 59% by the method of Holzinger 22). More recent twin studies (23–25), conducted with modern diagnostic criteria, validated semistructured interviews, and blinded assessments, confirm these earlier reports, although not without exception (26).

The results from the twin studies are consistent with a complex inheritance of these disorders. The reduced MZ concordance clearly suggests decreased penetrance of inherited susceptibility or the presence of phenocopies (nongenetic cases) among the MZ twins.

Table 1 Concordance Rates for Affective Illness in Twins

Ref.	Concordant pairs (total pairs %)			
	Monozygotic		Dizygotic	
Luxenburger, 1930 (14)	3/4	(75.0)	0/13	(0.0)
Rosanoff et al., 1935 (15)	16/23	(69.6)	11/67	(16.4)
Slater, 1953 (16)	4/7	(57.1)	4/17	(23.5)
Kallman, 1954 (17)	25/27	(92.6)	13/55	(23.6)
Harvald and Hauge, 1975 (18)	10/15	(66.7)	2/40	(5.0)
Allen et al., 1974 (19)	5/15	(33.3)	0/34	(0.0)
Bertelsen, 1977 (20)	32/55	(58.3)	9/52	(17.3)
Totals	95/146	(65.0)	39/278	(14.0)

Data not corrected for age. Diagnoses include bipolar and unipolar illness.

Among MZ twin pairs concordant for mood disorder, when one twin has a BP diagnosis, 20% of the ill cotwins have UP disorders (21). This observation supports the hypothesis that BP illness and UP disorders share some common genetic susceptibility factors. This observation has considerable clinical relevance. For example, it is a common practice for maintenance treatment of recurrent UP disorders to include the antidepressant drug that has helped the patient recover from episodes of UP disorders. For a patient with UP disorder who has a first-degree BP relative, preventive treatment with lithium is often helpful (27).

IV. ADOPTION STUDIES

Mendlewicz and Rainer (28) reported on a controlled adoption study of BP probands, including a control group of probands with poliomyelitis. The biological relatives of the BP probands had a 31% risk for BP or UP disorders, as opposed to 2% in the relatives of the control probands. The risk for affective disorder in biological relatives of adopted BP patients was similar to the risk in relatives of BP patients who were not adopted away (26%). Adoptive relatives do not show increased risk compared to relatives of control probands.

Wender et al. (29) and Cadoret (30) studied both UP and BP probands. Although evidence for genetic susceptibility was found, *adoptive* relatives of affective-disorder probands had a tendency to excess affective illness themselves, compared with the adoptive relatives of controls. Von Knorring et al. (31) did not find concordance in psychopathology between adoptees and biological relatives when examining the records of 56 adoptees with UP disorders. Heritable factors are more evident in BP syndromes than in UP disorders.

V. LINKAGE STUDIES

The complex inheritance of BP disorders raises difficulties in application of linkage techniques, because of genetic heterogeneity, variable age at onset, uncertain diagnostic boundaries, and reduced penetrance. These difficulties are not insurmountable, and substantial progress has been made recently. Before the recent progress is discussed, it is useful (from a historical perspective) to consider the earlier reports of BP linkage to two chromosomal regions, Xq28 and 11p15.

Cosegregation of BP disorder and clinically assessed color blindness in a single large kindred was described in 1969 (32). This report was followed by several confirmations employing clinically assessed color blindness and enzymatic determinations of G6PD deficiency (33–38). Linkage to both color blindness and G6PD deficiency is consistent because the G6PD locus is very near the red and green color vision loci on Xq28. These reports were on very few families in which BP disorder *and* G6PD deficiency or color blindness cosegregated. DNA markers for this region did not become widely available until the mid 1980s. All studies employing molecular (DNA marker genotyping) methods were not able to confirm this linkage (39–41). An initial report of Xq28 linkage in four Israeli kindreds (38), employing color blindness and G6PD deficiency, was not confirmed in those same pedigrees by molecular methods employing relevant Xq28 DNA markers (42). The dramatic decline from an initial lod score of 9 (38) to less than 2.5 (42) was due to several causes: new illness onsets, lack of information from the G6PD enzymatic assay, genotyping errors at the G6PD locus, and some G6PD genotypic determinations based solely on family history, a questionable method (43). It is noteworthy that no report of linkage to Xq28, using classic color blindness or G6PD deficiency, has been confirmed by molecular methods. There are no molecular linkage studies that support the presence of a BP susceptibility locus on Xq28.

The first report of BP linkage using molecular methods described evidence for a BP gene on 11p15.5 among the Old Order Amish (44). Decades of painstaking and elegant clinical research with the Old Order Amish by Professor Janice Egeland and colleagues has yielded some of the most carefully described BP kindreds in the world. Professor Egeland pioneered clinical methods of pedigree investigation that are now standard procedure throughout the field (45).

The original report of linkage on 11p15.5 (44) has been weakened by the failures to confirm the finding in numerous other pedigrees (46–52) and by evaluation of newly ascertained individuals in the original pedigree (53). The initial high enthusiasm for molecular genetic studies of BP disorders was dissipated by the failure of the Xq28 and 11p15 regions to yield definitive proof of major gene effects. In retrospect, given the complex inheritance pattern and phenotype of BP illness, expectations of common major gene effects (effects that increase or disease risk by a factor of 10 or more in a majority of patients) may have been naive. The necessary tools to genetically dissect a complex disease, such as BP disorder, became available only in the early 1990s.

Genetic linkage maps (54,55), consisting of thousands of highly polymorphic microsatellite loci (56), represent one such tool. These markers are amenable to semiautomated methods, allowing investigators to generate marker data for hundreds of loci for multiple families in short periods of time. Second, newer statistical methods to analyze such complex diseases at multiple loci were developed (57–59). These two sets of tools have provided investigators with the means to detect and confirm genes of minor or moderate effect. As investigators use these new tools in complex diseases, a flood of positive linkage reports for genes of minor effect can be expected. This situation has led mathematical geneticists to suggest guidelines for interpreting results of varying statistical significance (60–62). In these papers (60–62), one concept is paramount: independent confirmation. Loci for complex diseases must be confirmed by independent researchers before validity can be assumed, no matter what the initial statistical evidence for linkage. Recognition of the need for independent confirmation in genetically heterogeneous and complex disorders has led to mathematical treatments of confirmations.

Suarez (63) simulated initial detection of a susceptibility locus for a complex disorder caused in part by six equally frequent independent (unlinked) disease loci. He then studied the waiting time until a second simulated investigation detected the same susceptibility locus, as opposed to one of the five other loci. He found that a larger sample size and a long waiting time are needed for confirmation of a previously detected locus, compared to the size needed for initial detection of the first locus. This result may be expected intuitively, since sampling variation and population differences may allow for easier detection of other loci instead of the locus initially reported. Independent pedigree samples might detect one of the other five loci, as opposed to the one locus initially detected. The immediate result of these simulations (63) is the conclusion that universal agreement regarding reported linkages to BP illness with not be observed, even among those studies that have high power to detect loci of moderate to minor effects. Despite these caveats, when two or more independent investigators find significant evidence for linkage in independent series of pedigrees, it is reasonable to assume validity (60–62). Several groups have reported initial observations of BP susceptibility loci that have been confirmed independently.

Berrettini et al. (64,65) described a pericentromeric chromosome 18 BP susceptibility locus among Caucasian kindreds of European ancestry, using affected sibling pair (ASP) and affected pedigree member (APM) methods. With D18S53, S45, S37, and S40 marker data, multipoint APM and ASP yielded $p = ~10^{-5}$ (65). Independent confirmation on this pericentromeric chromosome 18 locus in BP kindreds of European ancestry was described by Stine et al. (66) at D18S37 ($p = 0.0002$), D18S53, and D18S40. Stine et al. (66) also reported linkage to 18q21 markers with both the lod score method (lod is 3.51 for D18S41) and the ASP method (0.00002 at D18S41). The data of Stine et al. (66) may be most consistent with a dominant 18q21BP susceptibility locus and a recessive pericentromeric locus (67).

Stine et al. (66,67) made a crucial observation that their evidence for linkage to 18q21 and the chromosome 18 pericentromeric region occurred in BP families in which disease alleles appeared to be *paternally* transmitted. When the data of Berrettini et al. (64,65) are analyzed by sex of the transmitting parent, the results clearly indicate that *paternal* kindreds explain the positive statistics, whereas no excess allele-sharing is observed among the families in which only *maternal* transmission has occurred (68). Pericentromeric evidence for linkage among *paternal* BP kindreds has been confirmed by Conrad Gilliam in an analysis of ~50 BP kindreds, in which a lod score of 2.68 among *paternal* kindreds was observed at D18S53 (69). Thus, there are three independent studies consistent with a pericentromeric chromosome 18 BP susceptibility locus in *paternal* kindreds.

In an observation that raises questions about the validity of nosological classification, Wildenauer and colleagues (70) at the University of Bonn have reported a lod score of ~3.5 at D18S53 among German and Israeli kindreds with schizophrenia and schizoaffective disorder. An analysis based on the sex of the transmitting parent was not reported. This observation by the Bonn group suggests that the pericentromeric chromosome 18 linkage may not be specific for BP disorder. One other linkage evaluation of this region with schizophrenia kindreds did not reveal evidence for a susceptibility locus (71).

Berrettini et al. (65) estimate that risk for BP disorder is increased by a factor of 1.5–2 for the chromosome 18 pericentromeric linkage. If this estimate is valid, attempts to confirm this linkage must be based on a minimum 100 affected sibling pairs (ASPs), because smaller sample sizes do not have sufficient power to detect a locus of such magnitude. For example, the data of Stine et al. (66,67) involved ~110 affected sibling pairs. Inadequate power to detect a locus of moderate effect may be the most cogent explanation for some negative attempts to confirm this locus (72). Moreover, it is strongly recommended that analysis of chromosome 18 marker data should proceed with the sex of the transmitting parent as a covariate. Some studies of adequate numbers of affected sibling pairs have failed to detect this locus (73,74), as would be expected, given the simulations of Suarez (63).

An observation relevant to the positive chromosome 18 reports is that *paternal* transmission is less frequent than expected in multiplex BP kindreds, as reported by McMahon et al. (75). This report of excess *maternal* transmission among multiplex BP kindreds has been confirmed by Gershon et al. (68). The relative dearth of *paternal* transmission may derive from genetic heterogeneity of BP disorder and in imprinting of specific BP susceptibility loci, such that paternally transmitted BP susceptibility alleles are expressed less frequently, or, conversely, *maternally* transmitted alleles express BP vulnerability more often.

Linkage of the phosphofructokinase (PFKL) locus on 21q21 to BP kindreds was reported by Straub et al. (76) in 1994. They described an extended BP pedigree with a lod score of 3.4. Moreover, among ~50 BP kindreds, APM analysis yielded data consistent with linkage ($p < 0.0003$ for PFKL). Confirmatory evidence has been reported by Gurling et al. (77), who conducted a two-locus analysis of genotypic data from 21q21 and 11p15.5 among Icelandic and English BP families. This 21q21 BP susceptibility locus also has been confirmed by Detera-Wadleigh et al. (78), who employed multipoint ASP analyses ($p < 0.001$). This latter evidence for linkage to chromosome 21q21 derives mostly from pedigrees in which disease alleles are *maternally* transmitted, suggesting that parent-of-origin may be a criterion by which to distinguish chromosome 21 BP kindreds from the chromosome 18 families.

A third region of interest for BP susceptibility is Xq26–27. Linkage to the factor IX (FIX) locus was reported by Mendlewicz et al. (79) in 1987 in a study of Belgian BP kindreds. The maximum lod score was 3.1 at 10 cM from FIX. Lucotte et al. (80) described a single large French BP family with a maximal lod score of ~3.5. Multipoint analysis suggested that the locus was centromeric to FIX. Two reports of cosegregation of FIX deficiency (hemophilia B) and BP disorder in single kindreds followed (81,82), lending further support for a BP susceptibility locus centromeric to FIX. However, these reports were less than convincing, because they involve either a single or a few DNA markers with low polymorphism content or clinically assessed FIX deficiency assessed in small numbers of affected individuals. Further evidence for BP linkage to this region (a lod score of 3.54 to DXS994) was reported by Pekkarinen et al. (83), who employed multiple microsatellite DNA markers in the region near HPRT (which is ~10 cM centromeric to F9) in a large Finnish BP kindred. The BP families originally described as linked to F9 (79–82) should be reanalyzed using microsatellite DNA markers near hypoxanthine phosphoribosyl transferase (HPRT).

This Xq26 BP susceptibility locus near HPRT cannot be seen as support for the prior positive color vision and G6PD reports (32–38), since the HPRT locus is ~50% recombination from the G6PD locus (84). All these positive Xq26–27 reports (79–83) used lod score methods. Confirmation of this Xq26 BP susceptibility locus should be attempted by X-linked nonparametric analysis methods as well (85).

Genome scans for linkage to BP disorders by several groups are proceeding toward completion, and initial positive observations have been published (86–88). Blackwood et al. (86) reported on a single large Scottish kindred that showed linkage (lod 4.1 at D4S394) to 4p DNA markers, near the alpha 2c adrenergic and D5 dopaminergic receptor genes. Weakly positive lod scores in several smaller kindreds of the same ethnic origins were reported. No mutations were found in mutation scanning of the dopamine D5 receptor gene. This report requires independent confirmation for validity.

A genomic scan of multiple kindreds from the Old Order Amish (87) included modest evidence for BP susceptibility loci on 6 (lod = 2.5 at D6S7), 13 (lod = 1.4 at D13S1), and 15 (lod = 1.1 at D15S45). Confirmation of these loci is required.

Freimer et al. (88) reported linkage disequilibrium studies of two extended Costa Rican BP pedigrees (with an apparent common founder). These authors found haplotype sharing for markers over a 10 cM region of 18q22 (chi-square statistic at D18S469 = 16, p = 0.0009; for D18S70, p = 0.0005). Lod score analysis of these markers yielded weakly positive statistics, and a joint linkage and association analysis suggested a BP susceptibility locus on 18q22. The BP susceptibility locus in the Costa Rican pedigrees is ~15 cM more telomeric than the 18q21 locus described by Stine et al. (66,67). The simplest and most conservative conclusion concerning these two reports is that the same locus has been detected, but the exact position of the locus, relative to genetically mapped markers, is imprecise. The ~15 cM location difference in evidence for linkage raises concern, but it should be recalled that the breast cancer locus, BRCA1, was characterized by a peak lod score (89) in 1990 at a location ~20 cM from the position at which it was cloned (90).

Linkage studies of BP disorders are entering a more mature phase of investigation. Independent investigators, using molecular methods, have convergent findings for several genomic regions. These provocative results will surely lead to disease-gene definition in the next several years.

VI. SUMMARY

Twin, family, and adoption studies of BP disorder are consistent with substantial heritability, which may be as high as 80%. Molecular linkage studies of BP illness, which have been confirmed independently in each case, are consistent with at least four BP susceptibility loci on 18p, 18q, Xq26, and 21q. Each of these loci represents genes of small to moderate effect, in that linkage is detectable in a minority of BP kindreds, and/or attributable risk is a small fraction of total familial risk. Gene identification will occur for at least one of these loci in the next several years, allowing for new insights into the pathophysiology of this common and complex disorder.

ACKNOWLEDGMENTS

A United States Public Health Service, National Institute of Mental Health, grant to WHB (MH 49181) supported the preparation of this chapter.

REFERENCES

1. McGuffin P, Katz R. The genetics of depression and manic-depressive disorder. Br J Psychiatry 1989; 155:294–304.
2. Rice J, Reich T, Andreasen NC, Endicott J, Van Eerdewegh M, Fisherman R, Hirschfield RMA, Klerman GL. The familial transmission of bipolar illness. Arch Gen Psychiatry 1987; 44:441–447.
3. Baron M, Gruen R, Anis L, Kane J. Schizoaffective illness, schizophrenia and affective disorders: morbidity risk and genetic transmission. Acta Psychiatrica Scand 1983; 65:253–262.
4. Winokur G, Tsuang MT, Crowe RR. The Iowa 500: affective disorder in relatives of manic and depressed patients. Am J Psychiatry 1982; 139:209–212.

5. Helzer JE, Winokur G. A family interview study of male manic-depressives. Arch Gen Psychiatry 1974; 31:73–77.

6. James, NM, Chapman CJ. A genetic study of bipolar affective disorder. Br J Psychiatry 1975; 126:449–456.

7. Johnson GFS, Leeman MM. Analysis of familial factors in bipolar affective illness. Arch Gen Psychiatry 1977; 34:1074–1083.

8. Angst J, Frey R, Lohmeyer R, Zerben-Rubin E. Bipolar manic depressive psychoses: results of a genetic investigation. Hum Gener 1980; 55:237–254.

9. Taylor MA, Berenbaum SA, Jampala VC, Cloninger CR. Are schizophrenia and affective disorder related?: preliminary data from a family study. Am J Psychiatry 1993; 150:278–285.

10. Winokur G, Coryell W, Keller M, Endicott J, Leon A. A family study of manic-depressive (bipolar I) disease: is it a distinct illness separable from primary unipolar depression? Arch Gen Psychiatry 1995; 52(5):367–373.

11. Maier W, Lichtermann D, Minges J, Hallmayer J, Heun R, Benkert O, Levinson DF. Continuity and discontinuity of affective disorders and schizophrenia: results of a controlled family study. Arch Gen Psychiatry 1993; 50:871–883.

12. Gershon ES, Hamovit J, Guroff JJ, Dibble E, Leckman JF, Sceery W, Targum SD, Nurnberger JI Jr, Goldin LR, Bunney WE Jr. A family study of schizoaffective, bipolar I, bipolar II, unipolar, and normal control probands. Arch Gen Psychiatry 1982; 39(10):1157–1167.

13. Weissman MM, Gershon ES, Kidd KK, Prusoff BA, Leckman JF, Dibble E, Hamovit J, Thompson WD, Pauls DL, Guroff JJ. Psychiatric disorders in the relatives of probands with affective disorder. Arch Gen Psychiatry 1984; 41:13–21.

14. Luxenburger H. Psychiatrisch-neurologische Zwillingspathologie. Zentralblatt fur die gesamte Neurologie und Psychiatrie 1930; 56:145–180.

15. Rosanoff AJ, Handy L, Plesset IR. The etiology of manic-depressive syndromes with special reference to their occurrence in twins. Am J Psychiatry 1935; 91:725–762.

16. Slater E. Psychotic and neurotic illness in twins. Medical Research Council Special Report Series no. 278. London: Her Majesty's Stationery Office, 1953.

17. Kallman F. In: Hoch PH, Zubin J, eds. Depression. New York: Grune & Stratton, 1954:1–24.

18. Harvald B, Hauge M. In: Neal JV, Shaw MW, Shull WJ, eds. Genetics and the Epidemiology of Chronic Diseases. PHS Publication no. 1163. Washington, DC: U.S. Department of Health, Education and Welfare, 1975:61–76.

19. Allen MG, Cohen S, Pollin W, Greenspan SI. Affective illness in veteran twins: a diagnostic review. Am J Psychiatry 1974; 131:1234–1239.

20. Bertelsen A, Harvald B, Hauge M. A Danish twin study of manic-depressive disorders. Br J Psychiatry 1977; 130:330–351.

21. Bertelsen A. In: Schou M, Stromgren E, eds. Origins, Prevention and Treatment of Affective Disorders. London: Academic Press, 1979:227–239.

22. Holzinger KJ. The relative effect of nature and nurture influences on twin differences. J Educational Psycho 1929; 20:241.

23. Kendler KS, Neale MC, Kessler RC, Health AC, Eaves LJ. A population based twin study of major depression in women: the impact of varying definitions of illness. Arch Gen Psychiatry 1992; 49:257–266.

24. Kendler KS, Petersen N, Johnson L, Neale MC, Mathe AA. A pilot Swedish twin study of affective illness, including hospital and population ascertained subsamples. Arch Gen Psychiatry 1993; 50:699–706.

25. McGuffin P, Katz R, Watkins S, Rutherford J. A hospital-based twin registry study of the heritability of DSM-IV unipolar depression. Arch Gen Psychiatry 1996; 53:129–136.

26. Andrews G, Stewart G, Allen R, Henderson AS. The genetics of six neurotic disorders: a twin study. J Affective Disord 1990; 19:23–29.

27. Souza FGM, Goodwin FK. Lithium treatment and prophylaxis in unipolar depression: a meta-analysis. Br J Psychiatry 1991; 158:666–675.

28. Mendlewicz, J, Rainer, JD. Adoption study supporting genetic transmission in manic-depressive illness. Nature 1977; 368(5618):327–329.

29. Wender H, Kety SS. Rosenthal D, Schulsinger F, Ortmann J, Lunde I. Psychiatric disorders in the biological and adoptive families of adopted individuals with affective disorders. Arch Gen Psychiatry 1986; 43:923–929.

30. Cadoret RJ. Evidence for genetic inheritance of primary affective disorder in adoptees. Am J Psychiatry 1978; 135(4):463–466.

31. Von Knorring AL, Cloninger, CR, Bohman M, Sigvardsson A. An adoption study of depressive disorders and substance abuse. Arch Gen Psychiatry 1983; 40:943–950.

32. Winokur G, Clayton PJ, Reich T: Manic-Depressive Illness. St. Louis: CV Mosby, 1969:112–125.

33. Mendlewicz J, Fleiss JL. Linkage studies with X-chromosome markers in bipolar manic-depressive and unipolar (depressive) illness. Biol Psychiatry 1974; 9:261–294.

34. Mendlewicz J, Linkowski P, Guroff JJ, Van Praag HM. Color blindness linkage to manic-depressive illness. Arch Gen Psychiatry 1979; 36:1442–1447.

35. Baron M. Linkage between an X-chromosome marker (deutan color blindness) and bipolar affective illness. Arch Gen Psychiatry 1977; 34:721–725.

36. Mendlewicz J, Linkowski P, Wilmotte J. Linkage between glucose-6-phosphate dehyrogenase deficiency and manic-depressive psychosis. Br J Psychiatry 1980; 137:337–342.

37. DelZompo M, Bochetta A, Goldin LR, Corsini GU. Linkage between X-chromosome markers and manic-depressive illness: two Sardinian pedigrees. Acta Psychiat Scand 1984; 70:282–287.

38. Baron M, Risch N, Hamburger R, Mandel B, Kushner S, Newman M, Drumer D, Belmaker RH. Genetic linkage between X-chromosome markers and bipolar affective illness. Nature 1987; 326:289–292.

39. Berrettini WH, Goldin LR, Gelernter J, Gejman PV, Gershon ES, Detera-Wadleigh S. X-chromosome markers and manic-depressive illness: rejection of linkage to Xq28 in nine bipolar pedigrees. Arch Gen Psychiatry 1990; 47:336–373.

40. Del Zompo M, Bocchetta A, Ruiu S, Goldin LR, Berrettini WH. Association and linkage studies of affective disorders. In: Racagni G, Brunello N, Fukuda T, eds. Biological Psychiatry. Vol 2. New York: Elsevier, 1991:446–448.

41. Smyth C, Kalsi G, Brynjolfsson J, Petursson H, Curtis D, Rifkin L, Murphy P, Moloney E, O'Neill J, Gurling HMD. A test of the Xq27–q28 linkage in bipolar and unipolar families selected for absent male-to-male transmission. Psychiatric Genet 1995; 5(suppl):S84.

42. Baron M, Freimer NF, Risch N, et al. Diminished support for linkage between manic-depressive illness and X-chromosome markers in three Israeli pedigrees. NatGenet 1993; 3:49–55.

43. Straub R, Gilliam C. Genetic linkage studies of bipolar affective disorder. Genome Analysis 1993; 6:77–99.

44. Egeland JA, Gerhard DS, Pauls DL, Sussex JN, Kidd KK, Allen CR, Hostetter AM, Housman DE. Bipolar affective disorder linked to DNA markers on chromosome 11. Nature. 1987; 325:783–787.

45. Egeland JA, et al. The impact of diagnoses on genetic linkage study for bipolar affective disorders among the Amish. Psychiatric Genet 1990; 1:5–18.

46. Detera-Wadleigh SD, Berrettini WH, Goldin LR, Boorman D, Anderson S, Gershon ES. Close linkage of c-Harvey-ras-1 and the insulin gene to affective disorder is ruled out in three North American pedigrees. Nature 1987; 325:806–808.

47. Detera-Wadleigh SD, Hsieh WT, Berrettini WH, Goldin LR, Rollins DY, Muniec D, Grewal R, Guroff JJ, Turner G, Coffman D, Barrick J, Mills K, Murray J, Donohue SJ, Klein DC, Sanders J, Nurnberger JI Jr, Gershon ES. Genetic linkage mapping for a susceptibility locus to bipolar illness: chromosomes 2,3,4,7,9,10p,11p,22, and Xpter. Neuropsychiatric Genet 1994; 54:206–218.

48. Coon H, Jensen S, Hoff M, Holik J, Plaetke R, Reimherr F, Wender P, Leppert M, Byerley W. A genome-wide search for genes predisposing to manic-depression assuming autosomal dominant inheritance. Am J Hum Genet 1993; 52:619–634.

49. Curtis D, Sherrington R, Brett P, Holmes DS, Kalsi G, Brynjolfsson J, Petursson H, Rifkin L, Murphy P, Moloney E, Melmer G, Gurling HMD. Genetic linkage analysis of manic-depression in Iceland. J Royal Soc Med 1993; 86:506–510.

50. Hodgkinson S, Sherrington R, Gurling HMD, Marchbanks RM, Reeders SST, Mallet J, Petursson H, Brunjolfsson J. Molecular evidence for heterogeneity in manic-depression. Nature 1987; 325:805–807.

51. Gill M, McKeon P, Humphries P. Linkage analysis of manic-depression in an Irish family using H-ras 1 and INS DNA markers. J Med Genet 1988; 25:634–637.

52. Mitchell P, Waters B, Morrison N, Shine J, Donald J, Eissman J. Close linkage of bipolar disorder to chromosome 11 markers is excluded in two large Australian pedigrees. J Affective Disord 1991; 20:23–32.

53. Kelsoe JR, Ginns EI, Egeland JA, Gerhard DS, Goldstein AM, Bale SJ, Pauls DL, Long RT, Kidd KK, Conte G, Housman DE, Paul SM. Re-evaluation of the

linkage relationship between chromosome 11p loci and the gene for bipolar affective disorder in the Old Order Amish. Nature 1989; 342:238–243.

54. Dib C, Faure S, Fizames C, Samson D, Drouot N, Vignal A, Millasseau P, Marc S, Hazan J, Seboun E, Lathrop M, Gyapay G, Morissette J, Weissenbach J. A comprehensive genetic map of the human genome based on 5264 microsatellites. Nature 1996; 380:152–154.

55. The Utah Marker Development Group. A collection of ordered tetranucleotide repeat markers from the human genome. Am J Hum Genet 1995; 57:619–628.

56. Weber JL, May PE. Abundant class of human DNA polymorphisms which can be typed using the polymerase chain reaction. Am J Hum Genet 1989; 44:388–396.

57. Weeks, DE, Lange K. A multilocus extension of the affected-pedigree-member method of linkage analysis. Am J Hum Genet 1992; 50:859–868.

58. Kruglyak L, Lander ES. A nonparametric approach for mapping quantitative trait loci. Genetics 1995; 139:1421–1428.

59. Goldgar DE, Lewis CU, Gholami K. Analysis of discrete phenotypes using a multipoint identity by descent method: application to Alzheimer's disease. Genet Epidemiol 1993; 10:383–388.

60. Lander E, Kruglyak L. Genetic dissection of complex traits: guidelines for interpreting and reporting linkage results. Nature Genet 1995; 11:241–247.

61. Thompson G. Identification of complex disease genes: progress and paradigms. Nature Genet 1994; 8:108–110.

62. Lander ES, Shork NJ. Genetic dissection of complex traits. Science 1994; 265:2037–2048.

63. Suarez B. In: Gershon ES, Cloninger CR, eds. Genetic Approaches to Mental Disorders. Proceedings of the 82nd Annual Meeting of the American Psychopathological Association, Inc. Washington, DC: American Psychiatric Press, 1994:63–76.

64. Berrettini WH, Ferraro TN, Goldin LR, Weeks D, Detera-Wadleigh S, Nurnberger JI Jr, Gershon ES. Chromosome 18 DNA markers and manic-depressive illness: evidence for a susceptibility gene. Proc Natl Acad Sci 1994; 91:5918–5921.

65. Berrettini WH, Ferraro TN, Choi H, Goldin LR, Detera-Wadleigh SD, Muniec D, Hsieh WT, Hoehe MR, Guroff JJ, Kazuba D, Nurnberger JI Jr, Gershon ES. Linkage studies of bipolar illness. Arch Gen Psychiatry. In press.

66. Stine OC, Xu J, Koskela R, McMahon FJ, Gschwend M, Friddle C, Clark CD, McInnis MG, Simpson SG, Breschel TS, Vishio E, Riskin K, Feilotter H, Chen E, Folstein S, Meyers DA, Botstein D, Marr TG, DePaulo JR. Evidence for linkage of bipolar disorder to chromosome 18 with a parent-of-origin effect. Am J Hum Genet 1995; 57:1384–1394.

67. Stine OC, Xu J, Koskela R et al. Evidence for linkage of bipolar disorder to HC 18 with a parent-of-origin effect. Biol Psychiatry 1996; 39:539.

68. Gershon ES, Badner JA, Ferraro TN, Detera-Wadleigh S, Berrettini WH. Maternal inheritance and chromosome 18 allele sharing in unilineal bipolar illness pedigrees. Am J Med Genet 1996; 67:202–207.

69. Gilliam TC, Knowles JA, Baron M. Genome wide search for genes predisposing to bipolar affective disorder. In: Function and Dysfunction in the Nervous System. Cold Spring Harbor, NY: Cold Spring Harbor Laboratory Press, 1996. In press.

70. Wildenauer DB, Albus M, Lerer B, Maier W. Searching for susceptibility genes in schizophrenia by genetic linkage analysis. In: Function and Dysfunction in the Nervous System. Cold Spring Harbor, NY: Cold Spring Harbor Laboratory Press, 1996. In press.

71. DeLisi LE, Lofthouse R, Lehner T, Morganti C, Vita A, Shields G, Bass N, Ott J, Crow TJ. Failure to find a chromosome 18 pericentromeric linkage in families with schizophrenia. Neuropsychiatric Genet. In press.

72. Pauls DL, Ott J, Paul SM, Allen CR, Fann CSJ, Carulli JP, Falls KM, Bouthillier CA, Gravius TC, Keith TP, Egeland JA, Ginns EI. Linkage analyses of chromosome 18 markers do not identify a major susceptibility locus for bipolar affective disorder in the Old Order Amish. Am J Hum Genet 1995; 57:636–643.

73. Smith C, Kalsi G, Brynjolfsson J, Sherrington RS, O'Neill J, Curtis D, Rifkin L, Murphy P, Petursson H, Gurling HMD. Linkage analysis of manic-depression (bipolar affective disorder) in Icelandic and British kindreds using markers on the short arm of chromosome 18. Arch Gen Psychiatry. In press.

74. Kelsoe JR, Sadovnick AD, Kristbjarnarson H, Bergesch P, Mroczkowski-Parker Z, Flodman P, Rapaport MH, Mirow AL, Egeland JA, Spence MA, Remick RA. Genetic linkage studies of bipolar disorder and chromosome 18 markers in North America, Icelandic and Amish pedigrees. Psychiatric Genetics 1995; 5:S17.

75. McMahon FJ, Stine OC, Meyers DA, Simpson SG, DePaulo JR. Patterns of maternal transmission in bipolar affective disorder. Am J Hum Genet 1995; 56:1277–1286.

76. Straub RE, Lehner T, Luo Y, Loth JE, Shao W, Sharpe L, Alexander JR, Das K, Simon R, Fieve RR, Endicott J, Gilliam TC, Baron M. A possible vulnerability locus for bipolar affective disorder on chromosome 21q22.3 Nature Genet 1994; 8:291–296.

77. Gurling H, Smyth C, Kalsi G, Moloney E, Rifkin L, O'Neill J, Murphy P. Linkage findings in bipolar disorder. Nature Genet 1995; 10:8–9.

78. Detera-Wadleigh SD, Badner JA, Goldin LR, Berrettini WH, Sanders AR, Rollins DY, Turner G, Moses T, Haerian H, Muniec D, Nurnberger JI Jr, Gershon ES. Analysis of linkage to bipolar illness on chromosome 21q. Am J Hum Genet 1996; 58:1279–1285.

79. Mendlewicz J, Simon P, Sevy S, Charon F, Brocas H, Legros S, Vassart G. Polymorphic DNA marker on X-chromosome and manic depression. Lancet 1987; i:1230–1232.

80. Lucotte G, Landoulsi A, Berriche S, David F, Babron MC. Manic depressive illnessis linked to factor IX in a French pedigree. Ann Genet 1992; 35:93–95.

81. Gill M, Castle D, Duggan C. Cosegregation of Christmas disease and major affective disorder in a pedigree. Br J Psychiatry 1992; 160:112–114.

82. Craddock N, Owen M. Christmas disease and major affective disorder. Br J Psychiatry 1992; 160:715.

83. Pekkarinen P, Terwilliger J, Bredbacka P-E, Lonnqvist J, Peltonen L. Evidence of a susceptibility locus for familial bipolar disorder on Xq26. Genome Research. In press.

84. NIH/CEPH Collaborative Mapping Group. A comprehensive genetic linkage map of the human genome. Science 1992; 258:67–86.

85. Cordell HJ, Kawaguchi Y, Todd JA, Farrall M: An extension of the maximum lod score method to X-linked loci. Ann Hum Genet 59:435–449, 1995.

86. Blackwood DHR, He L, Morris SW, et al. A locus for bipolar affective disorder on chromosome 4p. Nat Genet 1996; 12:427–430.

87. Ginns EI, Ott J, Egeland JA, et al. A genome-wide search for chromosomal loci linked to bipolar affective disorder in the Old Order Amish. Nat Genet 1996; 12:431–435.

88. Freimer NB, Reus VI, Escamilla MA et al. Genetic mapping using haplotype, association and linkage methods suggests a locus for severe bipolar disorder (BPI) at 18q22–q23. Nat Genet 1996; 12:436–441.

89. Hall JM, Lee MK, Newman B, Morrow JE, Anderson LE, Nuey B, King M-C. Linkage of early-onset familial breast cancer to chromosome 17q21. Science 1990; 250(4988):1684–1690.

90. Futreal PA, et al. BRCA1 mutations in primary breast and ovarian carcinomas. Science 1994; 266:120–122.

9

Toward an Integrated Biological Model of Bipolar Disorder

Charles L. Bowden
The University of Texas Health Science Center at San Antonio, San Antonio, Texas

I. INTRODUCTION

This chapter addresses the evidence from individual biological systems for biochemical or other etiopathological system evidence for a biological substrate for bipolar disorder. The main issue to be addressed here is evidence for possible cross-system links, which could come to provide an integrative understanding of the biopathophysiology of bipolar disorder and link this to the pharmacodynamic mechanisms of currently available treatments for bipolar disorder. This book includes up-to-date reviews of each currently recognized major biological system implicated in bipolar disorder. This chapter will only repeat and draw on those data insofar as there is some evidence linking two or more systems.

Additionally, because there is no suitable model system in vitro or in animals for bipolar disorder, I have largely limited the evidence for review here to that which emanates in part from studies of patients with the illness. This seems justified for two reasons. In the absence of data from patients with bipolar disorder, there is no adequate criterion to determine inclusion or exclusion of a result. Therefore, information would likely be included that is strictly speculative, possibly misleading, or just "noise." The second reason is that bipolar disorder is a uniquely promising disease for biological study in the late '90s, especially given a concatenation of developments. Because it is reliably diagnosed, one has great confidence that a patient diagnosed as having bipolar I disorder by a well-trained psychiatrist, using structured interview approaches such as the SADS or SCID, indeed has the disease. The main reason for this is the diagnostic specificity of a full manic episode, which is unlikely to be phenotypically mimicked by another disorder. In contrast, milder forms of the illness—e.g., hypomania, bipolar II disorder, or cyclothymia—may either escape detection or be identified as false-positive cases. Although these are important for study, especially in genetic or familial studies, the greater possibility of both false-positives and false-negatives argues against including them in most biological studies of bipolar disorder. Parenthetically, if a biological measure comes to have sufficient diagnostic utility, its use in addition to symptomatic and illness-course measures could allow more reliable studies of the spectrum of bipolar disorders (1).

Bipolar disorder thus stands in relatively sharp contrast to most other psychiatric disorders with a biological substrate but for which use of current diagnostic criteria may result in false-positive inclusion of subjects in samples. Bipolar disorder is also advantageous for biological study in that genetic transmissivity is high, allowing study of biological hypotheses, as well as highly promising recent studies of loci and paths of genetic transmission (2,3).

Bipolar disorder has early life onset, therefore allowing study in individuals not necessarily confounded by disorders of aging or their treatments. In almost all persons, the disease is high recurrent, usually (but not always) with relatively discrete episodes. This provides opportunities to study the illness prospectively within the same individual, thereby diminishing the variance inherent in studies limited to subjects in different groups assessed cross-sectionally. Finally, the presence of both manic and depressed episodes (and mixtures thereof) allows for comparisons with directional illness episodes, and, at least for depressed phase episodes, comparison with major depression as a control condition.

Additionally, two quite effective antimanic, mood-stabilizing drugs—lithium and valproate—allow potential testing of biological hypotheses in relationship to drug effect, including preclinical paradigms in which the investigator can exercise greater control over the variables under study. For this reason, I have included in this review information from preclinical studies of systems for which there is some evidence for diagnostic or illness state abnormality in bipolar disorder, or for pharmacodynamic effects of drugs that have antimanic, antidepressant, or mood-stabilizing properties. Unfortunately, although antidepressants have been extensively studied in major depression, both clinical trial and pharmacodynamic studies in specifically bipolar depressed patients are few in number, and nearly all have been limited to small samples.

II. ORGANIZING OBSERVATIONS

In all the systems reviewed here, life usually operates around the Kd. Phrased in the vernacular, quite low concentrations, relative to the concentration range possible for a compound, are usually effective functionally. Systems to reduce concentrations begin to come into play above the Kd, and in most of these systems there is some redundancy. This basic principle also fits in with signal amplification. Quite low concentrations of a compound may yield large effects. As an example, 10^{-10} M epinephrine yields a cyclic AMP signal of 10^{-6} M only several steps removed in signaling cascade—a signal amplification of 10,000-fold.

For most fundamental systems, controls are inherently multifactorial. This is a conservative strategy, but one that adds complexity to the study of a disease such as bipolar disorder. The conservative aspect is that the cell is always sensing a variety of inputs, rather than responding to one; therefore no single system disruption is likely to be fatal. This is why one does not see the dramatic biochemical findings of an inborn error of metabolism in bipolar disorder or other common, severe diseases. Were such the case, life, literally, would not be possible. Several biochemical tools are important because they fully obliterate a system, e.g., conotoxin and pertussis toxin. Such substances almost invariably have potentially fatal effects in nature. Cone mollusks stun their victims with conotoxin prior to eating them, and whooping cough, or pertussis, is a potentially fatal infectious disease.

The above concept of multifactorial inputs and controls does not mean that one should criticize the scientist who studies one relatively isolated system. One of the strengths of molecular biology has been the ability of scientists to ask questions that yield unequivocal answers, which means reducing, over time, alternative explanations for an event. However, there is now enough evidence in support of important roles for the processes described here that studies that examine two, three, or four systems now have the potential to advance our knowledge in epochal, not just incremental, ways.

Another implication of these studies is that inhibitory processes are generally more important than stimulatory ones. If low concentrations of a substance are sufficient for most processes, it is essential that there be systems to act antagonistically to the system if concentration rises beyond the zone of optimal activity. The role of presynaptic autoreceptors is a simple example of the former, Gi-proteins of the latter.

This leads to another little-discussed concept. Although we may describe numerous control points across systems, as well as within a single system, this does not mean that the value, or amplification potential, of each is equivalent. Thus for monoamines, control points include uptake blockade, autoreceptor agonism, heteroreceptor effects, and blockade of degradative enzymes (MAO, COMT). But inhibition of MAO has a much more robust effect than blockade of COMT and uptake inhibition is generally more robust than autoreceptor agonism. Most of the reasons for these important quantitative differences are known, but not germane to this chapter. This concept is almost certainly a factor in the existence of numerous mood-altering drugs that block uptake but few that act solely on the autoreceptor.

Methodological advances have revolutionized the study of diseases such as bipolar disorder over the past quarter century. Almost none of the information presented in this book was known in 1965, as can be recognized by the dates of the references. Nevertheless, methodological difficulties hamper progress. At the clinical level, there is some understandable bias toward studying chemicals that can be frozen, thus obtaining advantages of batching of sample, and potential shipment across centers. This is unfeasible for analyses that require live tissue, such as ionized calcium flux in response to agonist stimulation. Also, whereas some methods translate well from basic to clinical research—e.g., G-protein and monoamine metabolite measurement—others do not, e.g., patch clamp studies.

Experimental evidence regarding biochemical factors in the etiology and pathophysiology of bipolar disorder suffers from the small number of patients studied in most reports, and the small number of reports on a particular variable. To take as an example a variable among the most extensively studied, norepinephrine, the three open studies of lithium's effects on CSF MHPG were of 11, four and three patients, respectively (4,5). In addition to factors that pertain to most severe illnesses, such as the difficulty of studying patients free of effects of medications, mania adds an additional complication. Manic patients are often agitated, motorically hyperactive, emotionally volatile, and inconsistent in continuing consent and cooperation with study procedures. This especially interferes with repeat measures of a variable and procedures, such as 24-hour urine collection, that require active cooperation over a sustained period of time. Little of the evidence summarized here can be viewed as scientifically secure. It is more realistic to think of the data in this and the more detailed single-system chapters as being heuristically valuable. My preference is to give more credence to those findings for which there is convergent, supportive evidence from different perspectives. These perspectives may include diagnostic entity comparisons, changes with specific treatments, changes with illness state, changes in one system that are directly associated with those in another system, or clinical changes that are consistent with preclinical data.

Despite the limited experimental data base on which the information summarized here rests, the evidence is highly encouraging of several lines of investigation. The difficulty of study of bipolar-disordered patients is certain to continue, and even increase in some ways. For example, hospitalization is now generally limited to a more severely ill spectrum of patients, often with comorbid diagnoses, and, even for those patients, shorter in duration. Thus the setting most conducive to control of basic, important environmental variables, such as certainty of timing of dosing, diet, and physical activity, is often not available. Even investigative groups with clinical research units are likely to have small numbers of subjects and expertise in a limited number of systems. Therefore, progress may be quite limited unless collaborative ventures using protocols applied uniformly across centers are emphasized. Although these have heretofore largely been limited to clinical trials, both the NIMH Collaborative Programs on the biology and clinical features of depression provide encouraging operational and procedural models (6). Both have contributed greatly to our knowledge of bipolar disorder, including much of that summarized here on amine metabolism.

III. THE NEURON AND INTRANEURONAL SIGNAL TRANSDUCTION SYSTEMS

There is no single locus to start with in summarizing the data relevant to biological-system disturbances in bipolar disorder. A case can be made for focus on the CNS neuron, as a kind of Grand Central Station that receives messages from upstream, or presynaptic inputs, then amplifies this information into signals which may result in activation or inhibition of brain systems tied to arousal, reward, well-being, alertness, attention, aggression, and possibly other fundamental behavioral states that aggregate to yield the behaviors of which humans are capable. The number of intracellular systems that accomplish these changes is substantial; they include release of neurotransmitter or neurohumoral agents, alteration of protein phosphorylation, alteration of receptor number or sensitivity, alteration of substrate availability for chemical compounds intrinsic to signal cascades, alteration of permeability of ion channels, and alterations in RNA proteins. One dimension of which these several systems differ is temporal. In general, ion-channel changes are quickly occurring and transient, whereas changes in gene expression are slower and likely to be longer-lasting.

An additional advantage of focus at the level of the neuron is that some of the effects of several mood-stabilizing drugs at the neuronal level are known; therefore common and divergent effects across drugs can be compared. The two principal systems, both highly conserved across species and phylogenetically, are the phosphatidyl inositol (PI) pathway and the adenylyl cyclase pathway. There is important cross-linkage between these systems, which to date has been more a confound than a benefit in studies because it has often been difficult to ascertain whether an effect in response to a drug or other independent variable is primary or, rather, the consequence of other actions not directly assessed. The following section reviews signaling systems commencing with G-proteins. Ion channels are briefly discussed with neurotransmitters and membrane receptors.

A. G Proteins

Guanine nucleotide binding proteins (G-proteins), specifically the $G\alpha_s$, have been reported higher in brains from deceased bipolar patients than healthy controls (7). $G\alpha_s$-protein from leukocytes have similarly been reported to be elevated in bipolar patients compared to controls and greater in bipolar depressed than unipolar depressed patients (8). G-protein-related function in white blood cells was also greater in manic patients than controls (9). Both lithium and valproate at therapeutically relevant concentrations have been shown to reduce $G\alpha_s$ activity (9,10, Chapter 2). G-proteins act as molecular switches to regulate coupling to both the phosphoinositide (PI) and adenylate cyclase second-messenger systems. Adenylate cyclase in turn activates cyclic AMP and, thereby, PKC. PKC in platelet membranes of manic patients was increased compared to healthy control subjects (11). A possibility raised by Manji et al. (12) and others is that increased PKC activity could lead to increased $G\alpha_s$ activity. Both lithium and valproate reduce PKC at therapeutically relevant concentrations (12,13). Lithium and valproate selectively enhance DNA binding activity of the transcription factor AP1 (activator binding protein) (14). Furthermore, the effect of valproate appears to occur earlier than that of lithium, and may be greater in magnitude.

Taken together, these data suggest some increased signaling through selected G-protein pathways in bipolar disorder, with lithium and valproate (but not carbamazepine) causing attenuation in activation of the same select pathways. These effects appear to be specific to the type of agonist input and/or type of G-protein, since, for example, in the same brain areas under similar conditions forskolin-stimulated activity is increased, whereas β-adrenergic-stimulated activity is diminished (15).

It is therefore of interest to consider the evidence that ion channel activity and related change in the cytoskeleton of the plasma membrane affect G-protein activity. Lenox et al. (16) have demonstrated that a 45 kD protein and an 83 kD protein referred to as MARCKS protein is attenuated by PKC, and by lithium and valproate. One of the amino acids in MARCKS protein is involved in calcium-binding. Marcks also stabilizes actin. The possibility exists that MARCKS affects cytoskeletal integrity of calcium channels (17,18). There are no data on MARCKS protein activity in bipolar-disordered patients. Thus the pharmacodynamic effects of one or both of these mood-stabilizers may be proximal to this phosphorylation step in intra-cellular signaling.

B. Phosphatidyl Inositol

In the phosphatidyl inositol pathway, lithium has been conclusively demonstrated to inhibit myo-1-inositol phosphatase, thereby reducing the availability of inositol, which is a necessary substrate for the formation of PIP2 (19). It remains unclear whether this reduction is physiologically conse-quential under resting neuronal states, or only states in which neuronal activ-ity is stimulated. This is an important point since arguably the latter might characterize manic, but not other, mood states in bipolar disorders (20,21). PIP2 turnover is influenced by coupled receptors of several types (α_1, cholin-ergic, $5\text{-}HT_2$, $5\text{-}HT_{1C}$, D_1).

The inositol hypothesis both of the effects of lithium and of bipolar pathophysiology has been tested by addition of inositol to in vitro systems in the presence of lithium and to bipolar depressed patients. Lithium's effects on IP result in inositol depletion and consequent increase in diacyl glycerol (22). Manji et al. (9) have postulated that increased DAG by lithium could lead to increased degradation of PKC, but no experimental evidence is present. In vitro inositol may prevent the effects of lithium, but it does not reverse them (24). In bipolar depressed patients, lithium improved mood more in patients concurrently treated with inositol. The effects of inositol clinically must be interpreted recognizing that inositol does not readily cross the blood–brain barrier. However, 12 grams of inositol taken orally raised CSF levels of inositol by 70% (24).

Lithium reduces cyclic AMP activity in a variety of in vitro and animal studies (25), and in healthy humans (11). Cyclic AMP–stimulated phosphorylation of a 22 kD protein was greater in euthymic bipolar patients than in healthy controls (26). The primary locus of lithium's effect remains unknown, but may include alteration in G-proteins through crosstalk from, initially, PI system effects (27). The evidence that chronic lithium administration attenuates G-protein function is thoroughly reviewed by Young (Chapter 2) and elsewhere (9). The effects of lithium on G-proteins extends to messenger-RNA expression, an effect not present from carbamazepine (28).

Lithium has also been reported to activate NMDA receptors, which leads to glutamate release and calcium influx. However, the conditions of the study make it difficult to apply this action to bipolar disorder (29).

C. Calcium

Calcium has been studied in a small number of reports, but with relatively consistent results. Since IP3 activation may release calcium from intracellular stores, it is possible that PI-calcium-linked perturbation contributes to the pathophysiology of bipolar disorder (30–33).

Three groups of investigators have reported increased intracellular free calcium both at rest and in response to agonist stimulation in platelets of bipolar patients (31,34–36). The increased activity is not present in unipolar depression, and appears to persist in euthymic, lithium-treated patients, suggesting a trait characteristic. Other less functionally relevant indicators of calcium abnormalities have been consistently reported (30,33,37). However, samples have been small and methodologies varied; thus the data require confirmation in larger, methodologically more consistent studies to be viewed securely as being linked to bipolar pathophysiology. IP_3 specifically acts to release Ca^{2+} from endoplasmic reticulum to cytosol. Ca^{2+} acts synergistically with DAG to activate PKC. Ca^{2+} is also regulated by Ca ion channels and cyclic AMP (38). The ionized concentration of Ca^{2+} is generally 1/10,000th that of extracellular Ca (Chapter 2).

D. Consequences of Intracellular Signaling Disturbances

In the aggregate, the above data suggest that some key neuronal areas may be activated in persons with bipolar disorder, and that such activation may be more characteristic of manic states. What might be the downstream consequences of such activation? These include increased neurotransmitter release, increased neuroendocrine substance release, increased protein phosphorylation, and changes in early gene expression, which are reviewed in a later section. Signal transduction systems regulate the functional balance between neurotransmitter systems, thus providing one (but not the only) bridge system to account for imbalances across systems or, conversely, to provide target sites for drugs to rectify neurotransmitter imbalance (39,40).

What might be the upstream inputs that bias these neuronal systems toward altered levels of activation? These include the spectrum of neurotransmitters. The evidence supports specific roles for the following.

IV. AMINERGIC SYSTEMS

In addition to the general caveats discussed earlier about interpretation of results of the various systems reviewed here, an additional one applies particularly to aminergic systems. Although aminergic hypotheses of mood disorders have often been inclusive of bipolar disorder, the experimental evidence comes largely from studies of unipolar depressed patients.

A. Norepinephrine

Compared to healthy controls, manic patients, studied in the NIMH Collaborative Program on the Psychobiology of Depression, had elevated CSF MHPG and urinary NE, NM, and VMA, reflective of increased noradrenergic turnover. Urinary MET, reflective of increased epinephrine turnover, was higher among manic males (41). Jimerson et al. (33) reported that plasma MHPG in manic patients was higher than in controls. Bipolar patients also differed from unipolar depressed patients in response to the orthostatic challenge of change in posture from supine to standing, with lower basal but higher stimulated plasma NE in the bipolar patients (42–44). Compared with bipolar depressed patients, manics had higher CSF MHPG and HVA, and urinary NE. Potter et al. (45) also reported higher CSF MHPG in bipolar than unipolar depressed patients. Additionally, Post and coworkers (46) higher CSF NE in mania. Male bipolar depressed patients had lower CSF HVA and all bipolar depressed patients had higher NM, VMA, and MET than healthy controls (41). Swann et al. (4) reported that CSF MHPG levels correlated positively with dysphoric but not elated symptoms of mania. Post and colleagues (47) similarly reported a positive correlation of CSF NE with anxiety and dysphoria, but not mania; however, the basis for the behavioral assessments was not well described.

Two groups have reported data suggesting that an increased fractional release of NE compared to the amount of overall catecholamines synthesized may be a particularly strong characteristic of bipolar disorder. Urinary NE/TCS ratios were markedly higher in manics than in unipolar depressed and healthy control patients (48). Pretreatment urine MHPG/TCS ratios were significantly lower in manic patients who responded to lithium than in nonresponders ($R = 0.287 + 0.026$; NR = $0.513 + 0.003$; $p < 0.005$; $t = 4.4$; $df = 7$) (49). There was no overlap between responders and nonresponders. NR ratios were essentially similar to those of healthy controls. Manji and Potter (Chapter 1) analyzed aggregate data from NIMH intramural studies and reported an increased fractional excretion of NE in bipolar compared to unipolar depressed subjects and healthy controls.

With lithium treatment, CSF MHPG and urinary NE decreased significantly (50). Patients who responded to treatment with lithium had significantly smaller reductions in CSF MHPG and urinary NE than did nonresponders (51,52). Three other small studies also reported reduction of CSF MHPG with lithium treatment, with two reporting higher CSF MHPG in the patients at baseline (5). Lithium also reduced urinary Ne and metabolites in depressed patients (53).

Among bipolar depressed patients treated with tricyclic antidepressants, responders had less reduction in CSF MHPG than did nonresponders (51), with no differences in change in CSF 5-HIAA or HVA between responders and nonresponders. Bipolar depressed responders also had lower reductions than did nonresponders in urinary MET. Among bipolar depressed responders, urinary NE increased significantly (88%) and differed significantly from the reduction in nonresponders (−20%), with similar trends for NM. Urinary EPI change also differed significantly between responders and nonresponders, with an increase in responders and a reduction in nonresponders. This pattern of change differed from that seen in unipolar depressed patients (52).

In the aggregate, these data indicate an abnormality in noradrenergic activity in bipolar disorder, wherein relative NE output is higher in mania than in depression. Young et al. (53) have linked noradrenergic findings to G-protein changes in studies of postmortem brain from patients with bipolar disorder. The same brain samples that indicated increased GAS activity show increased NE turnover in cortical brain areas, without change in β-adrenoreceptors or adenylyl cyclase activity, when compared to the same brain regions from controls. This abnormality seems illness-state-dependent, since indices differ significantly between bipolar depressed and manic patients, and also differ over time in the small number of patients followed over successive bipolar mood episodes (54). The effects sizes of these differences are generally quite large, ranging from 0.5 to 1.8, with most greater than 0.8. The relationships to severity and to lithium effects, and the differential change in noradrenergic indices, further support a critical role for NE in the pathophysiology of bipolar disorder. Because NA can improve signal-to-noise ratios, the possibility exists that noradrenergic perturbations may be associated with increased signal sensitivity in mania and reduced sensitivity in depression (55).

B. Epinephrine

Although these findings clearly implicate norepinephrine and not epinephrine as being specific to the pathophysiology and illness state of bipolar disorder, there are indications that epinephrine may play a role in relationship to severity. E/NE ratios were higher in nonresponders than responders in both unipolar and bipolar depressed patients (56). E/NE and other adrenergic indices, but not noradrenergic indices, positively correlated with severity of manic syndrome and with anxiety and hostility in manic patients (49).

C. Dopamine and Serotonin

In contrast to compelling evidence for noradrenergic dysregulation as reviewed in Chapter 1 by Manji and Potter, studies of dopamine as well as serotonin have been largely negative and inconsistent. Manic women had increased CSF, HVA, and H-IAA compared to healthy controls, but these metabolites did not differ across diagnostic groups in men (41).

   Serotonergic inputs: 5-HT1 receptors are coupled to G-proteins. Several drugs mediate 5-HT1 activity, including buspirone and ipsapirone. 5-HT2 receptors are coupled to PIP2 and PI turnover. 5-HT3 receptors, limited to frontal brain areas, are coupled to ion channels. Antagonists to 5-HT3 receptors are ondansetron and granisetron, the former marked by some early evidence for benefits in anxiety states.

V. OTHER NEUROTRANSMITTERS AND NEUROMODULATORS

A. Glutamate

Both lithium and valproate result in increased glutamate release. Glutamate activates NMDA, leading to calcium influx (57). Substantial evidence indicates that glutamate, NMDA receptors, calcium channels, and sodium channels are intrinsically involved as a functional unit in intraneuronal signal transduction, as well as in crosstalk with G-protein and PI systems. Valproate and lithium activate NMDA receptors [see Hokin, Dixon, and Los abstract (29)]; with the exception of a modest amount of pharmacological data, none derives from study of bipolar disorder and therefore will not be reviewed further here.

B. Cortisol Activity

These data suggest a role for epinephrine linked clinically to mixed mania, and biologically to hypercortisolism. Mixed mania is generally more severe, and less responsive to lithium than pure mania (58). Mixed, but not pure, mania is associated with hypercortisolism in each of the three studies that have examined this relationship (59–61). CRF increases both NE and E in rats (62). Somatostatin, which has been reported as being low in unipolar depressed patients, also prevents the increase in E secondary to CRF, but not the increase in NE following CRF (63).

Therefore, a plausible hypothesis is that mixed mania will be associated with increased CRF, increased indices of cortisol activity, reduced somatostatin, and elevated E/NE ratios. Janowsky et al. (64) and Maas et al. (56) have presented evidence that stress may be linked to the relative activation of adrenergic in comparison to noradrenergic systems. Significant relationships between epinephrine and cortisol have been reported (65).

In contrast, pure mania will be associated with increased norepinephrine, but not with elevated adrenergic or hypothalamic-pituitary-adrenocortical activity. Furthermore, the presence of high E/NE ratios, increased CRF, or increased cortisol would be predicted to be associated with poor response to lithium. Since two studies report favorable results with valproate in mixed manic patients (66,67), one may speculatively predict that the above relationships will not be linked to valproate response, but the issue has not been experimentally tested. Although it is likely that increased noradrenergic activity alters the PI and adenyleal cydase system discussed earlier, this has not been studied in bipolar patients. Furthermore, efforts to complement amine and amine anetabolite studies have been compromised by methodological difficulties, including suitability of cells studied, freshness of tissue, and, specifically, methods employed (Chapter 1).

C. GABA

Results of studies of GABA in bipolar disorder are that plasma GABA levels were low in bipolar-disordered patients compared to controls before treatment, and increased with treatment in one study (68). Low pretreatment GABA levels were associated with greater improvement in manic symptoms with valproate therapy, but were unrelated to response to lithium. Additionally, the valproate-treated patients, but not lithium-treated patients, had significantly lower plasma GABA levels after 3 weeks of treatment. These data are consistent with those from two other studies of patients with epilepsy who were treated with valproate (69). Since valproate is known to augment GABA activity, possibly by several mechanisms, one explanation of such results is that GABA turnover is negatively related to functional activity on GABAergic systems, at least in patients with bipolar disorder and epilepsy.

VI. CHRONOBIOLOGICAL SYSTEMS: MELATONIN

Persons with bipolar disorder have greater reductions in melatonin following exposure to bright nocturnal light than do healthy controls, and appear to exhibit this difference as a trait characteristic rather than a function of mood state (70,71). Of note, the difficulties that apply to the study of manic patients in general interfered with the conduct of Nurnberger's study, in that it was difficult to get manic patients to sit in front of a lightbox, and the light exacerbated manic symptomatology. These differences are not characteristic of patients with major depression.

The effects of melatonin clinically have not been well studied, but morning melatonin tends to phase-delay circadian events (perhaps analogous to later rising of the sun). Conversely, evening melatonin tends to phase-advance, analogous to earlier setting of the sun (72). Seasonal affective disorder may be analogous to, and contributed to by, the later rising of the sun in the fall and winter, leading to phase-delay and depression. Earlier rising of the sun may contribute to phase-advance and mania or hypomania (73). Melatonin levels are higher in manic than depressed phases of bipolar disorder (74). So little experimental clinical data exist regarding this that the explanation must be considered speculative. However, one aspect of its appeal lies in part in its convergence with empirical observations regarding seasonal and circadian relationships to bipolar disorder and the more experimentally derived information on abnormalities of noradrenergic function in bipolar disorder. NE and 5-HT activity is highly correlated during the day but not at night, possibly suggesting a melatonin-linked disruption at night, although no direct test of this has been reported. Both NE and 5-HT levels fall during night in rats and humans (75). Also, because valproate has GABAergic activity, it would be expected to reduce melatonin activity, and thereby could exert some of its pharmacodynamic effects via this mechanism, although this possibility has not been experimentally examined.

An additional appeal of the concept of chronobiological disturbance as being fundamental to bipolar disorder pathophysiology is that it is compatible with the evidence of a weakened or altered signal-to-noise ratio for noradrenergic activity, both in terms of daily resetting, or entrainment, of the circadian pacemaker and because of the range of inputs that might contribute to increased "noise" (drugs, stress, bright nighttime light, jet travel across time zones, and age-related reductions in receptor responsivity). Furthermore, several of these assertions are suitable for immediate experimental assessment. Confirmation of the increased sensitivity of bipolar-disordered persons to the melatonin-suppressing effects of bright light could lead to a diagnostic test, could be coupled with assessments of other functionally involved systems (e.g., GABA, NE, cortisol), and could be tied to certain drug actions, especially valproate and other drugs with GABAergic effects (76).

VII. KINDLING MODELS

The work of Post and others on kindling behaviors and cocaine-induced behavioral sensitivity is of heuristic interest, but no direct experimental clinical evidence in bipolar patients exists. At present, its main appeal is to indicate different points in inter- and intracellular signaling that a) could be disrupted in the pathophysiology of bipolar disorder and b) could be subject to pharmacological intervention.

VIII. FUTURE DIRECTIONS[*]

The prediction of promising areas for further advances in understanding the biology of bipolar disorder is of limited value, but the following are arguable assertions. Studies of intracellular signaling will continue to be important, and will be of greater benefit to the degree to which they can be linked to brain circuitry, behavior, and neurotransmitter activity. Neurotransmitter activity is likely to be of renewed interest if it can be more specifically focused on receptor subtype. For example, studies of 5-HIAA as an indicator of the status of serotonergic activity are likely to be of limited value, given that at least 14 5-HT receptors have been identified. Coupling metabolite studies with techniques from molecular biology, or utilizing as pharmacological probes drugs with specificity for a particular receptor, offer good opportunities for solid advances.

Although I am skeptical of occasional molecular biological hubris, I also believe that studies of how genetic information encoded into cells is displayed in relationship to time and environments can be promising. In planning for studies, investigators need to remain cognizant of the lack of any animal model for bipolar disorder. This in turn further underscores the need to recognize the benefits of greater crosstalk between clinical and basic-science investigators.

REFERENCES

1. Angst J, Frey R, Lohmeyer R, Zerben-Rubin E. Bipolar manic depressive psychoses: results of a genetic investigation. Hum Genet 1980; 55:237–254.
2. McMahon FJ, Stine OC, Meyers DA, Simpson SG, DePaulo JR. Patterns of maternal transmission in bipolar affective disorder. Am J Hum Genet 1995; 56:1277–1286.
3. Berrettini WH, Ferrado TN, Goldin LR, Weeks DE, Detera-Wadleigh S, Nurnberger JI, Gershon ES. Chromosome 18 DNA markers and manic-depressive illness: evidence for a susceptibility gene. Proc Natl Acad Sci 1994; 91:5918–5921.
4. Swann AC, Koslow SH, Katz MM, Maas JW, Javaid J, Secunda SK, Robins E. Lithium carbonate treatment of mania: cerebrospinal fluid and urinary monoamine metabolites and treatment outcome. Arch Gen Psychiatry 1987; 44:345–354.
5. Wilk S, Shopsin B, Gershon S, Shul M. Cerebrospinal fluid levels of MHPG in affective disorders. Nature 1972; 235:440–441.
6. LaGuardia JG, Hirschfeld RMA. NIMH Depression Trials. In: Hertzman M, Feltner DE, eds. Clinical Trials in Central Nervous System Psychopharmacology. New York: New York University Press, 1997. In Press.
7. Young LT, Li PP, Kish SJ, Siu KP, Kamble A, Hornykiewicz O, Warsh JJ. Cerebral cortex Gsa protein levels and forskolin-stimulated cyclic AMP formation are increased in bipolar affective disorder. J Neurochem 1993; 61:890–898.
8. Young LT, Li PP, Kamble A, Siu KP, Warsh JJ. Mononuclear leukocyte levels of G proteins in depressed patients with bipolar disorder or major depressive disorder. Am J Psychiatry 1994; 151:594–596.
9. Manji HK, Chen G, Shimon H, Hsiao JK, Potter WZ, Belmaker RH. Guanine nucleotide-binding proteins in bipolar affective disorder—effects of long-term lithium treatment. Arch Gen Psychiatry 1995; 52:135–144.
10. Jope RS, Williams MB. Lithium and brain signal transduction systems. Biochem Pharmacol 1994; 47:429–441.

11. Friedman E, Wang HY, Levinson D, Connell TA, Singh H. Altered platelet protein kinase C activity in bipolar affective disorder, manic episode. Biol Psychiatry 1993; 33:520–525.

12. Manji H, Potter WA, Lenox RH. Molecular targets for lithium's actions. Arch Gen Psychiatry 1995; 52:543.

13. Chen G, Manji HK, Hawyer DB, Wright CB, Potter WZ. Chronic sodium valproate selectively decreases protein kinase C α and ε in vitro. J Neurochem 1994; 63:2361–2364.

14. Manji HK, Chen G, Hsiao JK, Masana MI, Potter WZ. Regulation of signal transduction pathways by mood stabilizing agents: implications for the delayed onset of therapeutic efficacy. J Clin Psychiatry 57(suppl 13):34–46, 1996.

15. Manji HK, Hsiao JK, Risby ED, et al. The mechanisms of action of lithium. Arch Gen Psychiatry 1991; 48:505–512.

16. Lenox RH, Watson DB, Patel J, Ellis J. Chronic lithium administration alters a prominent PKC substrate in rat hippocampus. Brain Res 1992; 570:333–340.

17. Warsh JJ, Mathews R, Young LT, Li PP. Brain Gaq/11 and phospholipase C-b$_1$ immunoreactivity in bipolar affective disorder (BD). Can J Physiol Pharmacol 1994; 72:545.

18. Aderem A. Signal transduction and the actin cytoskeleton: the roles of MARCKS and profilin. Trends Biochem Sci 1992; 17:438–443.

19. Hallcher LM, Sherman WR. The effects of lithium ion and other agents on the activity of myo-inositol-1-phosphatase from bovine brain. J Biol Chem 1980; 255:10896–10901.

20. Nahorski SF, Jenkinson, Challiss RAJ. Disruption of phosphoinositide signalling by lithium. Biochem Soc Transactions 1992; 20:430–434.

21. Berridge MJ, Downes CP, Hanley MR. Neural and developmental actions of lithium: a unifying hypothesis. Cell 1989; 59:411–419.

22. Brami BA, Leli U, Hauser G. Origin of the diacylglycerol produced in excess of inositol phosphates by lithium in NG108-15 cells. J Neurochem 1991; 57.

23. Kofman O, Belmaker RH. Biochemical, behavioral, and clinical studies of the role of inositol in lithium treatment and depression. Biol Psychiatry 1993; 34:839–852.

24. Levine J, Rapaport A, Lev L, Bersudsky Y, Kofman O, Belmaker RH, Shapiro J, Agam G. Inositol treatment raises CSF inositol levels. Brain Res 1993; 627:168–170.

25. Mork A, Geisler A. Effects of lithium ex vivo on the GTP-mediated inhibition of calcium-stimulated adenylate cyclase activity in rat brain. Eur J Pharmacol 1989; 168:347–354.

26. Perez J, Zanardi R, Mori S, Gasperini M, Smeraldi E, Racagni G. Abnormalities of cAMP-dependent endogenous phosphorylation in platelets from patients with bipolar disorder. Am J Psychiatry 1995; 152:1204–1206.

27. Lenox RH, Manji HK. Lithium. In: Schatzberg AF, Nemeroff CB, eds. The American Psychiatric Press Textbook of Psychopharmacology. 1st ed. Washington, DC: American Psychiatric Press, 1995:303–349.

28. Li PP, Young LT, Tam YK, Sibony D, Warsh JJ. Effects of chronic lithium and carbamazepine treatment on G protein subunit expression in rat cerebral cortex. Biol Psychiatry 1993; 34:167–170.

29. Hokin L, Dixon J, Los G. Lithium stimulates glutamate release and inositol 1,4,5-trisphosphate accumulation via activation of the N-methyl-D-aspartate receptor in monkey and mouse cerebral cortex slices [abstr]. 2nd International Conference on New Directions in Affective Disorders, Jerusalem 1995:S202.

30. Bowden CL, Huang LG, Javors MA, Johnson JM, Seleshi E, McIntyre K, Contreras S, Maas JW. Calcium function in affective disorders and healthy controls. Biol Psychiatry 1988; 23:367–376.

31. Tan CH, Javors MA, Seleshi E, Lowrimore PA, Bowden CL. Effects of lithium on platelet ionic intracellular calcium concentration in patients with bipolar (manic-depressive) disorder and healthy controls. Life Sci 1990 46:1175–1180.

32. Dubovsky SI, Franks RD, Allen S, Murphy J. Calcium antagonists in mania: a double blind study of verapamil. Psychiatry Res 1986; 18:309–320.

33. Jimerson DC, Insel TR, Reus VI, Kopin IJ. Increased plasma MHPG in dexamethasone-resistant depressed patients. Arch Gen Psychiatry 1983; 40:173–176.

34. Dubovsky SL, Murphy J, Thomas M, Rademacher J. Abnormal intracellular calcium ion concentration in platelets and lymphocytes of bipolar patients. Am J Psychiatry 1992; 149:118–120.

35. Dubovosky SL, Christiano J, Daniell LC, Franks RD, Murphy J, Adler L, Baker N, Harris RA. Increased platelet intracellular calcium concentration in patients with bipolar affective disorders. Arch Gen Psychiatry 1989; 46:632–638.

36. Kusumi I, Koyama T, Yamashita I. Serotonin-induced platelet intracellular calcium mobilization in depressed patients. Psychopharmacology 1994; 113:322–327.

37. Linnoila M, MacDonald E, Reinila M, Leroy A, Rubinow DR, Goodwin FK. RBC membrane adenosine triphosphatase activities in patients with major affective disorders. Arch Gen Psychiatry 1983; 40:1021–1026.

38. Sharma RK. Signal transduction: regulation of cAMP concentration in cardiac muscle by calmodulin-dependent cyclic nucleotide phosphodiesterase. Mol Cellular Biochem 1995; 149:240–247.

39. Bourne HR, Nicoll R. Molecular machines integrate coincident synaptic signals. Cell 1993; 72:65–75.

40. Ross EM. Signal sorting and amplification through G protein-coupled receptors. Neuron 1989; 3:141–152.

41. Koslow SH, Maas JW, Bowden CL, Davis JM, Hanin I, Javaid J. CSF and urinary biogenic amines and metabolites in depression and mania. Arch Gen Psychiatry 1983; 40:999–1010.

42. Rudorfer MV, Ross RJ, Linnoila M, Sherer MA, Potter WZ. Exaggerated orthostatic responsivity of plasma norepinephrine in depression. Arch Gen Psychiatry 1985; 42:1186–1192.

43. Rubin AL, Price LH, Charney DS. Noradrenergic function and the cortisol response to dexamethasone in depression. Psychiatry Res 1985; 15:5–15.

44. Veith RC, Barnes RF, Villacres E, Murburg MM, Raskind MA, Borson S, et al. Plasma catecholamines and norepinephrine kinetics in depression and panic disorder. In: Belmaker R, ed. Catecholamines: Clinical Aspects. New York: Alan R Liss, 1988:197–202.

45. Potter WZ, Rudorfer MV, Goodwin FK. Biological findings in bipolar disorders. In: Hales RE, Frances AJ, eds. American Psychiatric Association Annual Review. Washington, DC: American Psychiatric Press, 1987:32–60.

46. Post RM, Jimerson DC, Ballenger JC, Lake CR, Uhde TW, Goodwin FK. Cerebrospinal fluid norepinephrine and its metabolites is manic-depressive illness. In: Post RM, Ballenger JC, eds. Neurology of Mood Disorders. Baltimore: Williams and Wilkins, 1984:539–553.

47. Post RM, Rubinow DR, Uhde TW, Roy-Byrne PP, Linnoila M, Rosoff A, Cowdry R. Dysphoric mania: Clinical and biological correlates. Arch Gen Psychiatry 1989; 46:353–358.

48. Davis JM, Koslow SH, Gibbons RD, Maas JW, Bowden CL, Casper R, Hanin I, Javaid JI, Chang SS, Stokes PE. Cerebrospinal fluid and urinary biogenic amines in depressed patients and healthy controls. Arch Gen Psychiatry 1988; 45:705–717.

49. Swann AC, Secunda SK, Koslow SH, Katz MM, Bowden CL, Maas JW, Davis JM, Robins E. Mania: sympathoadrenal function and clinical state. Psychiatry Res 1991; 37:195–205.

50. Swann AC, Secunda SK, Katz MM, Koslow SH, Maas JW, Chang S, Robins E. Lithium treatment of mania: clinical characteristics, specificity of symptom change, and outcome. Psychiatry Res 1986; 18:127–141.

51. Bowden CL, Koslow SH, Hanin I, Maas JW, Davis JM, Robins E. Effects of amitriptyline and imipramine on brain amine neurotransmitter metabolites in cerebrospinal fluid. Clin Pharmacol Therapeutics 1985; 37:316–324.

52. Bowden CL, Koslow SH, Maas JW, Davis J, Garver DL, Hanin I. Changes in urinary catecholamines and their metabolites in depressed patients treated with amitriptyline or imipramine. J Psychiatric Res 1987; 21:111–128.

53. Young LT, Warsh JJ, Kish SJ, Shannak K, Hornykiewicz O. Reduced brain 5-HT and elevated NE turnover in bipolar affective disorder. Biol Psychiatry 1994; 35:121–127.

54. Goodwin FK, Jamison KR. Manic-Depressive Illness. New York: Oxford University Press, 1990.

55. Waterhouse BD, Woodward DJ. Interaction of norepinephrine with cerebrocortical activity evoked by stimulation of somatosensory afferent pathways in the rat. Experimental Neuro 1980; 67:11–34.

56. Maas JW, Katz MM, Koslow SH, Swann A, Davis JM, Berman N, Bowden CL, Stokes PE, Landis H. Adrenomedullary function in depressed patients. J Psychiatric Res 1994; 28:357–367.

57. Kofman O, Bersudsky Y, Levine J, Agam G, Benjamin J, Belmaker RH. Behavioural effects of inositol replenishment in lithium-treated animals and in patients with mood disorders [abstr]. 2nd International Conference on New Directions in Affective Disorders, Jerusalem, 1995:S204.

58. Secunda S, Katz MM, Swann A, Koslow SH, Maas JW, Chuang S, Croughan J. Mania: Diagnosis, state measurement and prediction of treatment response. J Affective Disord 1985; 8:113–121.

59. Swann AC, Stokes PE, Casper R, Secunda SK, Bowden CL, Berman N, Katz MM, Robins E. Hypothalamic pituitary-adrenocortical function in mixed and pure mania. Acta Psychiatrica Scandinavica 1992; 85:270–274.

60. Evans DA, Nemeroff CB. The dexamethasone suppression test in mixed bipolar disorder. Am J Psychiatry 1983; 140:615–617.

61. Krishnan RR, Maltbie AA, Davidson JR. Abnormal cortisol suppression in bipolar patients with simultaneous manic and depressive symptoms. Am J Psychiatry 1983; 140:203–205.

62. Brown MR, Fisher LA. Corticotropin-releasing factor: effects on the autonomic nervous system and visceral systems. Federation Proc 1985; 44:243–248.

63. Maas JW, Katz MM, Frazer A, Bowden CL, Koslow SH, Stokes PE, Swann AC, Davis JM, Casper R, Berman N. Current evidence regarding biological hypotheses of depression and accompanying pathophysiological processes: a critique and synthesis of results using clinical and basic research results. Integr Psychiatry 1991; 7:155–161.

64. Janowsky DS, Risch SC, Ziegler MG, Gillin JC, Huey L, Rausch J. Physostigmine-induced epinephrine release in patients with affective disorder. Am J Psychiatry 1986; 143:919–921.

65. Stokes PE, Koslow SH, Davis JM, Maas JW, Gurvits I, Stoll PM. Association of high cortisol and epinephrine release in depressive illness. In: Belmaker RH, Sandler M, Dahlstrom A, eds. Progress in Catecholamine Research. Part C. Clinical Aspects. New York: Alan R Liss, 1988:237–242.

66. Calabrese JR, Delucchi GA. Spectrum of efficacy of valproate in 55 patients with rapid-cycling bipolar disorder. Am J Psychiatry 1990; 147:431–434.

67. Bowden CL. Predictors of response to divalproex and lithium. J Clin Psychiatry 1995; 56:25–30.

68. Berrettini W, Nurenberger J, Narrow, et al. Cerebrospinal fluid studies of bipolar patients with and without a history of suicide attempts. In: Mann JJ, Stanley M, eds. Psychobiology of Suicidal Behavior. New York: New York Academy of Sciences, 1986.

69. Loscher W. Effects of the antiepileptic drug valproate on metabolism and function of inhibitory and excitatory amino acids in the brain. Neurochem Res 1993; 18:485–502.

70. Lewy AJ, Nurnberger JI, Jr., Wehr TA, Pack D, Becker LE, Powell RL, Newsome DA. Supersensitivity to light: possible trait marker for manic-depressive illness. Am J Psychiatry 1985; 142:725–727.

71. Nurnberger JI, et al. Supersensitivity to melatonin suppression by light in young people at high risk for affective disorder: a preliminary report. Neuropsychopharmacology 1988; 1:217–223.

72. Lewy AJ, et al. Melatonin shifts human circadian rhythms according to a phase-response curve. Chronobiol Int 1992; 9:380–392.

73. Rosenthal NE, et al. Seasonal affective disorder and phototherapy. Ann NY Acad Sci 1985; 453:260–269.

74. Lewy AJ, Wehr TA, Goodwin FK, Newsome DA, Markey SP. Light suppresses melatonin secretion in humans. Science 1980; 210:1267–1269.
75. Agren H, Oreland L. Early morning awakening in unipolar depressives with higher levels of platelet MAO activity. Psychiatry Res 1982; 7:245–254.
76. Joseph-Vanderpool JR, et al. Abnormal pituitary-adrenal responses to corticotropin-releasing hormone in patients with seasonal affective disorder: clinical and pathophysiological implications. J Clin Endocrinol Metab 1991; 72:1382–1387.

10

Is Bipolar Depression a Specific Biological Entity?

Alan C. Swann
University of Texas Medical School at Houston, Houston, Texas

I. DEVELOPMENT OF THE IDEA OF RECURRENT MOOD DISORDERS

Areteaus described a close relationship between depressed and manic states 2000 years ago, and there appear to be Biblical references to mixed states. Until Kraepelin (1921), however, recurrent mood disorder was not generally distinguished from schizophrenia. Only in the 1950s did the idea develop that different types of recurrent depressions could be distinguished by a history of manic episodes (Jackson, 1986).

I will review the basis for the relatively recent idea that there are two broad types of recurrent mood disorder based on the presence of manic episodes. Viewed as simply as possible, the questions of unipolar–bipolar specificity are

1. Are unipolar and bipolar depressed episodes different?
2. Regardless of characteristics of individual episodes, is some underlying characteristic of the patients different?
3. If the depressions are similar and no underlying differences exist, why do some individuals have manic episodes while others do not?

I will examine these questions in turn.

II. EVIDENCE FOR DIFFERENCES BETWEEN UNIPOLAR
AND BIPOLAR DEPRESSIONS

A. Can Episodes of Bipolar Depression Be Clinically
Distinguished from Unipolar Depression?

First, a word about nomenclature. Because mixed states exist in which severity of either depressive or manic syndromes can range widely and can vary
independently over time, the term *bipolar* is inaccurate and manic-depressive
illness is a more descriptive term for recurrent depressions and manias. For
convenience, however, we will use unipolar–bipolar terminology in this
review because it clearly distinguishes depressions with and without manias
and is in standard use. Unless specified otherwise, unipolar depression is
depression in an individual who has never experienced hypomania or mania.
Bipolar depression is depression in someone who has had at least one manic
or hypomanic episode, but it excludes mixed states.

Bipolar and unipolar depressions have been compared clinically as
isolated episodes. Bipolar depressions tend to have shorter duration (Angst
and Preisig, 1995) and are considered to be associated with more severe
psychomotor slowing and anergy (Katz et al., 1982; Leibenluft et al., 1995;
Thase et al., 1992). Some studies have found that bipolar depressions actually
have more psychomotor agitation (Mitchell et al., 1992), however, and there
is considerable overlap in all clinical characteristics. The most conservative
conclusion, therefore, is that clinical characteristics of unipolar and bipolar
depressive episodes overlap enough to make them essentially indistinguishable. It is impossible to differentiate unipolar from bipolar depressions clinically without information about the patient's course of illness (Cassano et al.,
1989, 1992).

B. Are There Biological Differences Between Bipolar
and Unipolar Depressive Episodes?

State-dependent biological changes during depression have been extensively
studied. There is, however, a disappointingly small amount of information
comparing bipolar and unipolar depressions, especially with a number of
patients adequate for firm statistical and clinical conclusions. Unipolar and
bipolar depressions could have different pathophysiological mechanisms
despite their overlapping phenomenology. Our focus is on areas with well-
documented direct comparisons between patients experiencing unipolar and
bipolar depressions, which unfortunately does not include some of the newest
areas of investigation. These include monoamine function, particularly nore-

pinephrine and serotonin, neuroendocrine function, particularly hypothalamic-pituitary-adrenocortical (HPA) axis function, and physiological changes including ion transport and neurophysiology.

Most neurotransmitter-based biological theories of mood disorders have implicitly accepted the Kraepelinian idea of a unitary recurrent affective disorder or have ignored the possibility of a distinct unipolar subtype. They have generally held that mania and depression are axial entities with opposing abnormalities in a biological system. For example, the original catecholamine hypothesis held that norepinephrine was increased in mania and reduced in depression; the serotonin-norepinephrine hypothesis combined the norepinephrine hypothesis with a general serotonergic deficit (Prange et al., 1974); the cholinergic-adrenergic hypothesis combined the norepinephrine idea with opposing changes in acetylcholine (Janowsky et al., 1972); the GABA hypothesis posits a general lowering of GABA in depression (Petty et al., 1993); and hypotheses based on second-messenger imbalances generally continue to propose depression-mania dichotomies (Lachman and Papolos, 1989; Wachtel, 1989).

1. Monoamine Function

The transmitters best studied with respect to comparisons of bipolar and unipolar disorders, or to comparison of manic and depressed phases of bipolar disorder, are norepinephrine, serotonin, acetylcholine, and GABA.

a. Norepinephrine

While the original catecholamine hypothesis for mood disorders was that norepinephrine was low in depression and high in mania, subsequent data have revealed a more complex picture.

Relationship to Mood State. Concentrations of norepinephrine and/or metabolites are higher in manic than in depressed phases of bipolar disorder, but during depression are not substantially different from those in non-depressed control subjects (Koslow et al., 1983; Azorin et al., 1990; Gerner et al., 1984; Greenspan et al., 1970). Increased norepinephrine may anticipate mood switches in cycling patients, but changes in sleep or activity patterns may be just as sensitive (Post et al., 1977). Sympathetic nervous system activity is elevated in depression, especially unipolar (Koslow et al., 1983; Lista, 1989). Concentrations of norepinephrine and its metabolites correlate significantly with severity of mania (Swann et al., 1987a) but not with depression (Redmond et al., 1986).

Catecholamine Metabolism. Depressed (Maas et al., 1987) and manic (Swann et al., 1987a) patients have abnormal catecholamine metabolism, with increased excretion of unmetabolized and O-methylated amines relative to deaminated metabolites, consistent with increased pulsatile release or decreased MAO activity. Unipolar and bipolar depressions, and manias, did not differ, suggesting a very broad abnormality across mood disorders. While some studies found no differences, other investigators have reported that platelet MAO activity is high in unipolar and low in bipolar depressed patients (Murphy and Weiss, 1972; Gershon et al., 1979). Further, platelet MAO activity appeared to correlate positively with severity of unipolar depression and negatively with severity of bipolar depression (Samson et al., 1985). A discriminant function based on NE and metabolite excretion was able to identify bipolar depressed patients prospectively, before their first manic episode (Schatzberg et al., 1989). The physiological basis of this difference has not been defined but may help to delineate differences between unipolar and bipolar depressions.

Receptor Binding and Function. Decreased postsynaptic α_2-receptor function, measured by growth hormone response to clonidine, has been reported in both manic and depressive episodes (Ansseau et al., 1987). Decreased β-receptor (β_1 and total) number was reported in brains of depressed suicides who were free of antidepressant drugs (De Paermentier et al., 1990), in rats with repeated stressors (Stone, 1987), and in lymphocytes from unipolar depressed patients (Jeanningros et al., 1991). The receptor changes may be state-dependent, because Young et al. (1994b) reported normal β-receptor binding in postmortem brain samples from individuals with bipolar disorder. β-receptor binding from lymphocytes of bipolar depressed patients responded normally to agonist (Berrettini et al., 1987a). Overall, the receptor-binding data are consistent with nonspecifically increased and poorly damped sympathetic nervous system activity during episodes, across affective disorders.

Relationship to Stressful Events. Animal models for depression have often been based on responses to uncontrollable stress (Overmier and Seligman, 1967; Maier and Seligman, 1976; Davies and Molyneux, 1982); generally, these could more accurately be considered models for single depressive episodes (or PTSD?) rather than recurrent unipolar or bipolar depressions. Bipolar and unipolar depressions may differ in their relationships between stressful events and catecholamines, with normal norepinephrine metabolism in unipolar and stress-related bipolar depressions and abnormal metabolism (consistent with low monoamine oxidase activity) in autonomous bipolar depressed episodes (Swann et al., 1990b).

Relationship to Pharmacological Agents. Low pretreatment indices of noradrenergic function selectively predict response to antidepressants that presumably work via norepinephrine in bipolar, but not unipolar, depressives (Maas et al., 1984). α_2-adrenergic antagonists, which increase norepinephrine release, can cause bipolar, but apparently not unipolar, depressed patients to switch to euthymia (Osman et al., 1989) or hypomania (Price et al., 1984). Bipolar depressions are similarly more sensitive to stimulants (Silberman et al., 1981). Antidepressant treatment can precipitate hypomania, mania, or rapid cycling in patients with bipolar disorder but only rarely, if at all, with unipolar or anxiety disorders (Sultzer and Cummings, 1989; Wehr and Goodwin, 1987).

In summary, the data support state-dependent noradrenergic alterations in patients with bipolar disorder, higher in manic- than in depressed-phase patients. Not only is norepinephrine increased in manic states, but patients with bipolar disorder appear more susceptible to norepinephrine-induced changes in affective state.

b. Serotonin

Low serotonin appears to be related to a broad general deficit in the modulation of aggressive, impulsive, consummatory, or other goal-directed behavior. It is unclear whether alterations in serotonergic function in some patients with affective disorders represent a low-serotonin behavior disturbance that cuts across many psychiatric disorders (Goodwin and Post, 1983), or whether a more specific serotonergic deficit is also present in certain affective disorders. Studies of metabolite levels, peripheral receptor binding or disposition, indirect central receptor function, and pharmacological effects have produced mixed results and have not always focused on distinguishing between bipolar and unipolar depressions.

Serotonin Metabolite Levels. Sometimes, but not consistently, lower metabolite levels have been reported in CSF from both manic and depressed patients; there are no consistent correlations with either depressive or manic symptoms (Koslow et al., 1983; Redmond et al., 1986; Swann et al., 1987a). Young et al. (1994c) reported serotonin and metabolite concentrations in postmortem brain consistent with reduced serotonin turnover in patients with affective disorder in general. CSF 5-HIAA appears to be related to stress (Swann et al., 1990b) and to treatment response (Maas et al., 1984) in unipolar but not bipolar patients, unlike norepinephrine, for which the converse is true.

Platelet Serotonin Uptake and Release. Platelet serotonin uptake may be higher in bipolar depressed patients than in controls, and lower in unipolar depressed patients (Jerushalmy et al., 1988; Modai et al., 1985). Results of reuptake site binding studies are inconclusive (Quintana, 1990).

Neuroendocrine Responses to Exogenous Serotonin Enhancers. Reduced neuroendocrine responses to serotonin agonists, precursors, or releasing agents have generally been reported in affective disorders, generally interpreted as consistent with reduced functional serotonin in affective disorders in general (Coccaro et al., 1989; Price et al., 1990a). Serotonin abnormalities appear similar in bipolar and unipolar depressed patients (Coccaro et al., 1989), and in the manic and depressive phases of bipolar disorder (Meltzer et al., 1984; Nurnberger et al., 1990). There is one report of blunted neuroendocrine responses to tryptophan in euthymic bipolar patients (Nurnberger et al., 1990).

Receptor Binding. Adaptation to low serotonin is consistent with the reported increase in 5-HT$_2$ binding in platelets from both unipolar and bipolar depressed patients (Yates et al., 1990; Pandey et al., 1991). Euthymic treated patients had normal binding (Yates et al., 1990; Biegon et al., 1990).

Pharmacological Effects. Lithium and tricyclic antidepressants may act in part via serotonin. Lithium transiently increases serotonergic function in depressed patients (Price et al., 1990b) and in normals (Glue et al., 1986). Two pharmacological effects on depression that appear to implicate serotonin—the reversible relapse of depression upon rapid plasma tryptophan depletion in patients responding to antidepressants (Delgado et al., 1990) and the augmentation by lithium of response to antidepressants (Demontigny et al., 1983)—occur in both unipolar and bipolar depressions.

In summary, studies using peripheral measures and neuroendocrine challenges have generally been consistent with reduced serotonergic activity in patients with affective disorders, especially in patients with increased risk of suicide (Roy et al., 1989). There may be a dimensional relationship between serotonergic function and impulsive-aggressive behavior that is independent of depression (Coccaro, 1992). While there is little consistent evidence for differences between unipolar and bipolar depressions, data on effects of stress and prediction of treatment response suggest a differential role in unipolar depressions.

c. Other Transmitters

Acetylcholine. There is little information about acetylcholine in affective disorders other than indirect pharmacological evidence. Drugs that increase acetylcholine increase depression (Janowsky et al., 1974) and decrease mania (Cohen et al., 1982). Bipolar depressed patients are more sensitive than controls to induction of REM sleep by the muscarinic cholinergic agonist arecoline (Nurnberger et al., 1989). Based on pharmacological or toxic effects of cholinergic agents, (Janowsky et al., 1972) have proposed a hypothesis for bipolar disorder based on norepinephrine-acetylcholine balance, with relatively increased norepinephrine and decreased acetylcholine in mania and the opposite in depression. Direct evidence for cholinergic abnormalities in any phase of any affective disorder is still lacking.

Gamma-Aminobutyric Acid (GABA). Low plasma- or CSF-free GABA levels have been reported in both depression and mania (Berrettini et al., 1982; Borsook et al., 1986; Lloyd et al., 1989). GABA levels did not correlate with severity and generally appeared unrelated to the type of affective disorder. Similar findings have been reported with respect to plasma GABA: about 30–40% of depressed patients, regardless of diagnosis or mood state, had plasma GABA more than about 1.5 standard deviations below the mean for healthy controls (Petty et al., 1990, 1993). Clinical or other biological differences between depressed patients with low and normal GABA have not been determined. CSF GABA was reported to be normal in euthymic bipolar patients (Berrettini et al., 1986). Serotonin enhances GABA activity, so a decrease in GABAergic activity may accompany relative serotonergic deficits (Afione et al., 1990). Overall, GABA appears likely to be low in affective episodes, regardless of type.

d. Summary

Transmitter studies support state-dependent roles for norepinephrine and acetylcholine within bipolar episodes, an episode-dependent but state-nonspecific role for GABA, and a state-nonspecific role for serotonin that could be related to susceptibility to mood cycles or to impulsivity. Postmortem brain data have been reported that were consistent with increased norepinephrine turnover in bipolar disorder and reduced serotonin turnover in affective disorders generally (Young et al., 1994c). Increased function of certain Gs-proteins in drug-free bipolar depressed subjects (Young et al., 1994a), which normalizes with successful lithium treatment (Schreiber et al., 1991), may be related to state-dependent transmitter changes. Bipolar and unipolar episodes have not always been clearly distinguished, and many studies have been limited to one type. Longitudinal information, including data from untreated euthymic subjects and high-risk subjects who have not yet developed full bipolar or unipolar depressive episodes, would be valuable in establishing the specificity of abnormal transmitter function.

2. Neuroendocrine and Peptide Function

a. The Hypothalamic-Pituitary-Adrenocortical System

The HPA system is overactive in many patients with unipolar and bipolar affective disorders, with elevated plasma cortisol, blurred diurnal variation, elevated CSF cortisol, and insensitivity to feedback suppression by dexamethasone (Stokes et al., 1984). Elevated HPA activity in mania may be related to mixed states (Evans and Nemeroff, 1983). Plasma, CSF, and urinary cortisol are normal in pure mania and correlate with severity of depressive symptoms in mixed states (Swann et al., 1992). Increased peripheral norepinephrine metabolite concentrations in patients with elevated HPA activity are consistent with a generalized increase in arousal stimulating both noradrenergic and HPA systems (Rubin et al., 1985), as is the increase in cortisol secretion after intravenous yohimbine, which stimulates norepinephrine release (Grunhaus et al., 1989). The HPA system appears to have a state-dependent relationship to depression, whether unipolar or bipolar.

b. Thyroid System

Depression and mania can accompany hypothyroid and hyperthyroid states (Josephson and MacKenzie, 1980), but there is little evidence linking thyroid function specifically to affective disorder. Plasma TSH may be increased in manic patients (Haggerty et al., 1987), with a blunted or absent nocturnal surge in TSH during bipolar depression (Souetre et al., 1988). Blunted TSH response to TRH can occur in depression but is not specific to bipolar disorder (Loosen and Prange, 1982).

Rapid cycling between manic and depressed states has been reported in hypothyroidism, and some rapid cyclers have responded to thyroid hormones (Cowdry et al., 1983). Most hypothyroid individuals, however, do not experience rapid mood cycling. The proportion of rapid cyclers who are hypothyroid is not known. Two groups reported an association between hypothyroid status and duration of lithium treatment but no relationship to rapid cycling (Cowdry et al., 1983; Joffe et al., 1988).

c. Peptides

There is relatively little information about function of peptidergic systems in bipolar disorder. Berrettini et al. (1987b) measured vasopressin, somatostatin, neurotensin, vasoactive intestinal peptide, corticotropin-releasing hormone, and ACTH in CSF from untreated and treated bipolar patients and healthy controls, and found no significant differences. Plasma LH was increased in recovered manics, suggesting a "state-independent abnormality" (Whalley et al., 1987), but it is difficult to interpret isolated findings without a physiological context.

3. Physiology

a. Sodium Transport

One of the oldest consistent biochemical findings in affective disorders is that cell [Na+] is increased (Coppen et al., 1966) and that Na,K-ATPase, the membrane enzyme system that transports Na+ out of the cell, is decreased. Increased cell Na+ could result in abnormal CNS excitability or arousal in mood disorders (Bunney et al., 1972; Whybrow and Mendels, 1969).

Na,K-ATPase Activity. Red blood cell Na,K-ATPase is decreased in depressed patients (Dagher et al., 1984; El-Mallakh, 1983; Nurnberger et al., 1982), whether unipolar or bipolar (Rybakowski and Lehmann, 1994), may fluctuate with mood state (Linnoila et al., 1983), and generally increases with recovery from depression (Strzyzewski et al., 1984) or with lithium treatment (Wood et al., 1989). In contrast to these largely state-dependent findings, we have found reduced Na,K-ATPase-mediated ion transport in lymphoblastoid cells from bipolar patients compared to their relatives or to healthy controls (Cherry and Swann, 1994).

Adaptive Response to Cell Na+. Na,K-ATPase from white blood cells of depressed patients does not respond to increased cell Na+, its normal physiological stimulus (Naylor and Smith, 1981; Wood et al., 1991). In the CNS, the result would be abnormal excitability and increased transmitter release (Stahl, 1986).

Na,K-ATPase activity is stimulated by catecholamines in rat brain and skeletal muscle (Swann, 1989), and in human skeletal muscle (Wood et al., 1990) and platelets (Turaihi et al., 1989). Catecholamines could therefore mediate state-dependent variation of Na,K-ATPase activity in bipolar disorder. Activity-dependent energy metabolism, and therefore the glucose or oxygen uptake measured in brain-imaging studies, largely represents Na,K-ATPase activity (Stahl, 1986), and Na,K-ATPase activity is regulated in part by electrical activity (Swann, 1991). Changes in energy use observed in functional brain-imaging studies are largely measures of Na,K-ATPase.

In summary, there is extensive evidence supporting decreased Na,K-ATPase activity in depression, consistent with abnormalities in arousal and transmitter release (Bunney et al., 1972; El-Mallakh and Wyatt, 1995; Whybrow and Mendels, 1969). Problems in interpreting the data include lack of information about specificity to bipolar disorder and the possibility of superimposed state- and trait-related properties. The regulation of Na,K-ATPase is complex and observed abnormalities could be secondary to changes in cation fluxes, neurotransmitter function, or second-messenger systems.

b. Lithium Transport

Lithium must enter cells in order to act. Lithium is more effective in bipolar than unipolar depressions (Joyce and Paykel, 1989; Bouman et al., 1986) and there appears to be a hereditary component to lithium responsiveness (Alda et al., 1994). Based on Donnan equilibrium, cell lithium should be higher than extracellular fluid lithium due to the negative resting membrane potential. However, this is not the case, owing to net lithium extrusion by an Na^+-Li^+ exchange system (Greil et al., 1977). Early reports that Na^+-Li^+ exchange was low in bipolar patients, leading to higher cell lithium (Rybakowski et al., 1990), have not been confirmed. For example, Hitzemann et al. (1989) reported no differences among many diagnostic groups with respect to RBC/ECF lithium ratios measured in vitro. A relatively high RBC/plasma lithium ratio early in treatment may predict ultimate lithium response (Swann et al., 1987b). Lithium transport rates correlate with catecholamine excretion and HPA activity (Swann et al., 1990a). The reported relationships between Na^+-Li^+ exchange and bipolar disorder may have resulted from differences in neuroendocrine or catecholamine function. Conversely, these factors could alter the efficacy of lithium treatment through their effects on Na^+-Li^+ exchange.

c. Calcium Transport

Calcium fluxes are strategic in transmitter release and signal transduction. Mechanisms include active efflux of calcium via Ca-ATPase, influx through receptor- and voltage-gated channels, and secondary passive transport through Na-Ca exchange (which is influenced in turn by Na,K-ATPase). There is only limited information about these systems in bipolar depression.

Intracellular [Ca^{2+}]. Platelet [Ca^{2+}] may be increased in bipolar depressed patients (Bowden et al., 1988; Dubovsky et al., 1989, 1991, 1992), but there are also negative reports (Bothwell et al., 1994; Tan et al., 1990). Increased cell [Ca^{2+}], like cell [Na^+], may be associated with increased or abnormally modulated arousal. Agonist-induced [Ca^{2+}] influx may be either increased (Bothwell et al., 1994) or decreased (Forstner et al., 1994) by lithium.

Ca-ATPase Activity. RBC Ca-ATPase was increased (although highly variable) in both depressed and manic bipolar patients compared to unipolar patients or controls (Bowden et al., 1988). This may be a physiological response to increased intracellular calcium. Lithium treatment increases Ca-ATPase and alters its response to calmodulin (Meltzer et al., 1988), but, like other reported biochemical effects of lithium, its relationship to the pathophysiology of bipolar disorder is not clear.

4. *Neurophysiological Arousal*

Whybrow and Mendels (1969) originally proposed that abnormal neuronal excitability was the pathophysiological basis for affective disorders. The basis for this idea was that patients with depression or mania had increased cell sodium, which would result in increased excitability and transmitter release but impaired recovery from electrical activity. Neurophysiological evidence supporting this idea has come largely from studies of evoked potentials and sensory physiology. Sensory gating abnormalities in mania appear to result from increased norepinephrine (Adler et al., 1990; Baker et al., 1990), unlike the case with schizophrenia. Bipolar depressed patients differ from unipolar depressed patients or controls in laterality of event-related potentials (Bruder et al., 1992) and of response to affective stimuli (Gruzelier and Davis, 1995). Time characteristics of event-related potentials were also different from those of unipolar depressed patients (John et al., 1994). The lateralization of the spatial pattern of the EEG differs between bipolar and unipolar disorders (Koles et al., 1994). P3 is abnormal in bipolar compared to unipolar depressions (Muir et al., 1991). Studies of lateralization generally have implicated a right-sided deficit in bipolar disorder. In addition, bipolar depressed patients are average evoked-response augmenters, while unipolar depressed patients tend to be reducers; evoked-response augmentation is associated with low MAO activity (Buchsbaum et al., 1977).

While it is difficult to define operationally, arousal as demonstrated by neurophysiological studies appears to be one of the most consistent areas in which individuals with bipolar and unipolar depressions differ. In a general sense, abnormal arousal is consistent with the differences in cation distribution that seem to exist between bipolar and unipolar depressions. The specific manner in which they are linked, however, is elusive. The many aspects of "arousal" that have been reported do not fit easily into a unitary scheme. The extent to which differences in arousal or in cation distribution are related to the depressed state or are underlying individual characteristics can also be ambiguous (Muir et al., 1991; El-Mallakh and Wyatt, 1995).

5. *Sleep*

Despite tantalizing relationships between affective disorders and sleep, unipolar and bipolar depressions have not always been clearly differentiated (Gillin, 1987). Depressed patients have decreased REM latency and abnormal sleep architecture, but anergic bipolar depressed patients may have abnormal sleep but normal REM latency (Thase et al., 1989). Sleep deprivation can improve unipolar or bipolar depression, and can increase the likelihood of manic episodes (Wehr et al., 1987).

Sleep-related neuroendocrine abnormalities include a reduced nocturnal surge of TSH secretion in bipolar depressed patients (Souetre et al.,
1988). Bipolar depressed patients have low baseline plasma melatonin levels
and decreased nocturnal suppression compared to unipolar patients and
healthy controls (Lam et al., 1990). Nocturnal melatonin was found to be
lower in the depressed phase and higher in the manic phase of a rapidly
cycling patient (Kennedy et al., 1989). Sleep effects may be related to
systems responding to light or to other diurnal factors, or may be an expression of an arousal disturbance.

6. Summary

Bipolar and unipolar depressions appear to differ in terms of some aspects of
norepinephrine system function, calcium distribution, and neurophysiological
arousal. Bipolar and unipolar depressions appear to be similar with respect to
serotonin, GABA, sodium transport, most neuroendocrine measures studied,
sleep, and some measures of arousal. It would be easier to understand possible biological differences between unipolar and bipolar depressions if more
studies compared the two groups rather than focusing on only one of them.
The most promising sources of biological specificity in bipolar depression
may lie outside the depressive episodes themselves.

III. ARE THERE DIFFERENCES BETWEEN PATIENTS WITH UNIPOLAR AND BIPOLAR DEPRESSIONS?

A. Epidemiology

Epidemiological or demographic differences between patients with unipolar
and bipolar disorder may reflect differences in biological susceptibility,
illness course, environmental risk factors, or effects of illness. Unipolar
disorder is five- to 10-fold more common than bipolar disorder. Bipolar and
unipolar disorders differ in gender distribution; individuals with bipolar
disorder have an even gender distribution while those with unipolar disorder
are more likely to be women. Age of onset is earlier in bipolar disorder and
recurrences are more frequent (Winokur et al., 1993). Socioeconomic status
is similar for patients with unipolar and bipolar disorder, but economic and
creative productivity appears to be greater in relatives of those with bipolar
than with unipolar disorder (Coryell et al., 1989; Richards et al., 1988;
Verdoux and Bourgeois, 1995). The greater frequency of episodes results in
greater socioeconomic burden in bipolar than unipolar disorder (Chakrabarti
et al., 1992).

B. Genetics

One would expect any meaningful biological difference between individuals with unipolar and bipolar depressions to have, ultimately, a genetic basis. Two broad classes of genetic studies have been carried out: family history studies and genetic linkage studies including candidate gene studies. Interpretation of genetic results is hampered by the fact that there is no objective test other than descriptive clinical criteria for the presence or absence of an affective disorder. The diagnosis of manic syndromes is quite reliable, but that of hypomania or of depression is less so (Dunner and Tay, 1993; Rice et al., 1986). Accurate diagnosis may require longitudinal assessment, which is usually not available. Nevertheless, the results of genetic studies of bipolar disorder have been quite tantalizing.

1. Family Studies

Affective disorders run in families: bipolar disorder is about 10 times as common in first-degree relatives of affected individuals; unipolar disorder is several times more common in relatives of those with unipolar depression (Andreasen et al., 1987; Kitamura et al., 1989; Gershon et al., 1982; Kupfer et al., 1988). Most studies have found that the rate of unipolar or bipolar disorder is not increased in relatives of those with the other (Kupfer et al., 1989; Andreasen et al., 1987; Heun and Maier, 1993; Maier et al., 1993; Rice et al., 1987; Stancer et al., 1987; Winokur et al., 1995), but increased unipolar disorder in families of bipolar disorder patients has also been reported (Gershon et al., 1982). Twin studies reflect greater concordance for bipolar disorder in monozygotic twins (Kendler et al., 1995b).

Family history appears to interact with age of onset. As age of onset becomes earlier, family loading increases (Strober et al., 1988; Kutcher and Marton, 1991; Geller et al., 1994).

Psychosis may be inherited independently of specific psychiatric syndromes. "Unipolar" and "bipolar" schizoaffective disorder appear to have distinct familial transmission analogous to unipolar and bipolar affective disorder (Van Eerdewegh et al., 1987). Family histories of schizophrenia and affective disorder seem to be independent (Taylor et al., 1993). Individuals with affective disorder who have psychotic family members are more likely than others to have psychotic symptoms themselves (Shenton et al., 1989; Kendler et al., 1993, 1995a).

Overall, the familial pattern for bipolar disorder appears stronger than that for unipolar. This may be related in part to the relatively high diagnostic reliability of mania. There is little evidence to support a continuum of psychotic or affective disorders; rather, studies of familial transmission suggest that schizophrenia, unipolar disorder, and bipolar disorder are distinct (Heun and Maier, 1993; Maier et al., 1993; Taylor et al., 1993).

2. Genetic Studies

The strong familial association with bipolar disorder has led to a search for more specific genetic abnormalities. This search has been complicated by the probable heterogeneity of bipolar disorder and the lack of reliable markers (Gershon et al., 1990; Gasperini et al., 1987; Gurling et al., 1988). Early suggestions of abnormal loci on chromosome 11 (Mendlewicz et al., 1991; Mitchell et al., 1991; Nanko et al., 1991) and the X chromosome (Baron, 1991; Berrettini et al., 1990; Gejman et al., 1990; Nanko et al., 1991) have proved negative, although a locus on the X chromosome has not been ruled out for some pedigrees (Mendelbaum et al., 1995). Advances in understanding the structure of the human genome have led to candidate gene strategies (Gurling, 1986), but, given the complexity and heterogeneity of bipolar disorder, it is perhaps not surprising that these studies have so far been negative, including a lack of association with genes for dopamine D_1 (Cichon et al., 1994), D_2 (Holmes et al., 1991; De Bruyn et al., 1994) and D_4 (De Bruyn et al., 1994) receptors, GABA-A receptor subunits (Coon et al., 1994), tyrosine hydroxylase (De Bruyn et al., 1994; Kawada et al., 1995), and monoamine-transporting proteins (Lesch et al., 1994, 1995). A promising recent development is the replication (Stine et al., 1995) of a linkage between susceptibility to manic-depressive illness and chromosome 18 (Berrettini et al., 1994). While this finding, combined with the results of most family studies, suggests genetic specificity for bipolar relative to unipolar disorder, Stine et al. (1995) observed that their data could not eliminate the possibility that the chromosome 18 abnormality also conferred increased susceptibility for unipolar disorder.

In summary, genetic and family studies suggest strongly that bipolar and unipolar disorder have distinct genetic transmissions, but so far provide no information about the specific nature of the distinction(s). A possible association between bipolar disorder and a locus on chromosome 18 is promising but, even after reliable genetic markers are established, their relationship to the pathophysiology of bipolar disorder must be established.

C. Course of Illness and Patterns of Recurrence

There is extensive evidence that the course of illness differs between bipolar and unipolar disorder, but other evidence for similarities. We will discuss onset of illness, frequency, and pattern of recurrence.

1. Onset of Illness

There is consistent evidence that the onset of bipolar disorder is earlier than that of unipolar disorder (Angst and Preisig, 1995; Winokur et al., 1993; Akiskal, 1995; Bashir et al., 1987). The relationship between early onset of illness and bipolar disorder appears to be so strong, and so consistently related to the presence of a family history of bipolar disorder, that any recurrent psychiatric illness with onset in adolescence or earlier and a family history of bipolar disorder may well be bipolar disorder (Geller et al., 1994; Kutcher and Marton, 1991; Akiskal et al., 1985; Bashir et al., 1987) including early-onset dysthymia (Kovacs et al., 1994), substance abuse (Akiskal et al., 1985), and conduct disorder (Kovacs and Pollock, 1995).

2. Frequency of Episodes

Patients with bipolar disorder, whether type I or II, have more episodes than do patients with unipolar disorder (Angst and Preisig, 1995; Brockington et al., 1991; Cassano et al., 1992; Coryell et al., 1987; Cutler and Post, 1982; Deister and Marneros, 1993; Angst, 1986; Goldberg et al., 1995). While the prognosis for a single episode of bipolar or unipolar depression is similar (Coryell et al., 1987), impairment and overall prognosis seem worse in bipolar disorder largely because of the higher number of episodes (Deister and Marneros, 1993; Goldberg et al., 1995). Individuals with apparently stable diagnoses of unipolar disorder who "switched" to bipolar disorder had more previous episodes of depression than those whose diagnosis remained unipolar (Winokur and Wesner, 1987).

3. Pattern of Recurrence

Frequency of recurrence accelerates in affective disorders, with successively briefer periods between episodes (Cutler and Post, 1982; Post et al., 1986; Kraepelin, 1921). Although unipolar and bipolar disorder differ in frequency of recurrence, they appear to share the acceleration of episode frequency, at least in a subset of patients.

In addition to increased frequency, successive episodes of affective disorders are progressively more autonomous relative to environmental stressors or negative events (Post et al., 1986; Swann et al., 1990b; Ambelas, 1987a). Bipolar and unipolar depressions share this characteristic (Swann et al., 1990b). There apparently are no differences between the role of stressors in bipolar and unipolar depressions, or depressive and manic episodes (Ambelas, 1987b).

About 15% of patients with bipolar disorder develop rapid cycling, or runs of four or more episodes per year. Rapid cycling is usually transient, sporadic, and nonfamilial (Coryell et al., 1992). The only reliable predictor of rapid cycling is past rapid cycling; no external characteristics not related to episodes of rapid cycling appear to distinguish patients with and without this characteristic (Maj et al., 1994). Although it is generally associated with bipolar illness, rapid cycling also occurs in unipolar disorder (Wolpert et al., 1990).

IV. SYNTHESIS

Einstein wrote that "things should be made as simple as possible but not simpler." Heeding his warning as closely as possible, a recurrent psychiatric disorder has two parts. The first is the content of the recurrent episodes. The second is the mechanism underlying the recurrence. Formulated in this manner, how are bipolar and unipolar depressions different?

A. Are Unipolar and Bipolar Depressive Syndromes Different?

Despite the oft-reported tendency for more psychomotor retardation and atypical features in bipolar depressions, there is so much clinical overlap between them that the only conservative conclusion is that there is no specificity in the phenomenology of unipolar and bipolar depressive syndromes. The depressive syndrome observed clinically is clearly a nonspecific final common pathway of many possible physiological mechanisms (Akiskal and McKinney, 1975).

Most biological abnormalities associated with depression are either similar in bipolar and unipolar depressions (such as hypothalamic-pituitary-adrenocortical function or decreased GABA) or lack sufficient data for a meaningful comparison. A disappointing number of biological hypotheses for abnormal affective states, including those positing abnormal second-messenger function, ignore the possibility of mixed states or do not distinguish bipolar from unipolar depressions (Lachman and Papolos, 1989; Wachtel, 1989).

The most consistent evidence for differences between bipolar and unipolar depressions are in noradrenergic systems and neurophysiology. Bipolar depressions are more likely to be characterized by relatively high excretions of unmetabolized or O-methylated catecholamines, low MAO activity, behavioral lability with respect to changes in norepinephrine, AER augmenting, and other abnormalities in event-related potentials and cortical electrical activity that suggest nondominant hemisphere dysfunction. In addition, there is evidence suggesting elevated concentrations of intracellular calcium and sodium. While these ionic abnormalities could well underlie abnormalities in neuronal excitability, it is extremely difficult to prove or to refute that such is actually the case.

B. Are Recurrent Unipolar and Bipolar Disorders Different?

Clinically, unipolar and bipolar depressions differ only in their frequency and onset. While bipolar depressions are more frequent than unipolar and have earlier onset, the overall form of their recurrence (accelerating course and dissociation from stressors) is similar.

Other than the timing of episodes, there is one prominent difference between unipolar and bipolar disorder that we have not discussed. By definition, bipolar depressions occur in individuals who have the potential for manic episodes (even during their depressions) while unipolar depressions do not. There are two ways in which manic episodes could be related to underlying biological differences between unipolar and bipolar disorders: 1) manic episodes may be a result of differences between unipolar and bipolar disorder or 2) manic episodes may cause differences between unipolar and bipolar disorders.

1. How Could the Biological Specificity of Bipolar Disorder Cause Manic Episodes?

Biological differences between depression and normal states, and their possible relationship to clinical state or behavior, tend to be subtle at best. This is not the case for mania, in which increased central and peripheral noradrenergic function are clearly related to severity of the manic state (Swann et al., 1987a; Post et al., 1989). Interestingly, catecholamine function is increased even more in mixed states than in pure mania (Swann et al., 1994). Manipulations that increase noradrenergic transmission, including stress, stimulants, yohimbine, and antidepressive agents, have the potential to precipitate mania in bipolar but not unipolar disorder. Therefore, part of the basic pathophysiology of bipolar disorder includes a deficiency in a system that normally either limits or damps noradrenergic activity or that opposes its effects. This deficiency may be a reflection of an arousal disturbance that may characterize bipolar disorder.

2. How Could Manic Episodes Cause the Apparent Specificity of Bipolar Disorder?

Manic episodes may be a random event in individuals with a recurrent affective disorder. Once a manic episode occurs, there is a surge of central noradrenergic and dopaminergic activity. This produces long-lasting changes in hippocampal neurophysiology (Dahl and Sarvey, 1989) and could result in effects similar to behavioral sensitization to exogenous stimulants in animals (Kalivas et al., 1993; Post and Weiss, 1989). The resulting destabilization might also make recurrences of depression more likely. Conditioning, analogous to place conditioning of stimulant self-administration in animals (Beninger and Herz, 1986), may result in increased likelihood of reproducing the behavior or circumstances associated with a manic episode. Within the same individual, recurrent manic episodes tend to occur in similar situations (Ambelas and George, 1988; Ambelas, 1987b) and seasons (Hunt et al., 1992) and to have similar prodromes (Molnar et al., 1988), although these characteristics vary widely from one individual to another. These characteristics strongly suggest a role for conditioning in recurrences of mania. Once a manic episode occurred for any reason, further recurrences would become more likely. The random occurrence of the first manic episode could generate an apparently distinctive course and biology of illness.

If this is the case, how does one account for the growing genetic evidence for distinctive unipolar and bipolar illnesses? Either there is no real genetic difference between unipolar and bipolar disorder, or there is a difference but it is not directly related to pathophysiology of the illness, or there is a difference and it is directly related to pathophysiology. The inheritance of affective disorders, even within bipolar disorder, is complex and heterogeneous. The pathophysiology of bipolar disorder is so potentially heterogeneous that one can easily see why its understanding has been elusive. The specificity of genes conferring susceptibility to bipolar disorder may lie in mechanisms related to recurrence or onset of episodes rather than the content of the episodes themselves.

In conclusion, despite extensive progress in investigating the properties and course of affective disorder, it is not easy to define the biological specificity of bipolar relative to unipolar disorder. While there appear to be some physiological and pharmacological differences between unipolar and bipolar depressive episodes, there are greater areas of similarity. The greatest differences appear to lie in the course of illness, with earlier onset and more episodes in bipolar disorder. Understanding of the pathophysiology of bipolar disorder will require the challenge of longitudinal studies and prospective investigation of individuals at risk.

REFERENCES

Adler LE, Gerhardt GA, Franks R, Baker N, Nagamoto H, Drebing C, Freedman R. Sensory physiology and catecholamines in schizophrenia and mania. Psychiatry Res 1990; 31:297–309.

Afione S, Duvilanski B, Seilicovich A, Lasaga M, Diaz MDC, Debeljuk L. Effects of serotonin on the hypothalamic-pituitary GABAergic system. Brain Res Bull 1990; 25:245–259.

Akiskal HS. Developmental pathways to bipolarity: are juvenile-onset depressions pre-bipolar? J Am Acad Child Adolesc Psychiatry 1995; 34:754–763.

Akiskal HS, McKinney WTJ. Overview of depression: integration of ten conceptual models into a comprehensive clinical frame. Arch Gen 1975; 32:285–305.

Akiskal HS, Downs J, Jordan P, Watson S, Daugherty D, Pruitt DB. Affective disorders in referred children and younger siblings of manic-depressives: mode of onset and prospective course. Arch Gen Psychiatry 1985 42:996–1003.

Alda M, Grof P, Zvolsky P, Walsh M. Mode of inheritance in families of patients with lithium-responsive affective disorders. Acta Psychiatrica Scandinavica 1994; 90:304–310.

Ambelas A. Life events and mania: a special relationship. Br J Psychiatry 1987a; 150:235–240.

Ambelas A. Causable mania (reactive, puerperal, secondary, life event related): the development of an idea. Acta Psychiatrica Scandinavica 1987b; 75:225–230.

Ambelas A, George M. Individualized stress vulnerabilities in manic depressive patients with repeated episodes. J Roy Soc Med 1988; 81:448–449.

Andreasen NC, Rice J, Endicott J, Coryell W, Grove WM, Reich T. Familial rates of affective disorder: a report from the National Institute of Mental Health Collaborative Study. Arch Gen Psychiatry 1987; 44:461–469.

Angst J. The course of affective disorders. Psychopathology 1986; 19:47–52.

Angst J, Preisig M. Course of a clinical cohort of unipolar, bipolar and schizoaffective patients: results of a prospective study from 1959 to 1985. Schweizer Archiv für Neurologie und Psychiatrie 1995; 146:5–16.

Ansseau M, von Frenckell R, Cerfontaine JL, Papart P, Franck G, Timsit Berthier M, Geenen V, Legros JJ. Neuroendocrine evaluation of catecholaminergic neurotransmission in mania. Psychiatry Research 1987; 22:193–206.

Azorin JM, Pupeschi G, Valli M, Joanny P, Raucoules D, Lancon C, Tissot R. Plasma 3-methoxy-4-hydroxyphenylglycol in manic patients: relationships with clinical variables. Acta Psychiatrica Scandinavica 1990; 81:14–18.

Baker NJ, Staunton M, Adler LE, Gerhardt GA, Drebing C, Waldo M, Nagamoto H, Freedman R. Sensory gating deficits in psychiatric inpatients: relation to catecholamine metabolites in different diagnostic groups. Biol Psychiatry 1990; 27:519–528.

Baron M. X-linkage and manic-depressive illness: a reassessment. Soc Biol 1991; 38:179–188.

Bashir M, Russell J, Johnson G. Bipolar affective disorder in adolescence: a 10-year study. Aus NZ J Psychiatry 1987; 21:36–43.

Beninger RJ, Herz RS. Pimozide blocks the establishment but not the expression of cocaine-produced environment-specific conditioning. Life Sciences 1986; 38:1425–1431.

Berrettini WH, Nurnberger JI, Hare T, Gershon ES, Post RM. Plasma and CSF GABA in affective illness. Br J Psychiatry 1982; 141:483–487.

Berrettini WH, Nurnberger JI, Hare TA, Simmons-Alling S, Gershon ES. CSF GABA in euthymic manic-depressive patients and controls. Biol Psychiatry 1986; 21:842–844.

Berrettini WH, Bardakjian J, Cappellari CB, Barnett AL, Albright A, Nurnberger JI, Gershon ES. Skin fibroblast beta-adrenergic receptor function in manic-depressive illness. Biol Psychiatry 1987a; 22:1439–1443.

Berrettini WH, Nurnberger JI, Zerbe RL, Gold PW, Chrousos GP, Tomai T. CSF neuropeptides in euthymic bipolar patients and controls. Br J Psychiatry 1987b; 150:208–212.

Berrettini WH, Goldin LR, Gelernter J, Gejman PV, Gershon ES, Detera-Wadleigh S. X-chromosome markers and manic-depressive illness: rejection of linkage to Xq28 in nine bipolar pedigrees. Arch Gen Psychiatry 1990; 47:366–373.

Berrettini WH, Ferraro TN, Goldin LR, Weeks DE, Detera-Wadleigh S, Nurnberger JI, Gershon ES. Chromosome 18 DNA markers and manic-depressive illness: evidence for a susceptibility gene. Proc Natl Acad Sci USA 1994; 91:5918–5921.

Biegon A, Essar N, Israeli M, Elizur A, Bruch S, Bar-Nathan AA. Serotonin 5-HT2 receptor binding on blood platelets as a state dependent marker in major affective disorder. Psychopharmacology 1990; 102:73–75.

Borsook D, Richardson GS, Moore-Ede MC, Brennan MJW. GABA and circadian timekeeping: implications for manic-depression and sleep disorders. Med Hypotheses 1986; 19:185–198.

Bothwell RA, Eccleston D, Marshall E. Platelet intracellular calcium in patients with recurrent affective disorders. Psychopharmacology 1994; 114:375–381.

Bouman TK, Niemantsverdriet van KJG, Ormel J, Slooff CJ. The effectiveness of lithium prophylaxis in bipolar and unipolar depressions and schizo-affective disorders. J Affective Disord 1986; 11:275–280.

Bowden CL, Huang LG, Javors MA, Johnson JM, Saleshi E, McIntyre K, Contreras S, Maas JW. Calcium function in affective disorders and healthy controls. Biol Psychiatry 1988; 23:367–376.

Brockington IF, Roper A, Copas J, Buckley M, Andrade CE, Wigg P, Farmer A, Kaufman C, Hawley R. Schizophrenia, bipolar disorder and depression: a discriminant analysis, using "lifetime" psychopathology ratings. Br J Psychiatry 1991; 159:485–494.

Bruder GE, Stewart JW, Towey JP, Friedman D, Tenke CE, Voglmaier MM, Leite P, Cohen P, Quitken FM. Abnormal cerebral laterality in bipolar depression: convergence of behavioral and brain event-related potential findings. Biol Psychiatry 1992; 32:33–47.

Buchsbaum MS, Haier RJ, Murphy DL. Suicide attempts, platelet monoamine oxidase and the average evoked response. Acta Psychiatrica Scandinavica 1977; 56:69–79.

Bunney WE, Goodwin FK, Murphy DL. The "switch process" in manic-depressive illness. III. Theoretical implications. Arch Gen Psychiatry 1972; 27:312–317.

Cassano GB, Akiskal HS, Musetti L, Perugi G, Soriani A, Mignani V. Psychopathology, temperament, and past course in primary major depressions. 2. Toward a redefinition of bipolarity with a new semistructured interview for depression. Psychopathology 1989; 22:278–288.

Cassano GB, Savino M, Perugi G, Musetti L, Akiskal HS. Major depressive episode: unipolar and bipolar II. Encephale 1992; 18:15–18.

Chakrabarti S, Kulhara P, Verma SK. Extent and determinants of burden among families of patients with affective disorders. Acta Psychiatrica Scandinavica 1992; 86:247–252.

Cherry LC, Swann AC. Cation transport mediated by Na,K-Adenosine triphosphatase in lymphoblastoid cells from patients with bipolar I disorder, their relatives, and unrealted control subjects. Psychiatry Res 1994; 53:111–118.

Cichon S, Nothen MM, Rietschel M, Korner J, Propping P. Single-strand conformation analysis (SSCA) of the dopamine D1 receptor gene reveals no significant mutation in patients with schizophrenia and manic depression. Biol Psychiatry 1994; 36:850–853.

Coccaro EF. Impulsive aggression and central serotonergic system function in humans: an example of a dimensional brain-behavior relationships. Int Clin Psychopharmacol 1992; 7:3–12

Coccaro EF, Siever LJ, Klar HM, Maurer G, Cochrane K, Cooper TB, Mohs RC, Davis KL. Serotonergic studies in patients with affective and personality disorders. Arch Gen Psychiatry 1989 46:587–599.

Cohen BM, Lipinsky JF, Altesmar RF. Lecithin in the treatment of mania. Am J Psychiatry 1982; 139:1162–1164.

Coon H, Hicks AA, Bailey ME, Hoff M, Holik J, Harvey RJ, Johnson KJ, Darlison, MG, Reimherr F, Wender P. Analysis of GABA-A receptor subunit genes in multiplex pedigrees with manic depression. Psychiatric Genet 1994; 4:185–191.

Coppen A, Shaw DM, Malleson A, Costain R. Mineral metabolism in mania. Br Med J 1966; i:71–75.

Coryell W, Andreasen NC, Endicott J, Keller M. The significance of past mania or hypomania in the course and outcome of major depression. Am J Psychiatry 1987; 144:309–315.

Coryell W, Endicott J, Keller M, Andreasen N, Grove W, Hirschfeld RM, Scheftner W. Bipolar affective disorder and high achievement: a familial association. Am J Psychiatry 1989; 146:983–988.

Coryell W, Endicott J, Keller M. Rapidly cycling affective disorder: demographics, diagnosis, family history, and course. Arch Gen Psychiatry 1992; 49:126–131.

Cowdry RW, Wehr TA, Zis AP, Goodwin FK. Thyroid abnormalities associated with rapid-cycling bipolar illness. Arch Gen Psychiatry 1983; 40:414–420.

Cutler NR, Post RM. Life course of illness in untreated manic-depressive patients. Comprehen Psychiatry 1982; 23:101–115.

Dagher G, Gay C, Brossard M, Feray JC, Olie JP, Garay RP, Loo H, Meyer P. Lithium, sodium, and potassium transport in erythrocytes of manic depressive patients. Acta Psychiatrica Scandinavica 1984; 69:24–36.

Dahl D, Sarvey JM. Norepinephrine induces pathway-specific long-lasting potentiation and depression in the hippocampal dentate gyrus. Proc Natl Acad Sci USA 1989; 86:4776–4780.

Davies CL, Molyneux SG. Routine determination of plasma catecholamines using reversed-phase, ion-paired high performance liquid chromatography with electrochemical detection. J Chromatog 1982; 231:41–51.

De Bruyn A, Mandelbaum K, Sandkuijl JA, Delvenne V, Hirsch D, Staner L, Mendlewicz J, Van Broeckhoven C. Nonlinkage of bipolar illness to tyrosine hydroxylase, tyrosinase, and D2 and D4 dopamine receptor genes on chromosome 11. Am J Psychiatry 1994; 151:102–106.

De Paermentier F, Cheetham SC, Crompton MR, Katona MLA, Horton RW. Brain beta-adrenergic binding sites in antidepressant-free depresed suicide victims. Brain Res 1990; 525:71–77.

Deister A, Marneros A. Predicting the long-term outcome of affective disorders. Acta Psychiatrica Scandinavica 1993; 88:174–177.

Delgado PL, Charney DS, Price LH. Serotonin function and the mechanism of antidepressant action—reversal of antidepressant-induced remission by rapid depletion of plasma tryptophan. Arch Gen Psychiatry 1990; 47:411–418.

Demontigny CM, Courmoyer G, Morisette B, Langlois R, Caille G. Lithium carbonate addition in tricyclic antidepressant-resistant depression: correlations with the neurobiologic actions of tricyclic antidepressant drugs and lithium ion on the serotonin system. Arch Gen Psychiatry 1983; 40:1327–1334.

Dubovsky SL, Christiano J, Daniell LC, Franks RD, Murphy J, Adler L, Baker N, Harris RA. Increased platelet intracellular calcium concentration in patients with bipolar affective disorders. Arch Gen Psychiatry 1989; 46:632–638.

Dubovsky SL, Lee C, Christiano J, Murphy J. Elevated platelet intracellular calcium concentration in bipolar depression. Biol Psychiatry 1991; 29:441–450.

Dubovsky SL, Murphy J, Thomas M, Rademacher J. Abnormal intracellular calcium ion concentration in platelets and lymphocytes of bipolar patients. Am J Psychiatry 1992; 149:118–120.

Dunner DL, Tay LK. Diagnostic reliability of the history of hypomania in bipolar II patients and patients with major depression. Comprehen Psychiatry 1993; 34:303–307.

El-Mallakh RS. The Na,K-ATPase hypothesis for manic-depression. I. General considerations. Med Hypotheses 1983; 12:253–268.

El-Mallakh RS, Wyatt RJ. The Na,K-ATPase hypothesis for bipolar illness. Biol Psychiatry 1995; 37:235–244.

Evans DA, Nemeroff CB. The dexamethasone suppression test in mixed bipolar disorder. Am J Psychiatry 1983; 140:615–617.

Forstner U, Bohus M, Gebicke-Harter PJ, Baumer B, Berger M, Van Calker D. Decreased agonist-stimulated Ca2+ response in neutrophils from patients under chronic lithium therapy. Eur Arch Psychiatry Clin Neurosci 1994; 243:240–243.

Gasperini M, Orsini A, Bussoleni C, Macciardi F, Smeraldi E. Genetic approach to the study of heterogeneity of affective disorders. J Affective Disord 1987; 12:105–113.

Gejman PV, Detera-Wadleigh S, Martinez MM, Berrettini WH, Goldin LR, Gelernter J, Hsieh WT, Gershon ES. Manic depressive illness not linked to factor IX region in an independent series of pedigrees. Genomics 1990; 8:648–655.

Geller B, Fox LW, Clark KA. Rate and predictors of prepubertal bipolarity during follow-up of 6- to 12-year old depressed children. J Am Acad Child Adolesc Psychiatry 1994; 33:461–468.

Gerner RH, Fairbanks L, Anderson GM, Young JG, Scheinin M, Linnoila M, Hare TA, Shaywitz BA, Cohen DJ. CSF neurochemistry in depressed, manic, and schizophrenic patients compared with that of normal controls. Am J Psychiatry 1984; 141:1533–1540.

Gershon ES, Targum SD, Leckman JF. Platelet monoamine oxidase (MAO) activity and genetic vulnerability to bipolar (BP) affective illness. Psychopharmacol Bull 1979; 15:27–30.

Gershon ES, Hamovit J, Guroff JJ, Dibble E, Leckman JF, Sceery W, Targum SD, Nurnberger JI, Goldin LR, Bunney WE. A family study of schizoaffective, bipolar I, bipolar II, unipolar and normal control probands. Arch Gen Psychiatry 1982; 39:1157–1167.

Gershon ES, Martinez M, Goldin LR, Gejman PV. Genetic mapping of common diseases: the challenges of manic-depressive illness and schizophrenia. Trends Genet 1990; 6:282–287.

Gillin JC. Sleep reduction: factor in the genesis of mania? Am J Psychiatry 1987; 144:1248–1249.

Glue PW, Cowen PJ, Nutt DJ, Kolakowska T, Grahame-Smith DG. The effect of lithium on 5-HT-mediated neuroendocrine responses and platelet 5-HT receptors. Psychopharmacology 1986; 90:398–402.

Goldberg JF, Harrow M, Grossman LS. Course and outcome in bipolar affective disorder: a longitudinal follow-up study. Am J Psychiatry 1995; 152:379–384.

Goodwin FK, Post RM. 5-hydroxytryptamine and depression: a model for the interaction of normal variance with pathology. Br J Clin Pharmacol 1983; 15:393S–405S.

Greenspan K, Schildkraut JJ, Gordon EK, Baer L, Aronoff MS, Durell J. Catecholamine metabolism in affective disorders. III. MHPG and other catecholamine metabolites in patients treated with lithium carbonate. J Psychiatric Res 1970; 7:171–183.

Greil W, Eisenreid F, Becker BF, Duhm J. Interindividual diferences in the Na+-dependent Li+ countertransport system and in the Li+ distribution across the red cell membrane among lithium-treated patients. Psychopharmacology 1977; 53:19–26.

Grunhaus L, Tiongco D, Zelnick T, Flegel P, Hollingsworth PJ, Smith CB. Intravenous yohimbine: selective enhancer of norepinephrine and cortisol secretion and systolic blood pressure in humans. Clin Neuropharmacol 1989; 12:106–114.

Gruzelier J, Davis S. Social and physical anhedonia in relation to cerebral laterality and electrodermal habituation in unmedicated psychotic patients. Psychiatry Res 1995; 56:163–172.

Gurling H. Candidate genes and favoured loci: strategies for molecular genetic research into schizophrenia, manic depression, autism, alcoholism and Alzheimer's disease. Psychiatric Dev 1986; 4:289–309.

Gurling HM, Sherrington RP, Brynjolfsson J, Potter M, McInnis M, Petursson H, Hodgkinson S. Molecular genetics and heterogeneity in manic depression. Mol Neurobiol 1988; 2:125–132.

Haggerty JJ, Sinmon JS, Evans DL, Nemeroff CB. Relationship of serum TSH concentration and antithyroid antibodies to diagnosis and DST response in psychiatric inpatients. Am J Psychiatry 1987; 144:1491–1493.

Heun R, Maier W. The distinction of bipolar II disorder from bipolar I and recurrent unipolar depression: results of a controlled family study. Acta Psychiatrica Scandinavica 1993; 87:279–284.

Hitzemann RJ, Mark C, Hirschowitz J, Garver DL. RBC lithium transport in the psychoses. Biol Psychiatry 1989; 25:296–304.

Holmes D, Brynjolfsson J, Brett P, Curtis D, Petursson H, Sherrington R, Gurling H. No evidence for a susceptibility locus predisposing to manic depression in the region of the dopamine (D2) receptor gene. Br J Psychiatry 1991; 158:635–641.

Hunt N, Sayer H, Silverstone T. Season and manic relapse. Acta Psychiatrica Scandinavica 1992; 85:123–126.

Jackson S. The various relationships of mania and melancholia. In: Depression and Melancholia: From Hippocratic Times to Modern Times. New Haven: Yale University Press, 1986:249–273.

Janowsky DS, El-Yousef MK, Davis JM, Sekerke HJ. A cholinergic-adrenergic hypothesis for mania and depression. Lancet 1972; ii:632–635.

Janowsky DS, Davis JM, El-Yousef MK. Acetylcholine and depression. Psychosom Med 1974; 36:248–257.

Jeanningros R, Mazzola P, Azorin JM, Samuelian-Massa C, Tissot R. Beta-adrenoceptor density of intact mononuclear leukocytes in subgroups of depressive disorders. Biol Psychiatry 1991; 29:789–798.

Jerushalmy Z, Modai I, Chachkes O, Mark M, Valewski A, Chachkes M, Tyano S. Kinetic values of active serotonin transport by platelets of bipolar, unipolar and schizophrenic patients at 2 and at 8 a.m.. Neuropsychobiology 1988; 20:57–61.

Joffe RT, Kutcher S, MacDonald C. Thyroid function and bipolar affective disorder. Psychiatry Res 1988; 25:117–121.

John ER, Prichep LS, Easton P. Standardized varimax descriptors of event related potentials: evaluation of psychiatric patients. Psychiatry Res 1994; 55:13–40.

Josephson AM, MacKenzie TB. Thyroxine-induced mania in hypothyroid patients. Br J Psychiatry 1980; 137:222–228.

Joyce PR, Paykel ES. Predictors of drug response in depression. Arch Gen Psychiatry 1989; 46:89–99.

Kalivas PW, Sorg BA, Hooks MS. The pharmacology and neural circuitry of sensitization of psychostimulants. Behav Pharmacol 1993; 4:315–334.

Katz MM, Robins E, Croughan J, Secunda S, Swann A. Behavioral measurement and drug response characteristics of unipolar and bipolar depression. Psychol Med 1982; 12:25–36.

Kawada Y, Hattori M, Fukuda R, Arai H, Inoue R, Nanko S. No evidence of linkage or association between tyrosine hydroxylase gene and affective disorder. J Affective Disord 1995; 34:89–94.

Kendler KS, McGuire M, Gruenberg AM, O'Hare A, Spellman M, Walsh D. The Roscommon Family Study. IV. Affective illness, anxiety disorders, and alcoholism in relatives. Arch Gen Psychiatry 1993; 50:952–960.

Kendler KS, McGuire M, Gruenberg AM, Walsh D. Examining the validity of DSM-III-R schizoaffective disorder and its putative subtypes in the Roscommon Family Study. Am J Psychiatry 1995a; 152:755–764.

Kendler KS, Pedersen NL, Neale MC, Mathe AA. A pilot Swedish twin study of affective illness including hospital- and population-ascertained subsamples: results of model fitting. Behav Genet 1995b; 25:217–232.

Kennedy SH, Tighe S, McVey G, Brown GM. Melatonin and cortisol "switches" during mania, depression, and euthymia in a drug-free bipolar patient. J Nerv Ment Disord 1989; 177:300–303.

Kitamura T, Takazawa N, Moridaira J. Family history study of major psychiatric disorders and syndromes. Int J Soc Psychiatry 1989; 35:333–342.

Koles ZJ, Lind JC, Flor-Henry P. Spatial patterns in the background EEG unerlying mental disease in man. Electroencephalogr Clin Neurophysiol 1994; 91:319–328.

Koslow SH, Maas JW, Bowden C, Davis JM, Hanin I, Javaid J. Cerebrospinal fluid and urinary biogenic amines and metabolites in depression, mania, and healthy controls. Arch Gen Psychiatry 1983; 40:999–1010.

Kovacs M, Pollock M. Bipolar disorder and comorbid conduct disorder in childhood and adolescence. J Am Acad Child Adolesc Psychiatry 1995; 34:715–723.

Kovacs M, Akiskal HS, Gatsonis C, Parrone PL. Childhood-onset dysthymic disorder: clinical features and prospective naturalistic outcome. Arch Gen Psychiatry 1994; 51:365–374.

Kraepelin E, Robertson GM, Barclay RB. Manic-depressive Illness and Paranoia. Edinburgh: E & S Livingston, 1921.

Kupfer DJ, Carpenter LL, Frank E. Is bipolar II a unique disorder? Comprehen Psychiatry 1988; 29:228–236.

Kupfer DJ, Frank E, Carpenter LL, Neiswanger K. Family history in recurrent depression. J Affective Disord 1989; 17:113–119.

Kutcher S, Marton P. Affective disorders in first-degree relatives of adolescent onset bipolars, unipolars, and normal controls. J Am Acad Child Adolesc Psychiatry 1991; 30:75–78.

Lachman HM, Papolos DF. Abnormal signal transduction: a hypothetical model for bipolar affective disorder. Life Sci 1989; 45:1413–1426.

Lam RW, Berkowitz AL, Berga SL, Clark CM, Kripke DF, Gillin JC. Melatonin suppression in bipolar and unipolar mood disorders. Psychiatry Res 1990; 33:129–134.

Leibenluft E, Clark CH, Myers FS. The reproducibility of depressive and hypomanic symptoms across repeated episodes in patients with rapid-cycling bipolar disorder. J Affective Disord 1995; 33:83–88.

Lesch KP, Gross J, Wolozin BL, Franzek E, Bengel D, Riederer P, Murphy DL. Direct sequencing of the reserpine-sensitive vesicular monoamine transporter complementary DNA in unipolar depression and manic depressive illness. Psychiatric Genet 1994; 4:153–160.

Lesch KP, Gross J, Franzek E, Wolozin BL, Riederer P, Murphy DL. Primary structure of the serotonin transporter in unipolar depression and bipolar disorder. Biol Psychiatry 1995; 37:215–223.

Linnoila M, MacDonald E, Rienila M, Leroy A, Rubinow DR, Goodwin FK. RBC membrane adenosine triphosphatase activity in patients with major affective disorders. Arch Gen Psychiatry 1983; 40:1021–1026.

Lista AL. Differential rates of urinary norepinephrine excretion in affective disorders: utility of a short time sampling procedure. Psychiatry Res 1989; 30:253–258.

Lloyd KG, Zivkovic B, Scatton B, Morselli PL, Bartholini G. The GABAergic hypothesis of depression. Prog Neuropsychopharmacol Biol Psychiatry 1989; 13:341–351.

Loosen PT, Prange AJ. Serum thyrotropin response to thyrotropin-releasing hormone in psychiatric patients: a review. Am J Psychiatry 1982; 139:405–416.

Maas JW, Koslow SH, Katz MM, Bowden CL, Gibbons RL, Stokes PE, Robins E, Davis JM. Pretreatment neurotransmitter metabolite levels and response to tricyclic antidepressant drugs. Am J Psychiatry 1984; 141:1159–1171.

Maas JW, Koslow SH, Davis JM, Katz MM, Frazer A, Bowden CL, Berman N, Gibbons R, Stokes PE, Landis DH. Catecholamine metabolism and disposition in healthy and depressed subjects. Arch Gen Psychiatry 1987; 44:337–344.

Maier SF, Seligman MEP. Learned helplessness: theory and evidence. J Exp Psychol 1976; 105:3–46.

Maier W, Lichtermann D, Minges J, Hallmayer J, Heun R, Benkert O, Levinson DF. Continuity and discontinuity of affective disorders and schizophrenia: results of a controlled family study. Arch Gen Psychiatry 1993; 50:871–883.

Maj M, Magliano L, Pirozzi R, Marasco C, Guarneri M. Validity of rapid cycling as a course specifier for bipolar disorder. Am J Psychiatry 1994; 151:1015–1019.

Meltzer HY, Umberkoman-Wiita B, Robertson A, Tricou BJ, Lowy M, Perline R. Effect of 5-hydroxytryptophan on serum cortisol levels in major affective disorders. I. Enhanced response in depression and mania. Arch Gen 1984; 41:366–374.

Meltzer HL, Kassir S, Goodnick PJ, Fieve RR, Chrisomalis L, Feliciano M, Szypula D. Calmodulin-activated calcium ATPase in bipolar illness. Neuropsychobiology 1988; 20:169–173.

Mendelbaum K, Sevy S, Souery D, Papadimitriou GN, De Bruyn A, Raeymaekers P, Van Broeckhoven C, Mendlewicz J. Manic-depressive illness and likage reanalysis in the Xq27–Xq28 region of chromosome X. Neuropsychobiology 1995; 31:58–63.

Mendlewicz J, Leboyer M, De Bruyn A, Malafosse A, Sevy S, Hirsch D, Van Broeckhoven C, Mallet J. Absence of linkage between chromosome 11p15 markers and manic-depressive illness in a Belgian pedigree. Am J Psychiatry 1991; 148:1683–1687.

Mitchell P, Waters B, Morrison N, Shine J, Donald J, Eisman J. Close linkage of bipolar disorder to chromosome 11 markers is excluded in two large Australian pedigrees. J Affective Disord 1991; 21:23–32.

Mitchell P, Parker G, Jamieson K, Wilhelm K, Hickie I, Brodaty H, Boyce P, Hadzi-Pavlovic D, Roy K. Are there any differences between bipolar and unipolar melancholia? J Affective Disord 1992; 25:97–105.

Modai I, Zemishlany Z, Jerushalmy Z. 5-hydroxytryptamine uptake by blood platelets of unipolar and bipolar depressive patients. Neuropsychobiology 1985; 12:93–95.

Molnar G, Feeney MG, Fava GA. Duration and symptoms of bipolar prodromes. Am J Psychiatry 1988; 145:1576–1578.

Muir WJ, St Clair, Blackwood DH. Long-latency auditory event-related potentials in schizophrenia and in bipolar and unipolar affective disorder. Psychol Med 1991; 21:867–879.

Murphy DL, Weiss R. Reduced monoamine oxidase activity in blood platelets from bipolar depressed patients. Am J Psychiatry 1972; 128:1351–1357.

Nanko S, Kobayashi M, Gamou S, Kudoh J, Shimizu N, Takazawa N, Kazamatsuri H, Furusho T. Linkage analysis of affective disorder using DNA markers on chromosomes 11 and X. Jap J Psychiatry Neurol 1991; 45:53–56.

Naylor GJ, Smith AHW. Defective genetic scontrol of sodium pump density in manic depressive psychosis. Psychol Med 1981; 11:257–263.

Nurnberger JI, Jimerson DC, Allen JR, Simmons S, Gershon E. Red cell ouabain-sensitive Na+-K+-adenosine triphosphatase: a state marker in affective disorder inversely related to plasma cortisol. Biol Psychiatry 1982; 17:981–992.

Nurnberger JI, Berrettini WH, Mendelson W, Sack DA, Gershon ES. Measuring cholinergic sensitivity. I. Arecoline effects in bipolar patients. Biol Psychiatry 1989; 25:610–617.

Nurnberger JI, Berrettini WH, Simmons-Alling S, Lawrence D, Brittain H. Blunted ACTH and cortisol response to afternoon tryptophan infusion in euthymic bipolar patients. Psychiatry Res 1990; 31:57–67.

Osman OT, Rudorfer MV, Potter WZ. Idazoxan: a selective α_2 antagonist and effective sustained antidepressant in two bipolar depressed patients. Arch Gen Psychiatry 1989; 46:958–959.

Overmier JB, Seligman MEP. Effects of inescapable shock on subsequent escape and avoidance learning. J Comp Physiol Psychol 1967; 63:28–33.

Pandey GN, Pandey SC, Janicak PG, Marks RC, Davis JM. Platelet serotonin-2 receptor binding sites in depression and suicide. Biol Psychiatry 1991; 28:215–222.

Petty F, Kramer GL, Dunnam D, Rush AJ. Plasma GABA in mood disorders. Psychopharmacol Bull 1990; 26:157–161.

Petty F, Kramer GL, Fulton M, Moeller FG, Rush AJ. Low plasma GABA is a trait-like marker for bipolar illness. Neuropsychopharmacology 1993; 9:125–132.

Post RM, Weiss SR. Sensitization, kindling, and anticonvulsants in mania. J Clin Psychiatry 1989; 50:23–30.

Post RM, Stoddard FJ, Gillin JC. Alterations in motor activity, sleep, and biochemistry in a cycling manic-depressive patient. Arch Gen Psychiatry 1977; 34:470–477.

Post RM, Rubinow DR, Uhde TW, Roy Byrne PP, Linnoila M, Rosoff A, Cowdry R. Dysphoric mania: clinical and biological correlates. Arch Gen Psychiatry 1989; 46:353–358.

Post RM, Rubinow DR, Ballenger JC. Conditioning and sensitization in the longitudinal course of affective illness. Br J Psychiatry 1986; 149:191–201.

Prange AJ, Wilson JC, Lynn CW, Alltop LB, Stikeleather RA. L-tryptophan in mania: contribution to a permissive hypothesis of affective disorders. Arch Gen Psychiatry 1974; 30:56–62.

Price LH, Charney DS, Heninger GR. Three cases of manic symptoms following yohimbine administration. Am J Psychiatry 1984; 141:1267–1268.

Price LH, Charney DS, Delgado PL, Goodman WK, Krystal JH, Woods SW, Heninger GR. Clinical studies of 5-HT function using I.V. L-tryptophan. Prog Neuropsychopharmacol Biol Psychiatry 1990a; 14:459–472.

Price LH, Charney DS, Delgado PL, Heninger GR. Lithium and serotonin function: implications for the serotonin hypothesis of depression. Psychopharmacology (Berlin) 1990b; 100:3–12.

Quintana Q. Platelet imipramine binding in endogenous depressed patients and controls: relationship to platelet MAO and 5HT uptake during successful imipramine treatment. Psychiatry Res 1990; 33:229–242.

Redmond DE Jr, Katz MM, Maas JW, Swann AC, Casper R, Davis JM. CSF biogenic amine metabolite relationships with behavioral measurements in depressed, manic, and healthy control subjects. Arch Gen Psychiatry 1986; 43:938–947.

Rice JP, McDonald Scott P, Endicott J, Coryell W, Grove WM, Keller MB, Altis D. The stability of diagnosis with an application to bipolar II disorder. Psychiatry Res 1986; 19:285–296.

Rice J, Reich T, Andreasen NC, Endicott J, Van Eerdewegh M, Fishman R, Hirschfeld RM, Klerman GL. The familial transmission of bipolar illness. Arch Gen Psychiatry 1987; 44:441–447.

Richards R, Kinney DK, Lunde I, Benet M, Merzel AP. Creativity in manic-depressives, cyclothymes, their normal relatives, and control subjects. J Abnorm Psychol 1988; 97:281–288.

Roy A, De Jong J, Linnoila M. Cerebrospinal fluid monoamine metabolites and suicidal behavior in depressed patients: a five year follow up study. Arch Gen Psychiatry 1989; 46:609–612.

Rubin AL, Price LH, Charney DS. Noradrenergic function and the cortisol response to dexamethasone in depression. Psychiatry Res 1985; 15:5–15.

Rybakowski JK, Lehmann W. Decreased activity of erythrocyte membrane ATPases in depression and schizophrenia. Neuropsychobiology 1994; 30:11–14.

Rybakowski JK, Amsterdam JD, Dyson WL, Winokur A, Kurtz J. Factors contributing to erythrocyte lithium-sodium countertransport activity in lithium-treated bipolar patients. Pharmacopsychiatry 1990; 22:16–20.

Samson JA, Gudeman JE, Schatzberg AF, Kizuka PP, Orsulak PJ, Cole JO, Schildkraut JJ. Toward a biolochemical classification of depressive disorders. VIII. Platelet monoamine oxidase activity in subtypes of depressions. J Psychiatric Res 1985; 19:547–555.

Schatzberg AF, Samson JA, Bloomingdale KL, Orsulak PJ, Gerson B, Kizuka PP, Cole JO, Schildkraut JJ. Toward a biochemical classification of depressive disorders. X. Urinary catecholamines, their metabolites, and D-type scores in subgroups of depressive disorders. Published erratum appears in Arch Gen Psychiatry 1989; 46(9):860. Arch Gen Psychiatry 1989; 46:260–268.

Schreiber G, Avissar S, Danon A, Belmaker RH. Hyperfunctional G proteins in mononuclear leukocytes of patients with mania. Biol Psychiatry 1991; 29:273–280.

Shenton ME, Solovay MR, Holzman PS, Coleman M, Gale HJ. Thought disorder in the relatives of psychotic patients [comments]. Arch Gen Psychiatry 1989; 46:897–901.

Silberman EK, Reus VI, Jimerson DC, Lynott AM, Post RM. Heterogeneity of amphetamine response in depressed patients. Am J Psychiatry 1981; 138:1302–1307.

Souetre E, Salvati E, Wehr TA, Sack DA, Krebs B, Darcourt G. Twenty-four-hour profiles of body temperature and plasma TSH in bipolar patients during depression and during remission and in normal control subjects. Am J Psychiatry 1988; 145:1133–1137.

Stahl WL. The Na,K-ATPase of nervous tissue. Neurochemistry 1986; 8:449–476.

Stancer HC, Persad E, Wagener DK, Jorna T. Evidence for homogeneity of major depression and bipolar affective disorder. J Psychiatr Res 1987; 21:37–53.

Stine OC, Xu J, Koskela R, McMahon FJ, Gschwend M, Friddle C, Clark CD, McInnis MG, Simpson SG, Breschel TS, Vishio E, Riskin K, Feilotter H, Chen E, Shen S, Folstein S, Meyers DA, Botstein D, Marr TG, DePaulo JR. Evidence for linkage of bipolar disorder to chromosome 18 with a parent-of-origin effect. Am J Hum Genet 1995; 57:1384–1394.

Stokes PE, Stoll PM, Koslow SH, Maas JW, Davis JM, Swann AC, Robins E. Pretreatment DST and hypothalamic-pituitary-adrenocortical function in depressed patients and comparison groups. Arch Gen Psychiatry 1984; 41:257–267.

Stone EA. Adaptation to stress and brain noradrenergic receptors. Neurosci Biobehav Rev 1987; 7:503–509.

Strober M, Morrell W, Burroughs J, Lampert C, Danforth H, Freeman R. A family study of bipolar I disorder in adolescence: early onset of symptoms linked to increased familial loading and lithium resistance. J Affective Disord 1988; 15:255–268.

Strzyzewski W, Rybakowski J, Potok E, Zelechowska-Ruda E. Erythrocyte cation transport in endogenous depression: clinical and psychophysiological correlates. Acta Psychiatrica Scandinavica 1984; 70:248–253.

Sultzer DL, Cummings JL. Drug-induced mania—causative agents, clinical characteristics and management: a retrospective analysis of the literature. Med Toxicol Adverse Drug Exp 1989; 4:127–143.

Swann AC. Noradrenaline and thyroid function regulate (Na+,K+)-ATPase independently in vivo. Eur J Pharmacol 1989; 169:275–283.

Swann AC. Brain Na,K-ATPase regulation in vivo: reduction in activity and response to sodium by intracerebroventricular tetrodotoxin. Brain Res 1991; 543:251–255.

Swann AC, Koslow SH, Katz MM, Maas JW, Javaid J, Secunda SK, Robins E. Lithium carbonate treatment of mania: cerebrospinal fluid and urinary monoamine metabolites and treatment outcome. Arch Gen Psychiatry 1987a; 44:345–354.

Swann AC, Berman N, Frazer A, Koslow SH, Secunda S. Lithium distribution in mania: plasma and red blood cell lithium, clinical state, and monoamine metabolites during lithium treatment. Psychiatry Res 1987b; 20:1–12.

Swann AC, Berman N, Frazer A, Koslow SH, Maas JW, Pandey GN, Secunda S. Lithium distribution in mania: single-dose pharmacokinetics and sympathoadrenal function. Psychiatry Res 1990a; 32:71–84.

Swann AC, Secunda SK, Stokes PE, Croughan J, Davis JM, Koslow SH, Maas JW. Stress, depression, and mania: relationship between perceived role of stressful events and clinical and biochemical characteristics. Acta Psychiatrica Scandinavica 1990b; 81:389–397.

Swann AC, Stokes PE, Casper R, Secunda SK, Bowden CL, Berman N, Katz MM, Robins E. Hypothalamic-pituitary-adrenocortical function in mixed and pure mania. Acta Psychiatrica Scandinavica 1992; 85:270–274.

Swann AC, Stokes PE, Secunda S, Maas JW, Bowden CL, Berman N, Koslow SH. Depressive mania vs agitated depression: biogenic amine and hypothalamic-pituitary-adrenocortical function. Biol Psychiatry 1994; 35:803–813.

Tan CH, Javors MA, Seleshi E, Lowrimore PA, Bowden CL. Effects of lithium on platelet ionic intracellular calcium concentration in patients with bipolar (manic-depressive) disorder and healthy controls. Life Sci 1990; 46:1175–1180.

Taylor MA, Berenbaum SA, Jampala VC Cloninger CR. Are schizophrenia and effective disorder related?: preliminary data from a family study. Am J Psychiatry 1993; 150:278–285.

Thase ME, Himmelhoch JM, Mallinger AG, Jarrett DB, Kupfer DJ. Sleep EEG and DST findings in anergic bipolar depression. Am J Psychiatry 1989; 146:329–333.

Thase ME, Mallinger AG, McKnight D, Himmelhoch JM. Treatment of imipramine-resistant recurrent depression. IV. A double-blind crossover study of tranylcypromine for anergic bipolar depression. Am J Psychiatry 1992; 149:195–198.

Turaihi MA, Khokher K, Barradas MA, Mikhalidis DP, Dandona P. 86Rb(K) influx and [3H]ouabain binding by human platelets: evidence for beta-adrenergic stimulation of Na,K-ATPase activity. Metabolism 1989; 38:773–776.

Van Eerdewegh MM, Van Eerdewegh P, Coryell W, Clayton PJ, Endicott J, Koepke J, Rochberg N. Schizo-affective disorders: bipolar-unipolar subtyping. Natural history variables: a discriminant analysis approach. J Affective Disord 1987; 12:223–232.

Verdoux H, Bourgeois M. Social class in unipolar and bipolar probands and relatives. J Affective Disord 1995; 33:181–187.

Wachtel H. Dysbalance of neuronal second messenger function in the aetiology of affective disorders: a pathophysiological concept hypothesizing defects beyond first messengers. J Neural Transm 1989; 75:21–29.

Wehr TA, Goodwin FK. Can antidepressants cause mania and worsen the course of affective illness? Am J Psychiatry 1987; 144:1403–1411.

Wehr TA, Sack DA, Rosenthal NE. Sleep reduction as a final common pathway in the genesis of mania—published erratum appears in Am J Psychiatry 1987; 144(4):542. Am J Psychiatry 1987; 144:201–204.

Whalley LJ, Kutcher S, Blackwood DH, Bennie J, Dick H, Fink G. Increased plasma LH in manic-depressive illness: evidence of a state-independent abnormality. Br J Psychiatry 1987; 150:682–684.

Whybrow P, Mendels J. Toward a biology of depression: some suggestions from neurophysiology. Am J Psychiatry 1969; 125:45–54.

Winokur G, Wesner R. From unipolar depression to bipolar illness: 29 who changed. Acta Psychiatrica Scandinavica 1987; 76:59–63.

Winokur G, Coryell W, Keller M, Endicott J, Akiskal HS. A prospective fullow-up of patients with bipolar and primary unipolar affective disorder. Arch Gen Psychiatry 1993; 50:457–465.

Winokur G, Coryell W, Keller M, Endicott J, Leon A. A family study of manic-depressive (bipolar I) disease: it is a distinct illness separable from primary unipolar depression? Arch Gen Psychiatry 1995; 52:367–373.

Wolpert EA, Goldberg JF, Harrow M. Rapid-cycling in unipolar and bipolar affective disorders. Am J Psychiatry 1990; 147:725–728.

Wood AJ, Brearley CJ, Aronson JK, Grahame Smith DG. The effect of oral salbutamol on cation transport measured in vivo in healthy volunteers. Br J Clin Pharmacol 1990; 30:383–390.

Wood AJ, Elphick M, Aronson JK, Grahame Smith DG. The effect of lithium on cation transport measured in vivo in patients suffering from bipolar affective illness. Br J Psychiatry 1989; 155:504–510.

Wood AJ, Smith CE, Clarke EE, Cowen PJ, Aronson JK, Grahame-Smith DG. Altered in vitro adaptive responses of lymphocyte Na+,K+-ATPase in patients with manic depressive psychosis. J Affective Disord 1991; 21:199–206.

Yates M, Leake A, Candy JM, Fairbairn AF, McKeith IG, Ferrier IN. 5HT-2 receptor changes in major depression. Biol Psychiatry 1990; 27:489–496.

Young LT, Li PP, Kamble A, Siu KP, Warsh JJ. Mononuclear leukocyte levels of G proteins in depressed patients with bipolar disorder or major depressive disorder. Am J Psychiatry 1994a; 151:594–596.

Young LT, Li PP, Kish SJ, Warsh JJ. Cerebral cortex beta-adrenoceptor binding in bipolar disorder. J Affective Disord 1994b; 30:89–92.

Young LT, Warsh JJ, Kish SJ, Shannack K, Hornykeiwicz O. Reduced brain 5-HT and elevated NE turnover and metabolites in bipolar affective disorder. Biol Psychiatry 1994c; 35:121–127.

11

Biological Models and Pharmacotherapy of Bipolar Disorder: Summary

L. Trevor Young and Russell T. Joffe
McMaster University, Hamilton, Ontario, Canada

I. INTRODUCTION

The importance of a broad range of specific biological factors in bipolar disorder has been addressed by individual authors in the preceding chapters. An integration of these diverse findings has been presented by Dr. Bowden in Chapter 9, followed by a discussion of their specificity to bipolar disorder by Dr. Swann. The aim of the present summary chapter is to discuss how these models relate to current and novel treatments for the disorder. This general question will be addressed from three separate perspectives: 1) how biological models relate to the mechanism of action of specific pharmacological agents, 2) their relevance to the treatment of specific phases of the disorder (i.e., mania, depression, and prophylaxis), and 3) consideration of their relevance to course of illness (i.e., rapid cycling; early versus late episodes). Although it is clear that we are far from having a complete understanding of the specific mechanisms that cause bipolar disorder, the body of evidence outlined in this volume provides clues that point to future directions for research. Furthermore, some intriguing hypotheses can be raised about what may be effective in the treatment of bipolar disorder.

II. HOW DO SPECIFIC BIOLOGICAL MODELS OF BIPOLAR DISORDER RELATE TO THE MECHANISM OF ACTION OF SPECIFIC PHARMACOLOGICAL AGENTS?

Typical antipsychotics, all classes of antidepressants, and benzodiazepines are widely prescribed in bipolar disorder. These agents, however, do not appear to have an action specific to this disorder as they are used widely in other disorders. On the other hand, drugs with proven efficacy as mood stabilizers (lithium and the anticonvulsants) may be more important in uncovering biological phenomena relevant to response to treatment (American Psychiatric Association, 1994). This is not intuitive given the diverse nature of these agents and the long-established prescribing of anticonvulsants in other CNS disorders prior to their use in bipolar disorder. As has been illustrated numerous times throughout this volume, many biological models of bipolar disorder are based on studies on the mechanisms of action of lithium, not only in patients but also in animal or cellular models.

Undoubtedly the most widely studied agent for bipolar disorder has been lithium carbonate. Discovery of this agent's efficacy in bipolar disorder was completely serendipitous and not based on any preconceived notion that this monovalent ion would have some particular utility for bipolar disorder (Cade, 1949). Each model has attempted to explore how lithium might bring about its effects by perturbing one of these biological systems. The large body of work attempting to correlate the effects of lithium on changes in the monoaminergic systems proposed to be relevant to bipolar disorder is reviewed in Chapter 1, by Drs. Manji and Potter. Their conclusion is that lithium's effects on the most well-understood monoaminergic systems— serotonin, noradrenaline, and dopamine—are not well established. It has been widely held, however, that the ability of lithium to modulate the serotonergic system may be important for its shared antidepressant properties and its ability to augment antidepressant treatments (Price et al., 1989). In addition, Manji and Potter have suggested that lithium's modulation of the dopaminergic system may also be important in its antidepressant effect. Some evidence suggests that lithium treatment may increase noradrenaline and its metabolite levels in CSF in patients who respond to their medication, although this is far from a well-replicated finding (Post et al., 1984).

Studying the effects of lithium on second-messenger systems has been more promising in generating hypotheses about the action of this drug, and to some extent has been consistent with findings in biological specimens from patients with bipolar disorder. Nonetheless, its effects on either G proteins or the phosphoinositide-generated second messenger are still some distance from fully explaining its mechanism of action (see Chapter 2). Some have argued that its effect on the protein kinase C system is even more important (Manji et al., 1995). Nevertheless, lithium does not appear to attenuate either G protein or calcium abnormalities, which appear to be quite consistently found in patients with bipolar disorder (Chapter 2). A larger question still remains about how to delineate the specific biological function important in the response of bipolar disorder to lithium, which is ubiquitously distributed when administered and would be expected to alter the function of multiple systems.

A very strong body of recent evidence has established that the anticonvulsants, particularly valproate, may be as effective as lithium, at least in treatment of mania (Bowden, 1995). This fact, in addition to the earlier literature demonstrating the role for carbamazepine in bipolar disorder (Post et al., 1987), raises an interesting question: how could lithium and two rather diverse anticonvulsants have very similar therapeutic responses in patients with bipolar disorder? This has led to a mostly unfruitful search—at least till the present—for a shared mechanism of action between these two classes of drugs. It has been close to impossible to find a shared effect by these agents on the monaminergic system (Chapter 1). Lithium has not been clearly shown to have effects on the GABAergic system, which is shared by these two anticonvulsant drugs. In many respects, lithium is a pro- rather than an anticonvulsant agent. There is some evidence of a similar effect of lithium and valproate on the glutaminergic system (Loscher, 1993) and also on downstream targets of protein kinase C (Manji et al., 1995; Chen et al., 1994). Given the differential responses to these different agents by specific patients, it would not be surprising if a common molecular mechanism is not elucidated (Bowden, 1995).

The basis for several other, less proven treatments for bipolar disorder has been described in detail elsewhere in this volume. For instance, there has long been interest in the role of thyroid hormone as a treatment for bipolar disorder (see Chapter 3). In contrast to what has been found in depression, thyroxine may reduce cycling and in some cases augment other mood-stabilizing agents. In major depression, thyroxine does not have such an effect, suggesting a different mechanism of action. Additionally, calcium channel blockers have been widely prescribed for bipolar disorder although their efficacy has not been well established (Dubovsky et al., 1986). There is considerable promise with a new agent, nimodipine. The administration of this class of drugs to bipolar patients is based on earlier findings of abnormalities in calcium metabolism in bipolar disorder and has been an interesting example of hypothesis-driven pharmacotherapy.

The very recent pilot work on novel anticonvulsants in the treatment of bipolar disorder, lamotrigine and gabapentin (Taylor, 1994), may lead to a re-examination of some of the earlier held hypotheses about how anticonvulsants work in bipolar disorder. As pointed out in Chapter 1, it is widely held that the anticonvulsant agents valproate and carbamazepine are less effective antidepressants that lithium. However, preliminary data have suggested that novel anticonvulsants may have both antidepressant and antimanic properties. This would set these agents apart from the more typical anticonvulsant agents, and suggest a broader spectrum of efficacy and possibly biological mechanisms. Speculation that these agents may have effects on the serotonergic system is supported by some very preliminary findings (Ben-Menachem et al., 1992). This might explain some of their possibly superior antidepressant properties and may eventually provide new clues to understanding the neurobiology of bipolar disorder. It will also be interesting to know whether these drugs are effective in major depressive disorder or whether this use will be confined to the depressive phase of bipolar disorder.

The last decade has witnessed a remarkable change in the pharmacotherapy of bipolar disorder with the introduction and demonstration of efficacy of several agents. It is hoped that in the coming years this expanding clinical knowledge will lead to novel approaches to further clarification of biological models underlying bipolar disorder.

III. WHAT DO BIOLOGICAL MODELS TELL US ABOUT PHASE-OF-ILLNESS-SPECIFIC TREATMENTS IN BIPOLAR DISORDER?

The treatment of bipolar disorder is conceptualized in three phases: the acute treatment of depression, the acute treatment of mania, and prophylaxis against relapses or recurrences of mood episodes. (Treatment of rapid cycling is a special case in the last category and will be addressed in the following section.) It has been very intriguing that this disorder presents with such diverse and almost opposite symptomatology. As illustrated very clearly in Chapter 10, by Dr. Swann, understanding the importance of depressive symptoms in mania has helped to reformulate our thinking about these two phases of the illness. A major challenge remains in formulating a pathophysiologic model that can incorporate both of these phases.

Depressive symptoms in bipolar disorder may respond to treatment with antidepressant agents from any of the major classes, including tricyclics, monoamine oxidase inhibitors, and the specific serotonin-reuptake inhibitors (SSRIs). There is, however, the well-established finding that tricyclic antidepressants as a class are more likely to up-regulate the noradrenergic system and the more likely to precipitate mania and destabilize bipolar disorder. This issue, well described in Chapter 1, is consistent with findings of increased noradrenergic function in bipolar subjects (Post et al., 1984). These authors also note that increased signaling through the dopaminergic system may also be important in precipitation of manic episodes. Nonetheless, the dopaminergic antidepressant bupropion may be among the antidepressants least likely to precipitate manic switches and be highly effective in bipolar disorder (Zornberg and Pope, 1994). It is becoming accepted practice to use the SSRIs, which may be less likely to precipitate mania, as a first-line treatment for depression in bipolar disorder (Peet, 1994). This is not consistent, however, with the lack of clear evidence of serotonergic abnormalities in bipolar disorder.

Consistent with the notion that specific agents may lead to a switch into mania or destabilization of bipolar disorder is the fact that antidepressants, particularly noradrenergic agents like desipramine, have been shown to increase coupling through the G-protein-coupled pathways (Ozawa and Rasenick, 1989), which may be up-regulated in bipolar disorder. These findings support avoiding these drugs in the treatment of bipolar disorder and may help in the design of novel agents. As noted above, the newer anticonvulsant agents such as lamotrigine and gabapentin appear to have novel antidepressant properties. Their molecular pharmacology is of great interest. The marked sensitivity of depressive symptoms in bipolar disorder to both light and changes in sleep suggests a strong link to chronobiological mechanisms which were also described in this volume, in Chapter 5, by Drs. Steiner and Ingram.

The clinical characteristics and treatment of mania are very different than for the depressed phase of bipolar disorder. It is therefore not surprising that different biological factors may be involved in this phase. The onset of mania is often rapid, with a marked severity, and can be associated with gross psychotic features (Goodwin and Jamison, 1990). As described by Dr. Swann, there are also marked differences between euphoric and dysphoric manias in both their clinical features and their treatment, and possibly in their biochemistry as well. The severity of mania can often be quickly reduced by inducing sleep and sedation. It can be precipitated quite rapidly by sleep deprivation or by administration of other substances. These factors have led many to wonder whether there is a biological "switch" for mania that can be turned on under a variety of clinical circumstances. This distinction has face validity with the phenomenon of pharmacological hypomania, which is often thought to suggest a predisposition to bipolar disorder without the actual diagnosis. Equally intriguing is the fact that a wide variety of agents, including typical and atypical antipsychotic agents, sedatives, and benzodiazepines, can all lead to marked improvement in the symptoms of mania. Specific agents such as lithium and sodium valproate, on the other hand, can also rapidly improve symptoms of the disorder and may have effects on a wide variety of symptoms, including psychosis and marked activation (Bowden, 1995). Since many of these effects also occur with drugs used to treat a variety of psychiatric disorders, it has been hard to elucidate what is specific in these drugs' effects to bipolar disorder. Models based both on neuroanatomical considerations and on receptor functionality have suggested increased activity in one or more CNS neurotransmitter pathways or second-messenger systems in mania (see Chapter 2). A dampening of this activity is thought to be important to its treatment.

The neurobiological basis of prophylaxis against relapses of mood episodes is an interesting and understudied question. It is becoming increasingly clear that drugs that effectively treat acute mood symptoms may not be effective prophylactically. This notion has not been adequately understood in the treatment of mood disorders but is generally accepted in many other areas of medicine. For example, in epilepsy, diazepam is used for status epilepticus but has few prophylactic properties. Calcium channel blockers and β-blockers are effective in prophylaxis against angina but are not necessarily used to treat acute chest pain. It is possible that focusing more specifically on the prophylactic properties of novel agents rather than on acute effects may lead to an improved understanding of the biological components of the relapsing nature of bipolar disorder.

IV. HOW CAN BIOLOGICAL MODELS HELP US TO UNDERSTAND COURSE-OF-ILLNESS DIFFERENCES IN RESPONSE TO TREATMENT FROM BIPOLAR DISORDER?

Clinical experience and recent follow-up data suggest that bipolar disorder may not respond as well to treatment at certain points in the course of the disorder. It is well known that a rapid-cycling course is notoriously difficult to treat and may require different pharmacological interventions than a non-rapid-cycling course (Goodwin and Jamison, 1990). Of more recent interest has been the fact that early intervention in the disorder, after only few mood episodes, may be much more effective than treating a disorder that is well established with multiple mood episodes (see Chapter 4 by Drs. Post and Weiss). These two examples illustrate the importance of continued focus on further clarification of the underlying neurobiological mechanisms in bipolar disorder. They will be discussed in turn.

Although some patients may have a long-standing pattern of rapid cycling that appears to be present for the course of their disorder, many appear to experience this phenomenon as a course modifier for a transient period of time, often several years (Coryell et al., 1992). Earlier reports had suggested that rapid cycling was associated with thyroid abnormalities whereas later reports have pointed out that female gender and young age at onset are much more important risk factors for rapid cycling (see Chapter 3, by Drs. Joffe and Sokolov). There is, moreover, a long-standing debate about the importance of past or current treatment with antidepressants in precipitating this course. It is generally conceptualized that the same phenomena that are important for switching a patient into mania may also be important for precipitating rapid cycling. One therefore could extrapolate that noradrenergic mechanisms may be more important in rapid cycling. Indeed, treatment with tricyclic antidepressants may be an important risk factor for the development of rapid cycling (Coryell et al., 1992). Furthermore, drugs of abuse, corticosteroids, and other agents are also thought to be important in the induction of rapid cycling, suggesting that other specific biological pathways may lead to this outcome. Hormonal factors may also be important in the development of rapid cycling since it is predominantly found in women. Treatment with sex steroid hormones may have some place in the management of this phenomenon, although this has not been proved beyond several case reports (see Chapter 5). Although an association of thyroid abnormalities with rapid cycling has not been a well-replicated finding, treatment with thyroxine is not uncommon.

In Chapter 4, Drs. Post and Weiss provide a comprehensive model of stress and episode sensitization and describe potential lasting neurobiological changes in bipolar disorder over time. Advances in understanding intraneuronal signaling pathways have led to specific hypotheses about signaling cascades, which are important because of their role in episode sensitization and a worsening of the course of this disorder. This model, and clinical experience, suggest that anticonvulsant treatments and possibly combination treatments may be more effective than lithium later in the course of the disorder. Lithium may be effective early in the course of disorder, especially if treatment is continuous without being withdrawn abruptly. The notion of change in the neurobiology underlying bipolar disorder over time is also supported by the findings that some patients in long-term follow-up appear to lose their prophylactic response to a mood stabilizer—in particular, lithium (Coryell et al., 1995). Therefore it is not inconceivable that the phenotype of the disorder interacting with other environmental factors over time may lead to biological changes that need to be taken into account in long-term treatment of the disorder. Post and others propose that if a clear understanding of these phenomena in bipolar disorder can be attained, it may lead to the development of treatment strategies that could reverse some or all of these phenomena and possibly bring back the disorder under pharmacological control.

V. CONCLUSION

In this volume, the reader will have found a clinically relevant description of current thinking about the biological systems thought to be important in the pathophysiology of bipolar disorder. These findings have already been useful in understanding the disorder and in making advances in the use of novel pharmacological agents. These models have also helped us to interpret the current response to medications with proven efficacy for this disorder, and have been useful in formulating ideas about how these medications may function. This brief concluding chapter offers a few examples of how a continued focus on understanding the neurobiology underlying bipolar disorder may ultimately be relevant to its response to specific treatments. Even as recently as over the past several years, many notions about what is acceptable for the treatment of bipolar disorders have changed. It is encouraging to see examples of what was called for by Dr. Bowden in Chapter 9: an interaction between clinical and basic science investigators in this field in order to promote our ultimate understanding of the treatment of this disorder. At present, careful clinical observation of the disorder with systematic analysis of treatment response is needed since all neurobiological models remain at the level of hypotheses, some of which can be tested in future investigations.

REFERENCES

American Psychiatric Association. Practice Guideline for the Treatment of Patients with Bipolar Disorder. Am J Psychiatry 1994; 151:51–536.

Ben-Menachem E, Persson LI, Hedner T. Selected CSF biochemistry and gabapentin concentrations in the CSF and plasma in patients with partial seizures after a single oral dose of gabapentin. Epilepsy Res 1992; 11:45–49.

Bowden CL. Predictors of response to divalproex and lithium. J Clin Psychiatry 1995; 56:25–30.

Cade JFJ. Lithium salts in the treatment of psychotic excitement. Med J Australia 1949; 36:349–352.

Chen G, Manji HK, Hawyer DB, Wright CB, Potter WZ. Chronic sodium valproate selectively decreases protein kinase C α and ε in vitro. J Neurochem 1994; 63:2361–2364.

Coryell W, Endicott J, Keller M. Rapid cycling affective disorder: demographics, diagnosis, family history, and course. Arch Gen Psychiatry 1992; 49:126–131.

Coryell W, Endicott J, Maser JD, Mueller T, Lavori P, Keller M. The likelihood of recurrence in bipolar affective disorder: the importance of episode recency. J Affect Disord 1995; 33:201–206.

Dubovsky SI, Franks RD, Allen S, Murphy J. Calcium antagonists in mania: a double blind study of verapamil. Psychiatry Res 1986; 18:309–320.

Fogelson DL, Bystritsky A, Pasnau R. Bupropion in the treatment of bipolar disorders: the same old story? J Clin Psychiatry 1992; 53:443–446.

Goodwin FK, Jamison KR. Manic depressive illness. New York: Oxford University Press, 1990.

Loscher W. Effects of the antiepileptic drug valproate on metabolism and function of inhibitory and excitatory amino acids in the brain. Neurochem Res 1993; 018:485–502.

Manji H, Potter WA, Lenox RH. Molecular targets for lithium's actions. Arch Gen Psychiatry 1995; 52:31–543

Ozawa H, Rasenick MM. Coupling of the stimulatory GTP-binding protein G_s to rat synaptic membrane adenylate cyclase is enhanced subsequent to chronic antidepressant treatment. Molec Pharmacol 1989; 36:803–808.

Peet M. Induction of mania with selective serotonin re-uptake inhibitors and tricyclic antidepressants. Br J Psychiatry 1994; 164:549–550.

Post RM, Jimerson DC, Ballenger JC, Lake CR, Uhde TW, Goodwin FK. Cerebrospinal fluid norepinephrine and its metabolites in manic-depressive illness. In: Post RM, Ballenger JC, eds. Neurology of Mood Disorders. Baltimore: Williams and Wilkins, 1984:539–553.

Post RM, Uhde TW, Roy-Byrne PP, Joffe RT. Correlates of antimanic responses to carbamazepine. Psychiatry Res 1987; 21:71–83.

Price LH, Charney DS, Delgado PL, Heninger GR. Lithium treatment and serotonergic function: neuroendocrine and behavioral responses to intravenous tryptophan in affective disorder. Arch Gen Psychiatry 1989; 46:13–19.

Taylor CP. Emerging perspectives on the mechanism of action of gabapentin. Neurology 1994; 44:S10–S16.

Zornberg GL, Pope HG. Treatment of depression in bipolar disorder: new directions for research. J Clin Psychopharmacol 1994; 13:397–408.

Index

Acetylcholine, 134, 260
ACTH (*see* Adrenocorticotropic hormone)
Activity protein-1 (AP-1), 49, 59–60, 67, 240
Adenylyl cyclase (AC)
  in bipolar disorders, 63
  in depression, 15
  signal transduction pathways, and, 42–56
ADP-ribosylation, 43, 56
Adrenal axis, 87
Adrenergic receptors
  α_2-adrenergic, 14–15
  β-adrenergic, 15–16
  blood, in, 13–16
Adrenocorticotropic hormone
  in depression, 17
  in mania, 163–164, 262
  response to CRF, 87
  in SAD, 145
AIF_4, 57
Aminergic system, 243–245
  dopamine, 245
  epinephrine, 245

[Aminergic system]
  norepinephrine, 243–245
  serotonin, 245
Amphetamine, 2, 25, 27
Anticonvulsant
  for bipolar disorders, 51, 288–290
  in depression, 5
  in kindling, 98–100
Anxiety, 17
Apomorphine, 22, 26
AP-1 (*see* Activity protein-1)
Arginine vasopressin (AVP), 163–164
ATF, 49
ATP, 43
AVP (*see* Arginine vasopressin)

β-adrenergic receptor (βAR)
  antidepressant drugs, and, 15–16
  desensitization, 60
  treatment of bipolar disorders, and, 51–53
βAR (*see* β-adrenergic receptor)
BDNF (Brain-derived neurotropic factor), 101

297

Benzodiazepines, 288
  diazepam
    kindled seizure, and, 98
    tolerance, 109–111
    triazolam, 146
Bipolar depressed, 67
Bipolar disorders (BD)
  biological models, 235, 287–294
  diagnosis, 235–237
  etiology, 237–239
  molecular pharmacology, 41
  nonrapid cyclers, 83–84
  rapid cyclers, 83–84
  treatment, 3–5, 288–294
Bipolar vs. unipolar
  acetylcholine, 260
  depressive episodes, 256–257
  epidemiology, 266
  family studies, 267
  GABA, 261
  genetics, 267–268
  neuroendocrine, 261–262
  neurophysiological arousal, 265
  norepinephrine, 257–259
  peptides, 261–262
  physiology, 263–265
  recurrence, 268–269
  serotonin, 259
  sleep, 265–266
  synthesis, 270
Blunted amplitude hypothesis, 132
Brain imaging
  emotions, neural substrate, 180–184
    basal ganglia-thalamocortical
      circuits, 181–183
    limbic system, 180–181
    paralimbic models, 184
  functional studies, 191–204
    cerebral blood flow (CBF),
      191–200
    primary depression, in, 197–200
  structural studies, 184
    computerized tomography (CT),
      184–185
    magnetic resonance imaging
      (MRI), 184–185

[Brain imaging]
  primary mood disorders, in,
    185–189
  secondary mood disorders, in,
    190
Bright artificial light therapy, 147–148
Bupropion, 4–5

Ca^{+2} channels, 64–65
Ca-ATPase, 264
Calcium
  in bipolar disorders, 242
  in mania, 64–65
  signal transduction pathways, and,
    42, 47–48
  transport rate, 264
  treatment of BD, and, 118
  in unipolar disorder, 64–65
Calcium channels, 45
Calcium channel blockers (CCBS),
    118, 289
Calmodulin, 48
cAMP-responsive element (CRE), 45,
    49, 67
cAMP-responsive element-binding
    protein (CREB), 45, 49
Carbachol, 59
Carbamazepine, 5, 51, 56, 59, 116,
    289–290
  cycle frequency, 5–6
  kindled seizure, and, 98
  lithium vs., 82
  mechanism of action, 51–59
  nimodopine, combination with, 118
  somatostatin, and, 166
  tolerance, 109–111
  treatment of bipolar disorders, 289–
    294
  treatment of depression, 82
  TRH and, 108, 110
  thyroid axis, 82
  valproate, combination with, 115–
    118
CBF (see Cerebral blood flow)
CCBs (see Calcium channel blockers)

CCK (*see* Cholecystokinin)
Cerebral Blood Flow (CBF), 191–200
c-Fos, 42, 49–51, 59, 98, 103
CGI (*see* Clinical global impression)
Cholecystokinin (CCK), 100, 168
Cholera toxin, 43
Chronesthesy, 146
Chronobiology
   hypothesis, 131–133
      blunted amplitiude, 132
      deficient process S, 132
      exogenous zeitgebers, 133
      internal desynchronization, 131
      kindling, 133
      phase advance, 132
   mood-related disorders, of, 127–133
Chronobiotics, 146
Circadian rhythms
   benzodiazepines, for, 147
   melatonin, 247
   mood disorders, and, 131–137
   normal physiology, 129, 137–139, 143
   NPY for, 168–169
   treatment, and, 145–148
   sleep and, 130
Circannual seasonal rhythms
   mood disorders, 144–145
   normal physiology, 143
   treatment, 145–148
c-Jun, 42, 49–51
Clinical global impression (CGI), 116
Clonidine, 15, 17–18, 258
CNPaseII, 59
Cocaine, 2, 93, 106
   sensitization, with, 103–108
Cold pressor test, 8
Cold stress, 19
Computerized tomography (CT), 184–185
COMT, 238
Corticotropin releasing factor (CRF), 87, 161–163, 246
Corticotropine-releasing hormone (CRH), 98, 145, 262

Cortisol, 17, 87, 193, 261, 246
CRE (*see* cAMP-responsive element)
CREB (*see* cAMP-responsive element-binding protein)
CREM, 49
CRF (*see* Corticotropin releasing factor)
CRH (*see* Corticotropine-releasing hormone)
CSF, 18, 261
CT (*see* Computerized tomography)
Cyclic AMP (cAMP)
   βAR and, 16
   blood levels, 16
   G-proteins, and, 52–53
   lithium, and, 242
   in mood disorders, 60–63
   signal transduction pathways, and, 42–49
Cyclic GMP, 44–45, 52–53
Cytochrome p450, 141

DAG (*see* Diacytylglycerol)
d-Amphetamine, 21
DARPP-32, 56
Deficient process S hypothesis, 132–133
Depression, 4
Desensitization, 62
Desipramine, 291
Dexamethasone nonsuppression, 87
Dexamethasone suppression, 87, 185, 262
Dexamethasone-suppression test (DST), 9, 163
Diacylglycerol (DAG), 42, 45, 47
Differential display PCR, 59
Dopamine
   antidepressant,and, 21–22
   cAMP modulation, 52
   HVA,and, 21
   in depression, 19, 21–24
   PET studies, 199-200
   serotonin,and, 245
Dynorphin, 98, 102, 106

Electroconvulsive therapy (ECT), 14,
    21, 28
Epinephrine, 237, 245–246
Exogenous Zeitgebers hypothesis, 133

Follicle-stimulating hormone (FSH),
    138
Forskolin, 63
FRAs (Fos related antigenes), 49, 103
FSH (*see* Follicle-stimulating
    hormone)

G-protein-coupled receptors, 48
G-proteins (guanine nucleotide-
    binding proteins), 27, 240–
    241
    GDP (guanosine diphosphate), 42–
    43
    GppNHp, 62
    GTP (guanosine triphosphate), 42–
    43, 53
    GTPγs, 57
GABA (*see* Gamma aminobutryic
    acid)
Gabapentin, 290
Gamma aminobutyric acid (GABA)
    anticonvulsant adaptation, 100
    in bipolar disorders, 246–247, 261
    circadian rhythms, and, 134
    hypothesis, 257
    plasma levels, 261
    receptors, 108
Gene expression, 106
    bipolar disorder, in, 58–59
    mood stabilizers, and, 58–59
    regulation, 49–51
Genetic studies
    adoption studies, 221
    family studies, 220
    linkage studies, 222–227
    twin studies, 219-221
Glucocorticoids, 16
Glutamate, 242, 245
Glutamine, 134
Gonadotropin-releasing hormone
    (GnRH), 137

Growth hormone (GH), 7,19, 81, 167–
    168, 193
Growth hormone-releasing hormone,
    17
Guanosine diphosphate (GDP), 43

5-HIAA (*see* 5-Hydroxy-indoleacetic
    acid)
Hormovanillic acid (HVA), 19–20,
    25–26, 28, 244
5-HT, 19, 22, 28, 51–52
5-Hydroxy-indoleacetic acid (5-
    HIAA), 19–20, 25–26, 28
Hyperthyroidism, 83, 86
Hypothyroidism, 81–83, 142
Hypothalamic-pituitary-adrenocortical
    axis (HPA axis), 129, 135,
    145, 162–165, 257, 261–262
Hypothalamic-Pituitary-Gonadal Axis
    (HPG Axis), 137, 139, 142

IEGs (*see* Immediate early genes)
Imidazoline, 15, 17
Imipramine, 22
Immediate early genes (IEGs), 97–100,
    103
IMPase (*see* Inositol monophosphate)
Inositol monophosphate (IMPase), 46,
    56–57, 64
Inositol polyphosphates, 42
Internal desynchronization hypothesis,
    131
Isradipine, 118

K-ATPase, 263
Kappa opiate receptors, 106
Kindling
    hypothesis, 133
    models, 248
    phenomenon, of, 93–103, 142
    stress sensitization and, 93–121
        complex combination therapy,
        117–121
        tolerance development, 93–96,
        109–114
        tolerance reduction, 114–117

L-dopa, 2
Lamotrigine, 5, 290
Late effector genes (LEGs), 97–100,
        103
Lateral ventricular enlargement, 185–
        187
LH (*see* Luteinizing hormone)
Lithium
    brain concentration, 202
    cycle frequency, and, 5
    in depression, 260
    G-proteins, and, 240–241
    mechanism of action, 51–59, 240–
        248
    rapid cyclers
        combination with sodium
            valproate, 115–116
    serotonin, and, 260
    signal transduction pathways and,
        41, 240–242
    somatostatin, and, 166
    transport rate, 264
    treatment of mood disorders,
        27–28, 63–64, 146, 288–
        294
    TRH, and, 88
    thyroid axis, and, 82–84
Luteinizing hormone (LH), 138

Magnetic resonance imaging (MRI),
        184–188
Magnetic resonance spectoscopy
        (MRS), 202–203
Mania, 4, 17
MAO (*see* Monoamine oxidase)
MAOIs (*see* Monoamine oxidase
        inhibitors)
MARCKS (*see* Myristolated alanine
        rich C kinase substrate)
MDD (major depression disorder), 62–
        63
Melatonin, 135, 143–144, 148, 247–
        248, 265
    mood disorders, and, 81, 88
Menstrual cycle, 137

3-Methoxy-4-hydroxyphenylglycol
        (MHPG)
    cerebrospinal fluid levels, 9
    depression in, 10
    dexamethasone suppressors, and, 7
    plasma levels, 7, 17
    urine levels, 11–13
Methyldopa, 2
MHPG (*see* 3-Methoxy-4-
        hydroxyphenylglycol)
MNLs (Mononuclear cells), 16
    in depression, 60
Monoaminergic, 22
Monoamines, 257
Monoamine oxidase (MAO), 238, 258
Monoamine oxidase inhibitors
        (MAOIs), 4–6, 22, 28, 290
Mood stabilizers
    mechanism of action
        gene expression, 58–59
        PI and, 56–58
        second messenger systems, 51–
            60
        treatment of BD, 51–60
MRI (*see* Magnetic resonance
        imaging)
MRS (*see* Magnetic resonance
        spectoscopy)
Myristolated alanine rich C kinase
        substrate (MARCKS), 47, 58,
        241

NAD (nicotanamide adenine
        dinucleotide), 43
NE (*see* Norepinephrine)
Neuroendocrine, 261
Neuropeptide Y (NPY), 168–169
Neuropeptides
    cholestokinin, 168
    corticotropin-releasing factor, 161–
        163
    growth hormone, 167–168
    neuropeptide Y, 168–169
    neurotensin, 165
    opioid peptides, 164–165
    somatostatin, 165–167

[Neuropeptides]
thyrotropin-releasing hormone, 169–170
vasopressin, 163–164
Neurotensin (NT), 165, 262
Neurotransmitters
interactions in brain, 24
monoaminergic, 41
neuropeptides, 161–170
βAR, agonists, 24
dopamine-serotonin, 25–26
5-HT, 24
norepinephrine-serotonin, 24
Neurotropin-3 (NT-3), 101
Nerve growth factor (NGF), 53
Nimodipine, 118, 121, 289
NMDA, 245–246
NMDA channels, 118
NMN (see Normetanephrine)
Noradrenergic, 2, 17
Noradrenergic receptors, 63
Norepinephrine (NE)
cAMP formation, and, 60
depression, and, 2, 10
dysphoric mania, and, 10
hypothesis, 257
in mood disorders, 18–19
interactions with dopamine, 24
interactions with serotonin, 24
MET, and, 243–245
MHPG, and, 7–9
cerebrospinal fluid levels, 7–9, 143–145
plasma levels, 143–144
NM and, 243
receptor binding, 258
stress, and, 258
unipolar vs. bipolar depression and, 257–259
urine levels, 11-14
VMA and, 243
Normetanephrine (NMN), 12–13, 18
NPY (see Neuropeptide Y)
NT (see Neurotensin)

Obsessive-compulsive, 17

Occipital cortex, 64
Opioid peptides, 164–165
Orthostatic stress, 19
Osteoporosis, 86

Panic disorder, 17
Para-aminoclodiline (PAC), 15
Paroxetine, 4
Partial sleep deprivation (PSD), 146
Peptides, 262
Pertussis toxin, 56
PET (see Positron emission tomography)
PGE, 60
Phase advance hypothesis, 131–132
Phenelzine, 22
Physostigmine, 2
PI (see Polyphosphoinositide)
Pilocarpine, 60
PIP2, 64
Pituitary hormones, 88
PKC (see Protein kinase C), 27, 43, 47, 50, 57–58, 64, 67, 240–241
Platelets, 56, 63
PLC (phospholipase C), 42, 45
PMDD (see Premenstural dysphoric disorder)
Polyphosphoinositide (PI), 45–47, 52, 56–58, 64, 240–241
Positron emission tomography (PET)
in healthy volunteers, 191–194
in primary mania, 200
in secondrary mood disorders, 200–201
Premenstural dysphoric disorder (PMDD), 140
Prevalence, 1, 82–84, 139, 190
Probenecid, 9
Prolactin, 81, 88, 93
Protein kinase C (PKC), 27, 43, 47, 50, 57–58, 64, 67, 240–241
PSD (partial sleep deprivation), 146

Quinpirole, 27

Rapid cyclers, 115, 141, 131

Receptor, 41
REM, 265
Reserpine, 1
Retinophypothalamic-pineal (RPH),
135

SAD (*see* Seasonal affective disorders)
Schizophrenia vs. mood disorders,
204–205
SCHs (*see* Subcortical hypertensities)
SCID, 236
SCN (*see* Suprachasmatic nucleus)
Seasonal affective disorders (SAD),
144–145, 147, 236
Secondary mood disorders, 190
Seizure, 93–100
Selective serotonin-reuptake inhibitors
(SSRIs), 141
Serotonin
blood levels, 259
cerebrospinal fluid levels, 19–21
dopamine and, 25–26, 245
5-HIAA, and, 19–20
HVA and, 19–20
metabolite levels, 259
neuroendocrine responses, 260
receptor binding, 260
Signal transduction systems
calcium, 242
cAMP, 43–45
G-proteins, 42–43, 240–241
gene expression, regulation, 49–51
interactions, 48–49
intracellular calcium, 47–48
mood stabilizers, and, 41–42
neuron and interaneuronal, 239–240
polyphosphoinositide (PI), 45–47,
241
Single photon emission computed
tomography (SPECT), 191,
199–201
Sodium transport, 263
Sodium valproate, 51, 240–241
carbamazepine, combination with,
117–118
cycle frequency, 5–6

[Sodium valproate]
G-proteins and, 240–241
lithium, combination with, 115–116
mechanism of action, 51–59
signal transduction pathways, 240–
241
treatment of mood disorders, 289–
294
Somatostatin, 17, 262
Somatostatin (SRIF), 165–167
SPECT (*see* Single photon emission
computed tomography)
Spillover rate, 8
SRE (Serum response element), 67
SRF (Serum-response factor), 51
Stress sensitization, 93, 106
Subcortical hyperintensities (SCHs),
188–189
Suprachasmatic nucleus (SCN), 129,
134–136
Synthesis, 270–272

TCAs (*see* Tricyclic antidepressants)
Thyroid
mood-stabilizing agents and, 82
T3, 82–85
thyroid axis, 81–85
thyroid hormone, 289
thyrotropin (TSH), 82–85, 262
thyrotropin-releasing hormone
(TRH), 82, 84, 98, 100, 169–
170, 262
thyroxine (T4), 82, 86, 289
treatment, in bipolar disorders, 85–
87
nonrapid cyclers, 86–87
rapid cyclers, 85–86
TRH receptors in depression, 108
Time-off-seizure, 111
Tolerance, 94–95
Tolerance reduction, 114–117
Total sleep deprivation (TSP), 146
TPA, 49–50
Transcription, 49
Transcription factors, 42, 49–51
Tranylypromine, 22

TRE, 50
Tricyclic antidepressants (TCA), 4–6,
     22, 28
   desipramine, 291
Tricyclics, 290
TSH (*see* Thyroid)

Unipolar, 60–62, 220–221

Vasoactive intestinal peptide, 262
Vasopressin, 163–164, 262
Ventricular brain ratio (VBR), 185
Verapamil, 118

Yohimbine, 17, 262

Zeitgeber, 142–147
Zif268, 98

About the Editors

L. Trevor Young is an Associate Professor in the Departments of Psychiatry and Biomedical Sciences as well as Director of the Mood Disorders Program, McMaster University, Hamilton, Ontario, Canada. The author or coauthor of over 60 journal articles and book chapters, he is a member of the Society for Neuroscience and Canadian College of Neuropsychopharmacology. Dr. Young received the M.D. degree (1983) from the University of Manitoba, Winnipeg, Canada, and the Ph.D. degree (1995) from the Institute of Medical Sciences, University of Toronto, Ontario, Canada. He is a Fellow of the Royal College of Physicians and Surgeons of Canada.

Russell T. Joffe is Professor in and Chair of the Department of Psychiatry, McMaster University, Hamilton, Ontario, Canada. The coeditor of several books, including *Anticonvulsants in Mood Disorders* (Marcel Dekker, Inc.) and the author or coauthor of over 175 professional papers, he is a Fellow of the Royal College of Physicians and Surgeons of Canada and the American Psychiatric Association as well as a member of the Canadian Psychiatric Association and the International Society of Psychoneuroendocrinology, among others. A Diplomate of the American Board of Psychiatry and Neurology, he received the M.B., B.Ch. degree (1977) from the University of Witwatersrand, Johannesburg, South Africa.